Central Nervous System: Role of Nutrition in Development, Maintenance and Aging

Central Nervous System: Role of Nutrition in Development, Maintenance and Aging

Editor: Kelly Turner

AMERICAN MEDICAL PUBLISHERS
www.americanmedicalpublishers.com

AMERICAN
MEDICAL PUBLISHERS
www.americanmedicalpublishers.com

Cataloging-in-Publication Data

Central nervous system : role of nutrition in development, maintenance and aging / edited by Kelly Turner.
p. cm.
Includes bibliographical references and index.
ISBN 978-1-63927-626-4
1. Central nervous system. 2. Central nervous system--Diseases--Nutritional aspects.
3. Central nervous system--Aging. 4. Central nervous system stimulants--Development.
I. Turner, Kelly.
QP370 .C46 2023
612.82--dc23

American Medical Publishers,
41 Flatbush Avenue,
1st Floor, New York,
NY 11217, USA

ISBN 978-1-63927-626-4 (Hardback)

Contents

Preface

The central nervous system (CNS) is the part of the nervous system that includes the spinal cord and brain. As a highly metabolic and specialized active organ, the brain relies on a consistent and adequate supply of nutrients. It is widely recognized that a balanced diet in terms of quantity and quality of nutrients is required for the regular functioning of the body, including the CNS at every stage of life from infancy to old age. Nutrition is crucial for neurodevelopment in teenagers, and preventing them from neurodegeneration during aging. The ability of nutrients to affect the CNS can be enhanced by incorporating food-derived supplements or whole foods. Understanding the mechanisms by which nutrients affect the brain is critical for utilizing nutrients to cure or prevent neurologic diseases. This book is a valuable compilation of topics, ranging from the basic to the most complex advancements in the study of central nervous system. It covers in detail the role of nutrition in development, maintenance and aging of the central nervous system. Those with an interest in this field would find this book helpful.

This book is the end result of constructive efforts and intensive research done by experts in this field. The aim of this book is to enlighten the readers with recent information in this area of research. The information provided in this profound book would serve as a valuable reference to students and researchers in this field.

At the end, I would like to thank all the authors for devoting their precious time and providing their valuable contribution to this book. I would also like to express my gratitude to my fellow colleagues who encouraged me throughout the process.

Editor

Equol Pretreatment Protection of SH-SY5Y Cells against Aβ (25–35)-Induced Cytotoxicity and Cell-Cycle Reentry via Sustaining Estrogen Receptor Alpha Expression

Meng-Chao Tsai [1,†], Shyh-Hsiang Lin [2,3,4,†], Kiswatul Hidayah [2] and Ching-I Lin [5,*]

1 Department of Psychiatry, Taoyuan General Hospital, Taoyuan 33004, Taiwan; mctsai1981@gmail.com
2 School of Nutrition and Health Sciences, Taipei Medical University, Taipei 11042, Taiwan; lin5611@tmu.edu.tw (S.-H.L.); kiswatul.hidayah@gmail.com (K.H.)
3 Master Program in Food Safety, Taipei Medical University, Taipei 11042, Taiwan
4 Research Center of Geriatric Nutrition, Taipei Medical University, Taipei 11042, Taiwan
5 Department of Nutrition and Health Sciences, Kainan University, Taoyuan 33857, Taiwan
* Correspondence: drcilin@gmail.com or cilin@mail.knu.edu.tw

† Meng-Chao Tsai and Shyh-Hsiang Lin equally contributed to this work.

Abstract: β-amyloid formation in the brain is one of the characteristics of Alzheimer's disease. Exposure to this peptide may result in reentry into the cell cycle leading to cell death. The phytoestrogen equol has similar biological effects as estrogen without the side effects. This study investigated the possible mechanism of the neuron cell-protecting effect of equol during treatment with Aβ. SH-SY5Y neuroblastoma cells were treated with either 1 μM S-equol or 10 nM 17β-estradiol for 24 h prior to 1 μM Aβ (25–35) exposure. After 24 h exposure to Aβ (25–35), a significant reduction in cell survival and a reentry into the cell cycle process accompanied by increased levels of cyclin D1 were observed. The expressions of estrogen receptor alpha (ERα) and its coactivator, steroid receptor coactivator-1 (SRC-1), were also significantly downregulated by Aβ (25–35) in parallel with activated extracellular signal-regulated kinase (ERK)1/2. However, pretreatment of cells with S-equol or 17β-estradiol reversed these effects. Treatment with the ER antagonist, ICI-182,780 (1 μM), completely blocked the effects of S-equol and 17β-estradiol on cell viability, ERα, and ERK1/2 after Aβ (25–35) exposure. These data suggest that S-equol possesses a neuroprotective potential as it effectively antagonizes Aβ (25–35)-induced cell cytotoxicity and prevents cell cycle reentry in SH-SY5Y cells. The mechanism underlying S-equol neuroprotection might involve ERα-mediated pathways.

Keywords: S-equol; 17β-estradiol; estrogen receptor alpha; cell cycle; β-Amyloid; Alzheimer's disease

---

1. Introduction

Neuronal cell death is an important feature of human neurodegenerative diseases such as Alzheimer's disease (AD). This cell death is considered to occur as a consequence of aberrant activation of the cell cycle in neurodegeneration [1]. Under normal conduction, the cell cycle is tightly controlled by specific regulatory proteins. For instance, cyclins and cyclin-dependent kinases (CDKs) are two key classes of regulatory molecules that determine a cell's progress in the cell cycle [2]. As a key regulator of the G1-S transition, cyclin D1 interacts with CDK4 to form the cyclin D1-CDK4 complex and moves to the nuclei, thereby promoting cell cycle progression. Normal adult neuron cells never reenter the cell cycle (but stay in the G_0 stage) and are thus recognized as permanently postmitotic cells [3]. Conversely, neurons reenter the cycle, undergo DNA replication, and die after they are exposed to DNA-damaging agents, oxidative stress, or certain neurotoxins such as beta-amyloid (Aβ) aggregates [3]. The Aβ peptide is the major component of senile plaque derived from the Aβ precursor protein (APP); this peptide is a neuropathological hallmark of AD [4]. There are numerous different Aβ species including Aβ (1–40), Aβ (1–42), and Aβ (25–35). The Aβ (25–35) fragment is universally used in research as it has been found to elicit profound toxic manifestations in elderly people and to physiologically play a role in AD [5]. It has been previously shown that cell cycle activation accompanied by the upregulation of cyclin D1 in primary cultured rat cortical neurons was observed in response to exposure to Aβ (25–35) and that such activation was followed by apoptotic neuronal death [6]. To elucidate the possible intracellular signaling pathway involved in the activation of the cell cycle by Aβ, extracellular signal-regulated kinase (ERK) 1/2-related pathways are the major focus of the present study because there is evidence of the involvement of ERK1/2 activation in Aβ-induced neuronal cell death [7]. It has been documented that activation of ERK 1/2 appears to be critical for G1 to S phase progression in cell cycle regulation [8]. A previous study showed that the overexpression of ERK 1/2 in cells exposed to Aβ was followed by an elevation in cyclin D1 expression, which resulted in changes in the cell-cycle distribution, particularly in the G1-S phase [9].

ERK1/2 is also the target of the regulatory action of estrogen and its regulation requires interaction with the known estrogen receptors (ERs), ERα and ERβ [10]. In addition to the reproductive system, both ERα and ERβ are broadly expressed in nonreproductive systems including the central nervous system [11]. Particularly, brain regions such as the hypothalamus, amygdala, and hippocampus appear to have distinct expression patterns of both ER subtypes [12]. Although it is recognized that ERβ is the predominant receptor in the hippocampus, where its absence has an impact on memory and cognitive function [13], ERα co-exists, and its coregulation may be important for ERβ to fulfill its cellular roles [14]. In other words, ERβ collaborating with ERα in its molecular actions is crucial for estrogen-mediated beneficial effects on hippocampus-dependent memory and cognition. The ERα subtype is of particular interest in the present study as it exhibits stronger transcription activity than ERβ and thus appears to be functionally superior to ERβ in the modulation of age-related memory decline [13–15]. It is noteworthy that ERα diminishing in the hippocampus with age leads to a decrease in the relative expression of ERα and ERβ, and nuclear ERα-mediated effects, all of which are putative molecular mechanisms for age-related memory decline in the presence of low estrogen levels [13]. In this regard, the molecular actions of both ER subtypes have been reported to be involved in the neuroprotection of estrogen against the pathogenic processes of AD [16]. Evidence suggests that estrogen is capable of protecting against Aβ-induced toxicity through ERα-mediated signaling pathways [17]. Moreover, the other major neuropathological hallmark of AD is intracellular aggregates of hyperphosphorylated Tau protein, which has recently been found to interact with ERα potentiating the reduction of ERα's transcriptional activity [18]. SRC-1 is one of the nuclear receptor coactivators which enhance the transcriptional activity of ERs to manipulate the relevant molecular events [19]. Studies performed in a human astrocytoma cell line demonstrated that estradiol treatment increased the cell number through the mediation of ERα, whereas the coactivator silencing by RNA interference of SRC-1 was able to block this effect [19].

Equol is a metabolite of daidzein, one of the major isoflavones in soybean food products, and is known as an ERs agonist [20]. Equol is capable of inducing transcriptional responses, especially through the binding of ERα [21]. The oral bioavailability of equol in humans seems to be high, resulting in a plasma concentration of 0.4~2 μM after taking a single bolus of 2 mg of equol [22]. Consumption of phytoestrogens has been found to avoid many side effects from estrogens [23]. Intriguingly, equol has been shown to be a promising neuroprotectant in in vitro models, and its neuroprotective effects are exerted through anti-neuroinflammatory mechanisms with the regulation of relevant signaling pathways at molecular levels [24]. However, whether the cell cycle regulatory event and ER-dependent signaling pathways involve the neuroprotective properties of equol remains an enigma. Thus, in this study, we investigated the effects of equol on protecting SH-SY5Y cells against

Aβ-induced perturbations and the cellular mechanisms underlying equol's neuroprotective action in cell cycle events and ER pathways.

2. Materials and Methods

2.1. Cell Culture

Human SH-SY5Y neuroblastoma cells were cultured at 37 °C and 5% CO_2 in Dulbecco's modified Eagle medium (DMEM) (Invitrogen™, Life Technologies, Grand Island, NY, USA) mixed with F12 (Invitrogen™, Life Technologies, Grand Island, NY, USA), 10% fetal bovine serum (FBS) (Biowest LLC, Miami, FL, USA), and glutamine (Biological Industries, Kibbutz Beit Haemek, Israel). The medium was changed twice per week. Cells were grown to 80% confluence before treatment.

2.2. Treatments

Aβ (25–35) (Sigma Aldrich, St. Louis, MO, USA) was dissolved in sterile distilled water at a concentration of 1 mM, then incubated in a capped vial at 37 °C for 5 days to allow formation of the aggregated form. It was then stored frozen at −20 °C until use. 17β-Estradiol, S-equol, and ICI-182,780 (all from Cayman Chemical, Ann Arbor, MI, USA) were dissolved in 99.5% ethanol to make stock solutions, which were used for experiments at a final concentration of 10 nM for estradiol and 1 μM for equol and ICI-182,780 in culture medium. It should be noted that no cytotoxic effect of the vehicle (99.5% ethanol) *per se* on cells was observed via the analysis of cell viability in our preliminary experiments that were conducted to determine the appropriate concentrations of the aforementioned treatments for the present study.

To induce cell death, cells were incubated with (Aβ) or without (C) 1 μM Aβ (25–35) for 24 h. To study the effects of estradiol (E2) and equol (Eq), cells were preincubated with estradiol (E2 + Aβ) or equol (Eq + Aβ) for 24 h prior to Aβ (25–35) exposure. Estradiol was used as a positive control and ICI-182,780 was used as an ER antagonist. It was added 1 h before the estradiol or equol treatment.

2.3. Cell Viability Analysis

Cell viability was assessed using a modified 3-[4,5-dimethylthiazol-2]-2,5 diphenyltetrazolium bromide (MTT) assay (Sigma, St. Louis, MO, USA). Cells were seeded in 24-well dishes at a seeding density of 2×10^5 cells/well. After treatment, 300 μL of the MTT solution (5 mg/mL) was added to each well and incubated at 37 °C for 3 h. After removing the culture medium, 250 μL of dimethyl sulfoxide (DMSO) was added to each well to dissolve the formazan, and then 200 μL of the solution was moved to a 96-well dish. The optical density was measured at 570 nm using a microplate reader. The absorbance of the control group was considered to have 100% cell viability.

2.4. Protein Extraction and Quantification

After treatment, cells were harvested, washed three times with PBS, and lysed using a cold RIPA lysis buffer supplemented with a protease inhibitor and an EDTA solution (Thermo, Hudson, NH, USA) at a ratio of 100:1:1, then centrifuged at 13,000 rpm and 4 °C for 30 min. The supernatant was collected, and the protein concentration was estimated with a BCA Protein Assay Kit (Sigma, St. Louis, MO, USA) using BSA as the standard.

2.5. Cell-Cycle Analysis

Cells (8×10^5) were seeded in 6-well dishes. After treatment, cells were trypsinized, washed in PBS, and centrifuged at 2000× *g* at 25 °C for 5 min, and then they were washed with PBS at least twice. Cells were fixed in 70% ethanol overnight. Before removing the ethanol, samples were centrifuged at 11 °C and 2200× *g* for 10 min. The pellet was then resuspended in 200 μL of DNA extraction buffer (containing 192 mL 0.2 M Na_2HPO_4 and 8 mL 0.1 M citric acid at pH 7.8) and incubated for 30 min at 37 °C. PI dye (200 μL, containing 0.1% Triton-X100, 100 μg/mL RNase-A, and 80 μg/mL PI in PBS) was added, gently mixed, and incubated for 30 min at room temperature in the dark. After removing the PI dye, samples were resuspended with 1 mL of cold PBS prior to analysis by flow cytometry.

2.6. Western Blot Analysis

A western blot analysis was performed to examine the expression levels of the proteins. Equal quantities (30 μg) of protein were separated by 10% sodium dodecyl sulfate polyacrylamide gel electrophoresis (SDS-PAGE) and then transferred onto nitrocellulose membranes. After transfer, membranes were blocked with Tris-buffered saline (TBS) containing 0.1% Tween-20 (TBST) and 5% non-fat-milk for 1 h. The membranes were then incubated with specific primary antibodies (Cell Signaling Technology, Danvers, MA, USA): Anti-cyclin D1 (1:1000), anti-p-ERK 1/2 (1:1000), anti-ERK 1/2 (1:1000), anti-ERα (1:1000), anti-SRC-1 (1:1000), and anti-β-actin (1:5000) overnight at 4 °C. After washing three times with TBST for 30 min, membranes were incubated with an anti-rabbit (1:80000) or anti-mouse (1:5000) immunoglobulin G (IgG) secondary antibody (Sigma) for 1 h, and then washed with TBST three times for 30 min. Immunoreactive proteins were detected by enhanced chemiluminescence (ECL) (Bionovas, Toronto, Canada) Western blot detection system.

2.7. Statistical Analysis

Data are shown as the mean and standard deviation (SD). Statistical comparisons were performed using SAS 9.3 (Cary, NC, USA). One-way analysis of variance (ANOVA) and least squared difference (LSD) post-hoc analysis of multiple comparisons were used. The statistical significance was accepted at $p < 0.05$.

3. Results

3.1. Cell Viability

As shown in Figure 1, the cell viability of the Aβ group decreased to 62.6% compared to the C group ($p < 0.05$), suggesting that Aβ (25–35) is cytotoxic to SH-SY5Y cells in the present study. After pretreatment with equol (Eq + Aβ), the cell viability was significantly increased by 9.6% compared to the Aβ group, and the same effect was observed in the E2 group which exhibited increased cell viability of up to 12.9% compared to the Aβ group ($p < 0.05$). No cytotoxic effect on cells was found from the treatments of 17β-estradiol (E2) and S-equol (Eq). These findings indicate that Eq, like E2, had the potential to provide the neuroprotective effects against Aβ cytotoxicity *in vitro*. Moreover, in order to confirm that the neuroprotective effects of S-equol and 17β-estradiol against Aβ (25–35) cytotoxicity are mediated by the estrogen receptors, cells were pretreated with 1 μM ER antagonist ICI-182,780 for 1 h prior to Eq or E2 treatment. In the presence of Aβ (25–35), pretreatment with ER antagonism of ICI-182,780 prior to Eq or E2 treatments significantly abolished their effects on SH-SY5Y cell viability ($p < 0.05$). These results suggest that Eq and E2 antagonized the reduced cell viability-induced by Aβ (25–35), at least in part, by mediating the ERs.

3.2. Estrogen Receptor Alpha (ERα) Protein Expression

Figure 2 shows that Aβ (25–35) alone markedly reduced the protein expression of ERα ($p < 0.05$), whereas pretreatments of Eq and E2 significantly attenuated the decreased protein expressions of ERα induced by Aβ (25–35) ($p < 0.05$). However, in the presence of ICI-182,780, the effects of the Eq and E2 pretreatments on ERα expression were significantly blocked ($p < 0.05$).

3.3. SRC-1 Protein Expression

Figure 3 shows the effects of the Eq and E2 pretreatments on the expression of the estrogen receptor coactivator SRC-1. Treatment of 1 μM Aβ (25–35) (Aβ) for 24 h significantly decreased the SRC-1 protein expression ($p < 0.05$). Pretreatment with either Eq or E2 significantly prevented Aβ (25–35)-induced reduction in SRC-1 protein expression ($p < 0.05$).

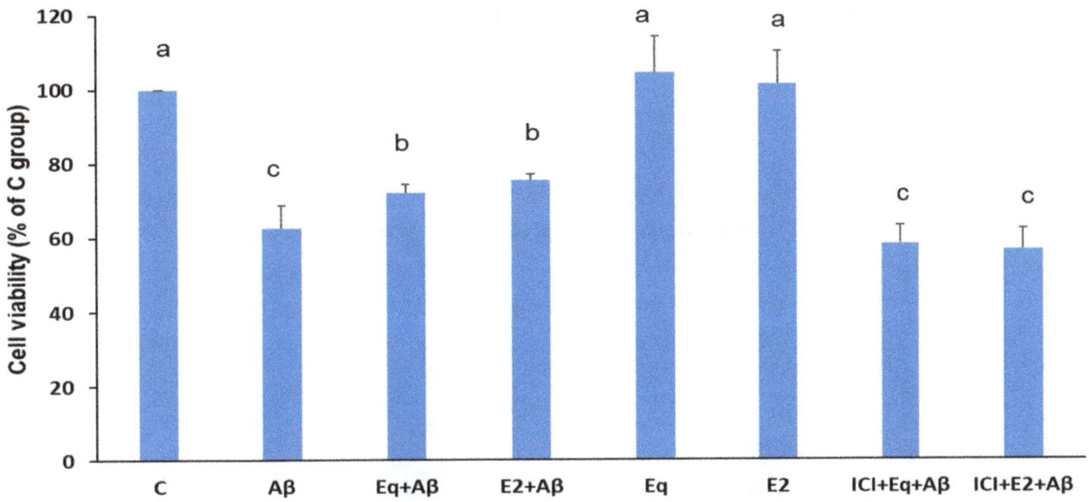

Figure 1. Cell viability of SH-SY5Y cells assessed with a modified 3-[4,5-dimethylthiazol-2]-2,5 diphenyltetrazolium bromide (MTT) assay. Data were analyzed by one-way ANOVA followed by the LSD post-hoc test and are representative of three independent experiments (n = 3). Values are presented as the mean + SD. Bars with different letters significantly differ at a level of $p < 0.05$. Eq, S-equol; E2, 17β-estradiol; ICI, ICI-182,780.

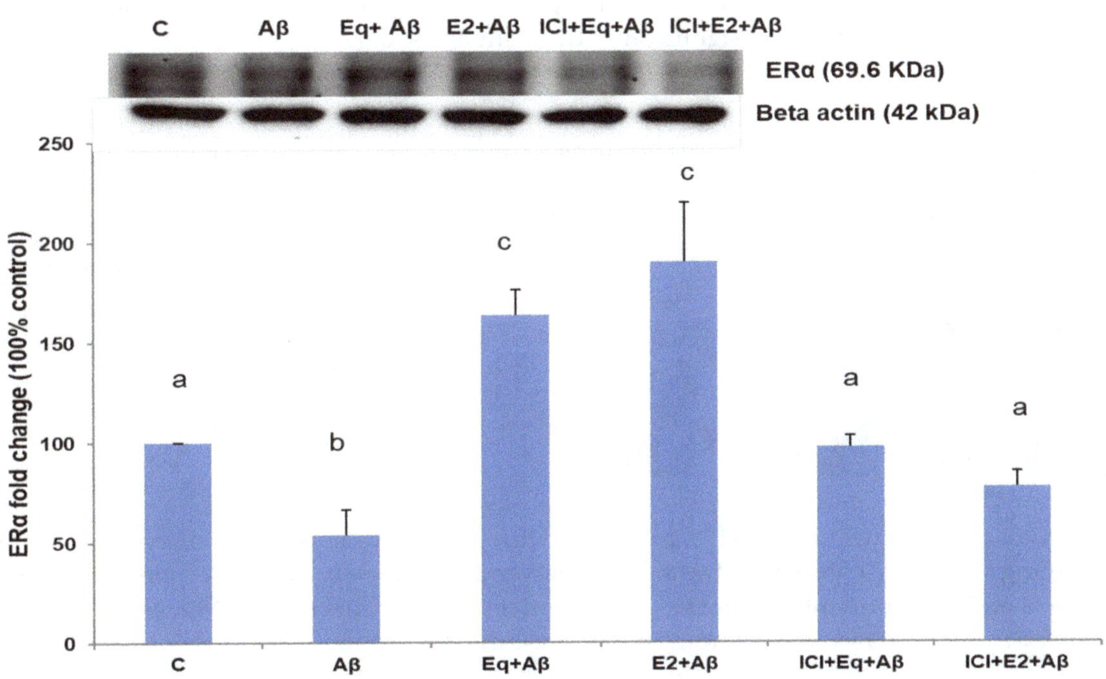

Figure 2. The estrogen receptor alpha (ERα) expressions of SH-SH5Y cells from different treatments. Data were analyzed by a one-way ANOVA followed by the LSD post-hoc test and are representative of three independent experiments (n = 3). Values are presented as the mean + SD. Bars with different letters are significantly different at $p < 0.05$.

3.4. Cell Cycle

Figure 4 shows the distribution of different phases of cell cycle. A significant increase of cells in the S phase in the Aβ group is observed compared to the C group as well as a concomitant reduction of cells in the G_2/M phases of the cycle (Figure 4). This result indicates that SH-SY5Y cells exposed to Aβ (25–35) escaped from the G_2/M phase. Pretreatment with either Eq (Eq + Aβ) or E2 (E2 + Aβ) showed a decreasing number of cells in the S phase and a significantly increasing number in the G_2/M phase compared to that in the Aβ group ($p < 0.05$). Cell cycle analysis showed that the cell cycle profiles were markedly altered by the treatment of Aβ (25–35), and pretreatment with Eq or E2 significantly blocked Aβ (25–35)-induced changes in the cell cycle profiles of the SH-SY5Y cells.

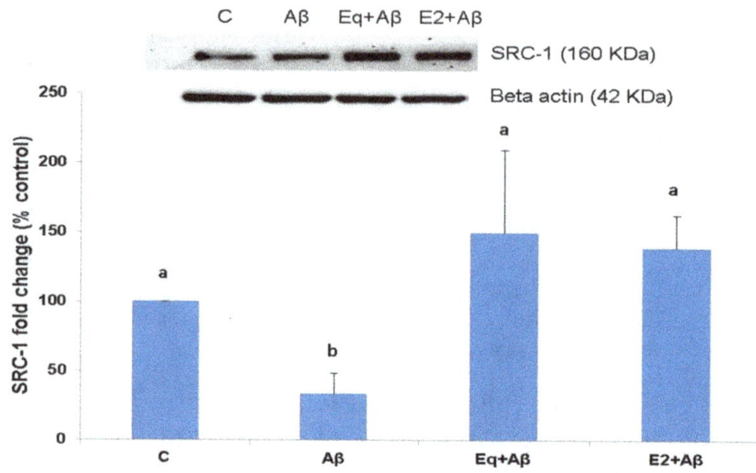

Figure 3. The SRC-1 expressions of SH-SH5Y cells from different treatments. Protein expressions were assessed by Western blotting. Data were analyzed by a one-way ANOVA followed by the LSD post-hoc test and are representative of three independent experiments ($n = 3$). Values are presented as the mean + SD. Bars with different letters are significantly different at $p < 0.05$.

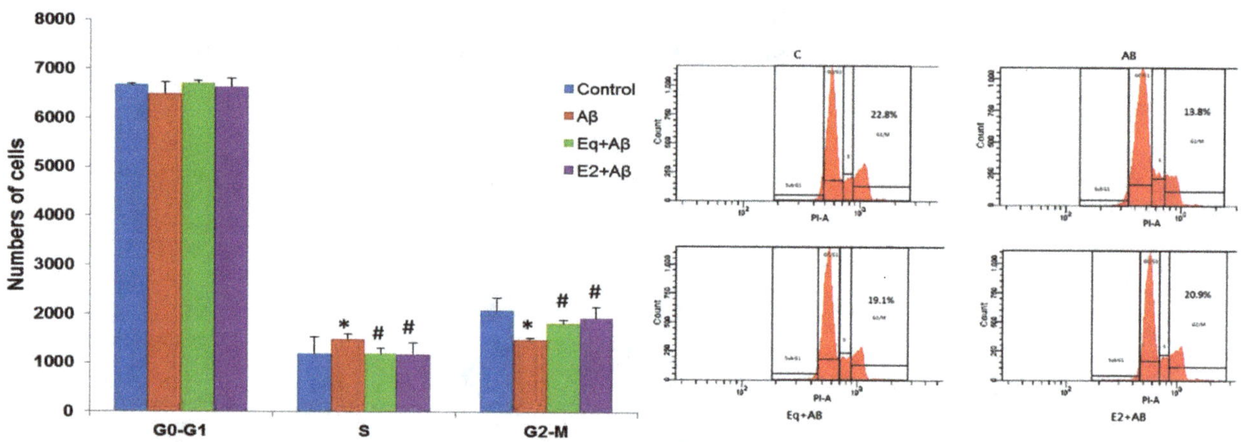

Figure 4. Cell cycle events of SH-SH5Y cells from different treatments. The cell cycle was assessed by PI staining with flow cytometry. Data were analyzed by one-way ANOVA followed by the LSD post-hoc test and are representative of three independent experiments ($n = 3$). Values are presented as the mean + SD. * $p < 0.05$ vs. the control; # $p < 0.05$ vs. the Aβ group.

3.5. *Cyclin D1 Protein Expression*

Figure 5 shows the relative expressions of cyclin D1, a protein marker for the G_0/G_1 phase, in different treatments. The relative expression increased markedly after cells were treated with Aβ (25–35) (Aβ group) in comparison to the untreated cells (C group). A decreased level of expression was observed in cells which underwent 24-h Eq or E2 pretreatment (Eq + Aβ group and E2 + Aβ group, respectively), compared to the Aβ group ($p < 0.05$).

3.6. *Activation of ERK 1/2*

Figure 6 shows that Aβ (25–35) treatment significantly increased the expression of phosphorylated (p)-ERK 1/2 ($p < 0.05$). The pretreatments of Eq and E2 significantly prevented the Aβ (25–35)-induced activation of ERK 1/2 ($p < 0.05$). On the other hand, when the ER activity was inhibited by ICI-182,780, the effect of Eq and E2 on deactivation of ERK 1/2 was significantly reduced ($p < 0.05$).

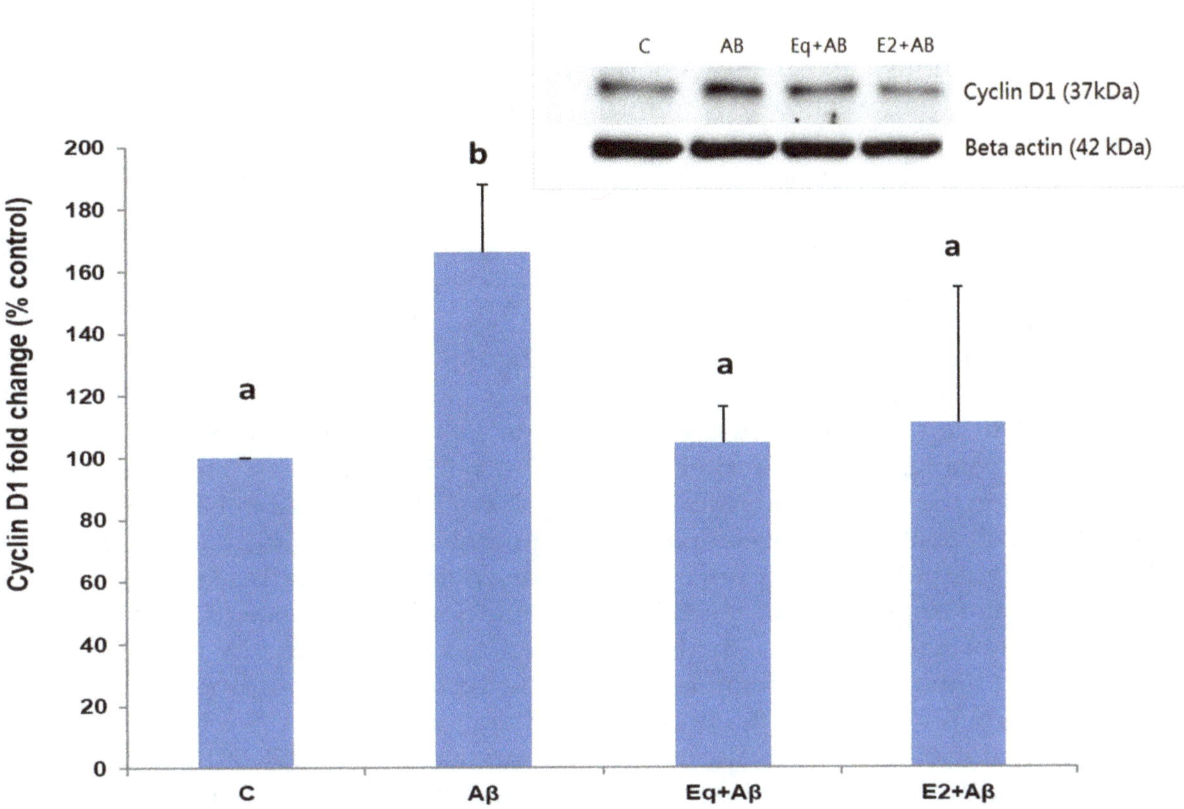

Figure 5. The cyclin D1 expressions of the SH-SH5Y cells from different treatments. Protein expressions were assessed by Western blotting. Data were analyzed by a one-way ANOVA followed by the LSD post-hoc test and are representative of three independent experiments (n = 3). Values are presented as the mean + SD. Bars with different letters are significantly different at $p < 0.05$.

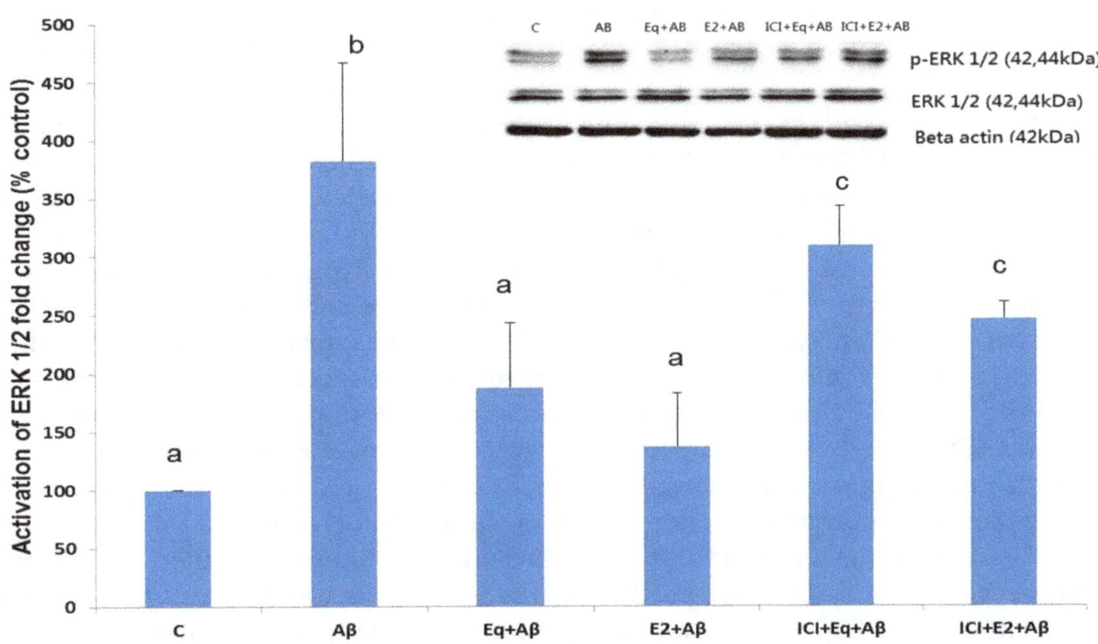

Figure 6. The phosphorylated (activated) ERK 1/2 expressions of SH-SH5Y cells from different treatments. Data were analyzed by a one-way ANOVA followed by the LSD post-hoc test and are representative of three independent experiments (n = 3). Values are presented as the mean + SD. Bars with different letters are significantly different at $p < 0.05$.

4. Discussion

Evidence from previous clinical and experimental studies showed that estrogen replacement therapy may have beneficial effects on AD in postmenopausal women [25,26]. However, the use of estrogen as treatment is known to have side effects, such as the development of breast and endometrial cancers in women [23]. Phytoestrogens may be an alternative treatment for AD with fewer side effects. A previous study showed that the phytoestrogen, α-zearanol, elevated the cell survival of Aβ (25–35)-induced PC-12 cells by attenuating oxidative stress and apoptotic cell death in a manner similar to 17β-estradiol [27]. In the present study, both S-equol and 17β-estradiol were also found to increase cell survival followed by Aβ (25–35) treatment. These results would predict that phytoestrogen, S-equol, possessed putative neuroprotective effects against Aβ (25–35)-induced cytotoxicity on SH-SH5Y cells analogous to those of 17β-estradiol [28,29]. In addition, the result of the inhibition of ER with antagonist ICI-182,780 prior to the Eq and E2 treatments suggested that ER may have a role in the neuroprotection of S-equol and 17β-estradiol against Aβ (25–35) cytotoxicity. The critical roles of ERs have been implicated in the cognitive function [14]. The loss of ERα expression has been noted to more likely contribute to AD-related memory impairment and amyloidogenesis [30,31]. Our observations showed the downregulation of ERα protein expression in SH-SH5Y cells exposed to Aβ (25–35) alone, emphasizing the importance of the ERα functional role in response to Aβ (25–35)-induced cytotoxicity. Under normal conditions, the ERα function can be enhanced by its coactivators, such as SRC-1, for efficient transcriptional regulation [32]. The decreased SRC-1 protein expression in the Aβ (25–35)-treated group was seen in the present study showing the Aβ (25–35)-induced disruption of the SRC-1 coactivator. These results support the notion that Aβ (25–35)-induced perturbation of ERα was further evident from the corresponding decrease in the expression of SRC-1. Furthermore, S-equol or 17β-estradiol pretreatments efficiently attenuated the effects of Aβ (25–35) in the current study, demonstrating that to provide a neuroprotective effect, equol binds with ERα and recruits SRC-1 to enhance its effect. On the other hand, the actions of both compounds were blocked by anti-estrogen ICI-182,780 in the present study, observing that ERα is required for the neuroprotective response of S-equol or 17β-estradiol to Aβ (25–35) cytotoxicity.

17β-estradiol binding to ERα is able to trigger transcriptional regulation of target genes, such as cyclin D1 [33]. In this regard, a recent study has reported that 17β-estradiol bound ERα has a role in controlling cell cycles [34]. In the present data, we presume that downregulated ERα expression in the presence of Aβ (25–35) might partially contribute to aberrant cell cycles. In normal conditions, neuron cells are postmitotic and stay in the G_0 phase, as indicated by the downregulation of proteins related to the cell cycle [35]. For instance, cyclin D1, a protein marker of the G_0/G_1 phase, is expressed at the beginning of the G1 phase and continually accumulates in the nucleus during the G1 phase in the presence of the cell cycle reactivation [36]. When the cells progress into the S phase, cyclin D1 can secrete into the cytoplasm and its overexpression can reduce cell sizes and shorten the G1 phase resulting in the accelerated entry into the S phase [37]. Likewise, our results showed that Aβ (25–35) caused cells to leave the postmitotic phase and reenter the cell cycle in parallel with the increasing level of cyclin D1. This finding is in line with previous studies which found that Aβ (25–35) toxicity induces cell-cycle reentry [9,38]. However, only a tendency toward a decrease in cell number of the G1 phase in the Aβ-treated group was observed in this study. Such observation might be ascribed to a more rapid cell cycle progression in response to a higher level of cyclin D1 followed by Aβ treatment as mentioned above. Alternatively, it is plausible that there is a high degree of variability in the G1-phase progression due to the differences in nature between cells, which indicates that the cell itself may enter into G1 or exit from G1 at different time points from its neighboring cells [39]. In presenilin (PS)-1 familial AD brains, the presence of cyclin D1 accumulation was observed to be linked to cell-cycle activation and subsequently led to cell death [40]. Our results are in accordance with previous findings showing that when exposed to 25 μM Aβ (25–35), SH-SY5Y cells accumulated in the S phase, indicating that they did not progress beyond the S phase accompanied by apoptosis [9,41]. Taken together, we speculate that changes in ERα and cyclin D1 expressions concomitantly occurring with aberrant cell cycle reentry appear likely to underlie the cytotoxic mechanisms of Aβ (25–35). Thus, apoptotic neuronal death is presumably the consequence of Aβ (25–35)-induced cytotoxicity [42]. However, it is noteworthy that more recent evidence indicates neuronal cell death triggered by a cell cycle reentry event could be independent of an apoptotic mechanism in AD [43]. More in-depth investigation is warranted to resolve this discrepancy. Nevertheless, S-equol prevented Aβ (25–35)-induced changes in the cell-cycle behavior, ERα, and cyclin D1 expressions, indicative of the neuroprotective potential of S-equol.

A common target for estrogen signaling and Aβ neurotoxicity is ERK 1/2 [9,10,44]. It was shown that ERK 1 and 2 are expressed in the pooled cerebrospinal fluid (CSF) of patients with AD, and elevated levels of ERK 1/2 in CSF are accompanied by increased levels of tau protein and the Aβ42 peptide [45]. Rapid activation of ERK 1/2 was reported in SH-SY5Y neuroblastoma cells exposed to Aβ (25–35) [9] and in mature hippocampal neurons [46]. Aberrant activation of ERK 1/2 was correlated with an elevated level of cyclin D1 that has been shown to be responsible for cell cycle reentry in neurons under Aβ-induced toxicity conditions, thereby potentiating the neuronal apoptosis responses [38]. The present data showed that Aβ (25–35) triggered ERK 1/2 activation, and pretreatments of S-equol and 17β-estradiol were able to prevent this response. In contrast, treatment with ICI-182,780 appeared to diminish the protective effects of S-equol and 17β-estradiol. These observations led us to propose that the neuroprotective mechanisms of the actions of S-equol and 17β-estradiol against Aβ (25–35) cytotoxicity might be mediated by the ERK1/2 pathways via ERα. Previous studies have shown that estrogen prevents cytotoxic effects of Aβ by activating MAPK which regulates ERK 1/2 expression and cyclin D1 to control cell cycle reentry [9,29]. Herein, we have shown that S-equol exhibited neuroprotective effects that mimicked the action of 17β-estradiol on Aβ (25–35)-treated SH-SY5Y cells through preventing cell cycle reentry downregulating cyclin D1 and ERα-mediated ERK 1/2 expressions, all of which might have involved suppression of Aβ (25–35)-induced cell cycle reentry by S-equol or 17β-estradiol pretreatments in the current study.

5. Conclusions

This study concludes that Aβ (25–35) caused diminished ERα levels, which mediated estrogen actions to disrupt normal cell cycle regulation and thus potentiates cell death. S-equol might act as a putative neuroprotective agent against Aβ (25–35) cytotoxicity, and its neuroprotective role might be, at least in part, attributed to its estrogenic potency. The observed putative neuroprotective effects of equol were associated with sustaining ERα levels and cell survival in our cell models. Furthermore, the molecular mechanism underlying this putative neuroprotection of S-equol is shown to involve the suppression of cell cycle reentry which might be synergized with ERα-involved activation of ERK 1/2 along with the prevented activation of cyclin D1.

Author Contributions: Conceptualization, M.-C.T., S.-H.L., K.H., and C.-I.L.; methodology, S.-H.L., K.H., and C.-I.L.; software, S.-H.L. and K.H.; validation, M.-C.T., S-H.L., K.H., and C.-I.L.; formal analysis, S.-H.L. and K.H.; resources, M.-C.T. and S-H.L.; data curation, S.-H.L., K.H., and C.-I.L.; writing—original draft preparation, review, and editing, C.-I.L.; supervision, M.-C.T. and S.-H.L.; project administration, M.-C.T. and C.-I.L.; funding acquisition, M.-C.T.

References

1. Nagy, Z. Cell cycle regulatory failure in neurones: Causes and consequences. *Neurobiol. Aging* **2000**, *21*, 761–769. [CrossRef]
2. Frade, J.M.; Ovejero-Benito, M.C. Neuronal cell cycle: The neuron itself and its circumstances. *Cell Cycle* **2015**, *14*, 712–720. [CrossRef] [PubMed]
3. Herrup, K. The involvement of cell cycle events in the pathogenesis of Alzheimer's disease. *Alzheimer's Res. Ther.* **2010**, *2*, 13. [CrossRef] [PubMed]

4. Querfurth, H.W.; LaFerla, F.M. Alzheimer's disease. *N. Engl. J. Med.* **2010**, *362*, 329–344. [CrossRef] [PubMed]
5. Clementi, M.E.; Marini, S.; Coletta, M.; Orsini, F.; Giardina, B.; Misiti, F. Abeta(31–35) and Abeta(25–35) fragments of amyloid beta-protein induce cellular death through apoptotic signals: Role of the redox state of methionine-35. *FEBS Lett.* **2005**, *579*, 2913–2918. [CrossRef] [PubMed]
6. Wang, J.; Zhang, Y.J.; Du, S. The protective effect of curcumin on Abeta induced aberrant cell cycle reentry on primary cultured rat cortical neurons. *Eur. Rev. Med. Pharmacol. Sci.* **2012**, *16*, 445–454. [PubMed]
7. Frasca, G.; Carbonaro, V.; Merlo, S.; Copani, A.; Sortino, M.A. Integrins mediate beta-amyloid-induced cell-cycle activation and neuronal death. *J. Neurosci. Res.* **2008**, *86*, 350–355. [CrossRef] [PubMed]
8. Mebratu, Y.; Tesfaigzi, Y. How ERK1/2 activation controls cell proliferation and cell death: Is subcellular localization the answer? *Cell Cycle* **2009**, *8*, 1168–1175. [CrossRef]
9. Frasca, G.; Chiechio, S.; Vancheri, C.; Nicoletti, F.; Copani, A.; Angela Sortino, M. Beta-amyloid-activated cell cycle in SH-SY5Y neuroblastoma cells: Correlation with the MAP kinase pathway. *J. Mol. Neurosci.* **2004**, *22*, 231–236. [CrossRef]
10. Mannella, P.; Brinton, R.D. Estrogen receptor protein interaction with phosphatidylinositol 3-kinase leads to activation of phosphorylated Akt and extracellular signal-regulated kinase 1/2 in the same population of cortical neurons: A unified mechanism of estrogen action. *J. Neurosci.* **2006**, *26*, 9439–9447. [CrossRef]
11. Paterni, I.; Granchi, C.; Katzenellenbogen, J.A.; Minutolo, F. Estrogen receptors alpha (ERalpha) and beta (ERbeta): Subtype-selective ligands and clinical potential. *Steroids* **2014**, *90*, 13–29. [CrossRef] [PubMed]
12. Jung, M.E.; Gatch, M.B.; Simpkins, J.W. Estrogen neuroprotection against the neurotoxic effects of ethanol withdrawal: Potential mechanisms. *Exp. Biol. Med.* **2005**, *230*, 8–22. [CrossRef] [PubMed]
13. Foster, T.C. Role of estrogen receptor alpha and beta expression and signaling on cognitive function during aging. *Hippocampus* **2012**, *22*, 656–669. [CrossRef] [PubMed]
14. Bean, L.A.; Ianov, L.; Foster, T.C. Estrogen receptors, the hippocampus, and memory. *Neuroscientist* **2014**, *20*, 534–545. [CrossRef] [PubMed]
15. Carroll, J.C.; Pike, C.J. Selective estrogen receptor modulators differentially regulate Alzheimer-like changes in female 3xTg-AD mice. *Endocrinology* **2008**, *149*, 2607–2611. [CrossRef]
16. Zhao, L.; Wu, T.W.; Brinton, R.D. Estrogen receptor subtypes alpha and beta contribute to neuroprotection and increased Bcl-2 expression in primary hippocampal neurons. *Brain Res.* **2004**, *1010*, 22–34. [CrossRef]
17. Kim, H.; Bang, O.Y.; Jung, M.W.; Ha, S.D.; Hong, H.S.; Huh, K.; Kim, S.U.; Mook-Jung, I. Neuroprotective effects of estrogen against beta-amyloid toxicity are mediated by estrogen receptors in cultured neuronal cells. *Neurosci. Lett.* **2001**, *302*, 58–62. [CrossRef]
18. Wang, C.; Zhang, F.; Jiang, S.; Siedlak, S.L.; Shen, L.; Perry, G.; Wang, X.; Tang, B.; Zhu, X. Estrogen receptor-alpha is localized to neurofibrillary tangles in Alzheimer's disease. *Sci. Rep.* **2016**, *6*, 20352. [CrossRef]
19. Gonzalez-Arenas, A.; Hansberg-Pastor, V.; Hernandez-Hernandez, O.T.; Gonzalez-Garcia, T.K.; Henderson-Villalpando, J.; Lemus-Hernandez, D.; Cruz-Barrios, A.; Rivas-Suarez, M.; Camacho-Arroyo, I. Estradiol increases cell growth in human astrocytoma cell lines through ERalpha activation and its interaction with SRC-1 and SRC-3 coactivators. *Biochim. Biophys. Acta* **2012**, *1823*, 379–386. [CrossRef]
20. Mueller, S.O.; Simon, S.; Chae, K.; Metzler, M.; Korach, K.S. Phytoestrogens and their human metabolites show distinct agonistic and antagonistic properties on estrogen receptor alpha (ERalpha) and ERbeta in human cells. *Toxicol. Sci.* **2004**, *80*, 14–25. [CrossRef]
21. Setchell, K.D.; Clerici, C. Equol: Pharmacokinetics and biological actions. *J. Nutr.* **2010**, *140*, 1363s–1368s. [CrossRef] [PubMed]
22. Setchell, K.D.; Zhao, X.; Shoaf, S.E.; Ragland, K. The pharmacokinetics of S-(-)equol administered as SE5-OH tablets to healthy postmenopausal women. *J. Nutr.* **2009**, *139*, 2037–2043. [CrossRef] [PubMed]
23. Morabito, N.; Crisafulli, A.; Vergara, C.; Gaudio, A.; Lasco, A.; Frisina, N.; D'Anna, R.; Corrado, F.; Pizzoleo, M.A.; Cincotta, M.; et al. Effects of genistein and hormone-replacement therapy on bone loss in early postmenopausal women: A randomized double-blind placebo-controlled study. *J. Bone Miner. Res.* **2002**, *17*, 1904–1912. [CrossRef] [PubMed]
24. Subedi, L.; Ji, E.; Shin, D.; Jin, J.; Yeo, J.H.; Kim, S.Y. Equol, a Dietary Daidzein Gut Metabolite Attenuates Microglial Activation and Potentiates Neuroprotection In Vitro. *Nutrients* **2017**, *9*, 207. [CrossRef]
25. Merlo, S.; Spampinato, S.F.; Sortino, M.A. Estrogen and Alzheimer's disease: Still an attractive topic despite disappointment from early clinical results. *Eur. J. Pharmacol.* **2017**, *817*, 51–58. [CrossRef]

26. Christensen, A.; Pike, C.J. Age-dependent regulation of obesity and Alzheimer-related outcomes by hormone therapy in female 3xTg-AD mice. *PLoS ONE* **2017**, *12*, e0178490. [CrossRef]
27. Dong, Y.; Yang, N.; Liu, Y.; Li, Q.; Zuo, P. The neuroprotective effects of phytoestrogen alpha-zearalanol on beta-amyloid-induced toxicity in differentiated PC-12 cells. *Eur. J. Pharmacol.* **2011**, *670*, 392–398. [CrossRef]
28. Zhao, L.; Mao, Z.; Brinton, R.D. A select combination of clinically relevant phytoestrogens enhances estrogen receptor beta-binding selectivity and neuroprotective activities in vitro and in vivo. *Endocrinology* **2009**, *150*, 770–783. [CrossRef]
29. Valles, S.L.; Borras, C.; Gambini, J.; Furriol, J.; Ortega, A.; Sastre, J.; Pallardo, F.V.; Vina, J. Oestradiol or genistein rescues neurons from amyloid beta-induced cell death by inhibiting activation of p38. *Aging Cell* **2008**, *7*, 112–118. [CrossRef]
30. Hwang, C.J.; Yun, H.M.; Park, K.R.; Song, J.K.; Seo, H.O.; Hyun, B.K.; Choi, D.Y.; Yoo, H.S.; Oh, K.W.; Hwang, D.Y.; et al. Memory Impairment in Estrogen Receptor alpha Knockout Mice Through Accumulation of Amyloid-beta Peptides. *Mol. Neurobiol.* **2015**, *52*, 176–186. [CrossRef]
31. Tang, Y.; Min, Z.; Xiang, X.J.; Liu, L.; Ma, Y.L.; Zhu, B.L.; Song, L.; Tang, J.; Deng, X.J.; Yan, Z.; et al. Estrogen-related receptor alpha is involved in Alzheimer's disease-like pathology. *Exp. Neurol.* **2018**, *305*, 89–96. [CrossRef] [PubMed]
32. Tetel, M.J.; Acharya, K.D. Nuclear receptor coactivators: Regulators of steroid action in brain and behaviour. *J. Neuroendocrinol.* **2013**, *25*, 1209–1218. [CrossRef]
33. Cicatiello, L.; Addeo, R.; Sasso, A.; Altucci, L.; Petrizzi, V.B.; Borgo, R.; Cancemi, M.; Caporali, S.; Caristi, S.; Scafoglio, C.; et al. Estrogens and progesterone promote persistent CCND1 gene activation during G1 by inducing transcriptional derepression via c-Jun/c-Fos/estrogen receptor (progesterone receptor) complex assembly to a distal regulatory element and recruitment of cyclin D1 to its own gene promoter. *Mol. Cell. Biol.* **2004**, *24*, 7260–7274. [CrossRef] [PubMed]
34. JavanMoghadam, S.; Weihua, Z.; Hunt, K.K.; Keyomarsi, K. Estrogen receptor alpha is cell cycle-regulated and regulates the cell cycle in a ligand-dependent fashion. *Cell Cycle* **2016**, *15*, 1579–1590. [CrossRef] [PubMed]
35. Negis, Y.; Unal, A.Y.; Korulu, S.; Karabay, A. Cell cycle markers have different expression and localization patterns in neuron-like PC12 cells and primary hippocampal neurons. *Neurosci. Lett.* **2011**, *496*, 135–140. [CrossRef]
36. Sumrejkanchanakij, P.; Tamamori-Adachi, M.; Matsunaga, Y.; Eto, K.; Ikeda, M.A. Role of cyclin D1 cytoplasmic sequestration in the survival of postmitotic neurons. *Oncogene* **2003**, *22*, 8723–8730. [CrossRef]
37. Quelle, D.E.; Ashmun, R.A.; Shurtleff, S.A.; Kato, J.Y.; Bar-Sagi, D.; Roussel, M.F.; Sherr, C.J. Overexpression of mouse D-type cyclins accelerates G1 phase in rodent fibroblasts. *Genes Dev.* **1993**, *7*, 1559–1571. [CrossRef]
38. Modi, P.K.; Komaravelli, N.; Singh, N.; Sharma, P. Interplay between MEK-ERK signaling, cyclin D1, and cyclin-dependent kinase 5 regulates cell cycle reentry and apoptosis of neurons. *Mol. Biol. Cell* **2012**, *23*, 3722–3730. [CrossRef]
39. Jackman, J.; O'Connor, P.M. Methods for synchronizing cells at specific stages of the cell cycle. *Curr. Protoc. Cell Biol.* **2001**. [CrossRef]
40. Malik, B.; Currais, A.; Andres, A.; Towlson, C.; Pitsi, D.; Nunes, A.; Niblock, M.; Cooper, J.; Hortobagyi, T.; Soriano, S. Loss of neuronal cell cycle control as a mechanism of neurodegeneration in the presenilin-1 Alzheimer's disease brain. *Cell Cycle* **2008**, *7*, 637–646. [CrossRef]
41. Copani, A.; Condorelli, F.; Caruso, A.; Vancheri, C.; Sala, A.; Giuffrida Stella, A.M.; Canonico, P.L.; Nicoletti, F.; Sortino, M.A. Mitotic signaling by beta-amyloid causes neuronal death. *FASEB J.* **1999**, *13*, 2225–2234. [CrossRef] [PubMed]
42. Millucci, L.; Ghezzi, L.; Bernardini, G.; Santucci, A. Conformations and biological activities of amyloid beta peptide 25–35. *Curr. Protein Pept. Sci.* **2010**, *11*, 54–67. [CrossRef] [PubMed]
43. Barrio-Alonso, E.; Hernandez-Vivanco, A.; Walton, C.C. Cell cycle reentry triggers hyperploidization and synaptic dysfunction followed by delayed cell death in differentiated cortical neurons. *Sci. Rep.* **2018**, *8*, 14316. [CrossRef] [PubMed]
44. Fitzpatrick, J.L.; Mize, A.L.; Wade, C.B.; Harris, J.A.; Shapiro, R.A.; Dorsa, D.M. Estrogen-mediated neuroprotection against beta-amyloid toxicity requires expression of estrogen receptor alpha or beta and activation of the MAPK pathway. *J. Neurochem.* **2002**, *82*, 674–682. [CrossRef] [PubMed]
45. Spitzer, P.; Schieb, H.; Kamrowski-Kruck, H.; Otto, M.; Chiasserini, D.; Parnetti, L.; Herukka, S.K.; Schuchhardt, J.; Wiltfang, J.; Klafki, H.W. Evidence for Elevated Cerebrospinal Fluid ERK1/2 Levels in Alzheimer Dementia. *Int. J. Alzheimer's Dis.* **2011**, *2011*, 739847. [CrossRef] [PubMed]

2

Dietary Sialyllactose Does Not Influence Measures of Recognition Memory or Diurnal Activity in the Young Pig

Stephen A. Fleming [1,2], Maciej Chichlowski [3], Brian M. Berg [3,4], Sharon M. Donovan [4,5] and Ryan N. Dilger [1,2,4,*]

1 Piglet Nutrition and Cognition Laboratory, Department of Animal Sciences, University of Illinois, Urbana, IL 61801, USA; sflemin2@illinois.edu
2 Department of Animal Sciences, University of Illinois, Urbana, IL 61801, USA
3 Mead Johnson Pediatric Nutrition Institute, Evansville, IL 61142, USA; maciej.chichlowski@rb.com (M.C.); dr.brianberg@gmail.com (B.M.B.)
4 Division of Nutritional Sciences, University of Illinois, Urbana, IL 61801, USA; sdonovan@illinois.edu
5 Department of Food Science and Human Nutrition, University of Illinois Urbana-Champaign, Urbana, IL 61801, USA
* Correspondence: rdilger2@illinois.edu

Abstract: Sialic acid (SA) is an integral component of gangliosides and signaling molecules in the brain and its dietary intake may support cognitive development. We previously reported that feeding sialyllactose, a milk oligosaccharide that contains SA, alters SA content and diffusivity in the pig brain. The present research sought to expand upon such results and describe the effects of feeding sialyllactose on recognition memory and sleep/wake activity using a translational pig model. Pigs were provided ad libitum access to a customized milk replacer containing 0 g/L or 380 g/L of sialyllactose from postnatal day (PND) 2–22. Beginning on PND 15, pigs were fitted with accelerometers to track home-cage activity and testing on the novel object recognition task began at PND 17. There were no significant effects of diet on average daily body weight gain, average daily milk intake, or the gain-to-feed ratio during the study (all $p \geq 0.11$). Pigs on both diets were able to display recognition memory on the novel object recognition task ($p < 0.01$), but performance and exploratory behavior did not differ between groups (all $p \geq 0.11$). Total activity and percent time spent sleeping were equivalent between groups during both day and night cycles (all $p \geq 0.56$). Dietary sialyllactose did not alter growth performance of young pigs, and there was no evidence that providing SA via sialyllactose benefits the development of recognition memory or gross sleep-related behaviors.

Keywords: pig; nutrition; brain; development; sialyllactose; sialic acid; oligosaccharide; cognition

---

1. Introduction

Human milk has been shown to have numerous benefits in comparison to infant formula in stimulating the growth and development of gastrointestinal and immune systems [1]. A recent meta-analysis suggests that breastfeeding promotes cognitive development [2], but the mechanisms and strength of the relationship are unclear [3]. There is mounting evidence that components of human milk such as DHA [4], choline [5], and gangliosides [6] support brain development, and emerging research suggests milk oligosaccharides (ranging from 3–32 monosaccharide units in length [7]) may contribute to brain development as well [8]. Some milk oligosaccharides may act as prebiotics [8], and we recently demonstrated that pigs fed a combination of prebiotics demonstrated increased exploratory behavior and improved recognition memory [9]. Milk oligosaccharides are a heterogeneous group of oligosaccharides with diverse functions largely related to immunity and gut physiology [8]. The composition of human milk oligosaccharides is 10–20% sialylated [8]. As sialic acid (SA) is present at relatively high concentrations in the brain as a part of gangliosides and signaling molecules that regulate neurodevelopment [6], the impact of sialylated oligosaccharides such as sialyllactose (SL) is of interest as they may support brain development.

Supplementation with SA-containing ingredients, including complex milk lipids [10], gangliosides [11], casein glycomacropeptide (cGMP) [12], lactoferrin [13], and SL [14], has been shown to improve cognition or alter stress-related behaviors. In a young adult mouse model investigating possible anxiolytic effects of SL, both 3′ and 6′ isomers reduced anxiety-related measures and restored performance to control levels when mice were introduced to a social stressor. Furthermore, SL attenuated stress-related sleep disruptions in adult rats [15] and tended to increase performance on spatially-based behavioral tasks [16]. A recent study demonstrated that pigs fed SL-supplemented formula for 21 days had greater total SA concentrations in the corpus callosum when fed milk containing 2 g/L of either 3′- or 6′-SL compared with pigs provided formula containing no SL or 4 g SL/L milk [17]. Similarly, a previous study from our lab showed that of a range of doses of SL, ranging from 55–779 mg SL/L of formula, a moderate dosage of 429 mg SL/L increased free-to-bound hippocampal SA, reduced bound SA in the prefrontal cortex, and increased mean, axial, and radial diffusivity in the corpus callosum [18]. Taken together with the findings of Jacobi and colleagues [17], these results show that feeding SL results in dose-dependent, structural, and region-specific increases in brain SA, but it remains to be shown whether this has functional consequences for behavior. Accordingly, our hypothesis in the present study was that supplementation with a moderate dosage of 380 mg SL/L would improve the performance of pigs on the novel object recognition task and influence measures of sleep/wake activity. We chose to supplement the diet at 380 mg SL/L, which is within the concentration range found in mature human milk [19].

2. Materials and Methods

2.1. Animals and Housing

All animal care and experimental procedures were in accordance with the National Research Council Guide for the Care and Use of Laboratory Animals and approved by the University of Illinois at Urbana-Champaign Institutional Animal Care and Use Committee. Approval for this research project was verified on 3 March 2015 and is identified as IACUC 15034 at the University of Illinois Urbana-Champaign. Beginning on postnatal day (PND) 2, naturally-farrowed, intact male pigs ($n = 36$) were artificially-reared through PND 22. The trial was completed in one replicate with 18 pigs per diet, selected from 9 L to control for genetics (same sire and related dams between litters) and initial bodyweight. All pigs were provided a single subcutaneous 5 mL dose of *Clostridium perfringens* antitoxin C and D (Colorado Serum Company, Denver, CO, USA) on PND 2. If health status appeared compromised (i.e., diarrhea, lethargy, elevated body temperature), an additional 5 mL dose of *C. perfringens* antitoxin C and D was administered orally until symptoms resolved; a total of seven pigs were given additional doses of antitoxin. Housing, temperature, and lighting were conducted as described previously [18]. Two pigs were euthanized prior to the conclusion of the study due to insufficient weight gain and failure-to-thrive ($n = 1$/diet). Data from the remaining 34 pigs ($n = 17$/diet) were used for subsequent analyses and are presented herein.

2.2. Dietary Groups

All diets were produced by Mead Johnson Nutrition (Evansville, IN, USA) using a proprietary blend of nutrients formulated to meet the nutritional needs of growing pigs. Pigs were provided one of two custom diets from PND 2–22. The control diet (Control) included docosahexaenoic acid (DHA, 87 mg/100 g milk replacer powder; DSM, Heerlen, The Netherlands), arachidonic acid (ARA, 174 mg/100 g milk replacer powder; DSM, Heerlen, The Netherlands), galactooligosaccharide (GOS,

1.0 g/100 g milk replacer powder; FrieslandCampina, Zwolle, The Netherlands), and polydextrose (PDX, 1.0 g/100 g milk replacer powder; Danisco, Terre Haute, IN, USA). The experimental diet (Sialyllactose) was formulated using the Control diet as the base and supplemented with bovine-derived modified whey enriched with SL (SAL-10; Arla Foods Ingredients, Aarhus, Denmark) to provide a final SL concentration of 190 mg SL/100 g milk replacer powder.

Milk replacer powder was reconstituted fresh each day at 200 g of dry powder per 800 g of water. At this reconstitution rate, all diets provided equal concentrations of DHA (174 mg/L), ARA (348 mg/L), and PDX/GOS (each at 2 g/L). The reconstituted milk replacers were formulated to contain 0 mg SL/L (Control) or 380 mg SL/L (Sialyllactose). Pigs were fed ad libitum using an automated milk replacer delivery system that dispensed milk from 10:00 to 06:00 the next day. Leftover milk from the previous day and individual pig bodyweights were recorded daily. The remaining volume of milk was subtracted from the initial volume provided to quantify milk disappearance following the 20-h feeding period, which will henceforth be referred to as milk intake. Milk intake from PND 21 was omitted from analyses as pigs were fasted overnight prior to the end of study on PND 22. An electrolyte solution (Swine Bluelite, Tech Mix, Stewart, MN, USA) was provided to all pigs from PND 2–5 to help maintain electrolyte balance and avoid dehydration.

2.3. *Behavioral Testing*

2.3.1. Novel Object Recognition

The novel object recognition (NOR) task was used to assess object recognition memory. Testing consisted of a habituation phase, a sample phase, and a test phase. During the habituation phase, each pig was placed in an empty testing arena for 10 min each day for two days leading up to the sample phase. In the sample phase, the pig was placed in the arena containing two identical objects and given 5 min for exploration. After a delay of 48 h, the pig was returned to the arena for the test phase. During the test phase, the pig was placed in the arena containing one object from the sample phase as well as a novel object and allowed to explore for 5 min. Between trials, objects were removed, immersed in hot water with detergent and rubbed with a towel to mitigate odor, and the arena was sprayed with water to remove urine and feces. Objects chosen had a range of characteristics (i.e., color, texture, shape, and size); however, the novel and sample objects only differed in shape and size. Only objects previously shown to elicit a null preference were used for testing. Habituation trials began at PND 17 and testing on the NOR task began at PND 19. The amount of time exploring objects and distance moved was measured using a combination of automated procedures using Ethovision (Ethovision XT 11®, Noldus Information Technology, Wageningen, The Netherlands) and manual tracking (for a review of each measure assessed, see Fleming and Dilger [20]). The recognition index, the proportion of time spent with the novel object compared to total exploration of both objects, was used to measure recognition memory. A recognition index significantly above 0.50 demonstrates a novelty preference and, thus, recognition memory. Trials were removed from analyses if experimental/technical errors existed or pigs explored either object for less than 2 s during the sample or test trial. If pigs did not explore either object for greater than 2 s during the sample trial, they were also removed from analysis during the test trial regardless of performance. Two and five pigs provided the Control and SL diets, respectively, did not meet the above criteria and were removed from the final analysis (final n = 15, Control; n = 12, Sialyllactose).

2.3.2. Activity Analysis

Accelerometers (Actiwatch 2, Philips Respironics, Bend, OR, USA) were secured to collars and fastened around each pig's neck between PND 15 and 22 (n = 12 per diet) and were set to sample movement every 15 s. Only periods where full day and night cycles were recorded were used for analysis (PND 15 and 22 were omitted as collars were only on for part of the day, for a remaining total of six full cycles between PND 16 and 21). When pigs were found without collars, the collar was re-applied and the time was noted. After study completion, home-cage video was used to verify that periods of complete inactivity were due to the loss of the collar, and these times were also removed from analysis. For the analysis of sleep/wake outcomes, specialized software (Actiware 6.0.7, Philips Respironics, Murrysville, PA, USA) was used to calculate a unique wake threshold value (used to determine if the pig was asleep or awake based on movement during 2-min periods before and after a single 15-s epoch) for each pig and quantify the total activity count and percent time asleep. Data were collected for six consecutive days and sleep outcomes were assessed as averages across that period.

A preliminary analysis was conducted to assess the validity of sleep scores in pigs from actigraphy data. Approximately one hour of activity data collected from six pigs was scored by actigraphy software as compared to the manual scoring of recorded video. Video was split into 15-s epochs, for a total of 247 epochs, and manually analyzed. If a pig was visually-assessed as asleep for more than 50% of a single 15-s epoch, that epoch was classified as a "sleep" epoch. Epochs were chosen by selecting for periods of apparent transition between sleep and wakefulness as these are the most difficult to classify and appeared to be most variable between manual and automatic scoring methods.

2.4. Statistical Analysis

All data generated as part of this study were subjected to an analysis of variance (ANOVA) using the MIXED procedure of SAS Enterprise Guide 5.1 (SAS Institute Inc., Cary, NC, USA). Depending on the outcome, one of two statistical models was used: (1) data collected at a single time-point (e.g., average body weight gain over the entire study, performance in the NOR test trial) were analyzed by one-way ANOVA; and (2) data collected from the same animal on more than one occasion (e.g., diurnal activity) were analyzed using two-way repeated-measures ANOVA. Litter was included as a random effect in both statistical models. For NOR testing, a one-tailed t-test was conducted to assess if recognition index was greater than 0.5 (i.e., random chance). In all instances statistical significance was considered at $p < 0.05$.

3. Results

3.1. Diet Composition

Analytical assessment conducted after study completion showed levels of SL in the experimental diets were close to formulated levels (374 mg SL/L vs. 380 mg SL/L in the Sialyllactose diet). However, the Control diet contained 58 mg SL/L due to endogenous SL in the bovine milk ingredients. Energy, macronutrient, and micronutrient composition were comparable between Control and Sialyllactose diets (see Table 1 for analyzed nutrient composition).

Table 1. Analyzed nutrient composition of experimental diets.

Nutrient per Liter	Control	Sialyllactose
Sialyllactose, mg	58	374
Energy and macronutrients		
Total calories, kcal	1049	1020
Carbohydrate, g	57	58
Fat, g	64	60
Protein, g	61	62
Minerals		
Calcium, mg	2233	2178
Chlorine, mg	1141	1158
Copper, µg	1640	1505
Iodine, µg	274	271
Iron, mg	19	19
Magnesium, mg	227	241

Table 1. *Cont.*

Nutrient per Liter	Control	Sialyllactose
Manganese, µg	2305	2159
Phosphorus, mg	1621	1673
Potassium, mg	2255	2349
Selenium, µg	65	68
Sodium, mg	1708	1708
Zinc, mg	17	17
Vitamins and other nutrients		
Vitamin A, IU	4572	4112
Vitamin D_3, IU	761	795
Vitamin E, IU	30	31
Vitamin K, µg	321	362
Thiamin, µg	1322	1588
Riboflavin, µg	2608	2780
Niacin, µg	13,366	11,132
Vitamin B_6, µg	1210	1414
Folic acid, µg	211	237
Vitamin B_{12}, µg	6	7
Pantothenic acid, µg	9216	8170
Biotin, µg	74	74
Choline, mg	352	394
Polydextrose, g	1.8	1.9
Galactooligosaccharide, g	2.1	1.7
Arachidonic acid, mg	318	288
Docosahexaenoic acid, mg	155	141

3.2. *Growth Performance and Health Status*

No differences were observed for average daily body weight gain, average daily milk intake, or the feed efficiency ratio (i.e., gain-to-milk intake) between diets across the duration of the study (all $p \geq 0.11$, Table 2, Figure 1). Additionally, daily health checks revealed low incidence of loose stool in pigs and no differences in pig health status or compliance to consume experimental dietary treatments. Thus, all pigs remained healthy throughout the study duration and both dietary treatments were equally well tolerated by pigs as evident in the observed trajectory of body weight gain.

Table 2. Effects of dietary sialyllactose supplementation on the growth performance of pigs over the duration of the feeding study [1].

	Diet [2]		Pooled	
Measure [3]	Control	Sialyllactose	SEM	*p*-Value [4]
ADG, g/day	311	306	14	0.69
ADMI, g milk/day	1220	1347	62	0.11
ADMI, g solids/day	244	269	12	0.11
G:F, g BW:kg milk	255	234	11	0.16

[1] Abbreviations: SEM, standard error of the mean; BW, body weight; kg, kilogram; ADG, average daily body weight gain; ADMI, average daily milk intake; G:F, gain-to-feed ratio (i.e., feed efficiency); [2] $n = 17$ per diet; [3] Calculations reflect a milk reconstitution rate of 20% solids; [4] *p*-values derived from mixed model ANOVA.

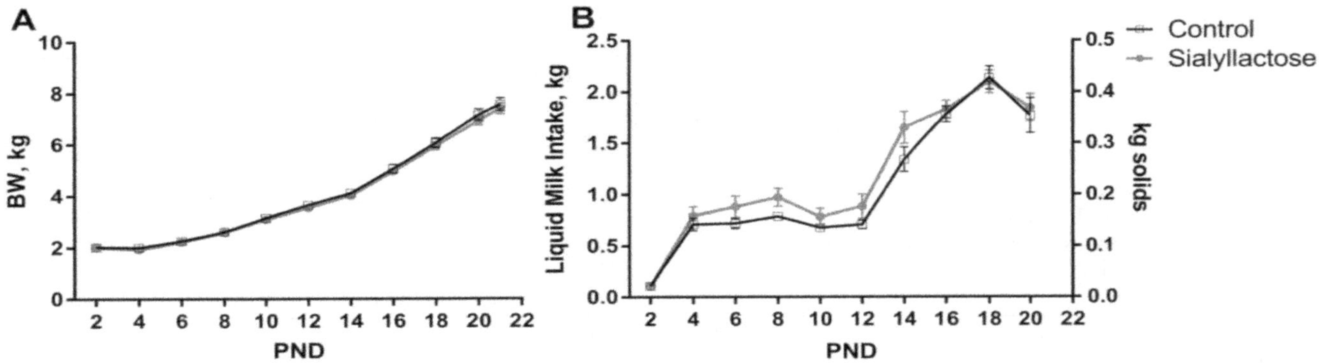

Figure 1. Body weight (BW) (**A**) and liquid milk intake (**B**) during the trial. No differences in average daily body weight gain, average daily milk intake, or the feed efficiency ratio (i.e., body weight gain:feed intake ratio) were observed between groups ($p \geq 0.11$). Data for milk intake on postnatal day (PND) 22 are not shown as piglets were fasted overnight prior to the end of study.

3.3. Novel Object Recognition

Regardless of dietary treatment, all pigs were able to display recognition memory in the NOR test trial ($p < 0.01$, Table 3). However, there were no differences between dietary treatment groups for measures of exploratory behavior, most notably time spent investigating objects, number of object visits, and mean time spent per object visit (all $p \geq 0.11$, Table 4). Although some pigs were removed due to non-compliance, ultimately our study was powered to capture an effect size of 0.89 with a power of 0.80 when evaluating differences in the NOR recognition index.

Table 3. Ability of pigs to display a recognition index score above 0.50 as a measure of recognition memory in the NOR test trial [1].

Diet	*n*	Mean	SEM	*p*-Value [2]
Control	15	0.65	0.046	<0.01
Sialyllactose	12	0.66	0.047	<0.01

[1] Abbreviations: NOR, novel object recognition; SEM, standard error of the mean; [2] *p*-Value derived from one-tailed *t*-test for a recognition index above 0.50.

Table 4. Effect of dietary sialyllactose supplementation on exploratory behavior during the test trial of the NOR task [1].

	Diet					
	Control		Sialyllactose		Pooled	
Measure	*n*	Mean	*n*	Mean	SEM	*p*-Value [2]
Recognition index	15	0.66	12	0.65	0.05	0.94
Novel object visit time, s	15	56.63	12	42.05	7.77	0.18
Number of novel object visits	15	8.33	12	6.78	1.07	0.25
Mean novel object visit time, s	15	6.19	11	6.41	1.12	0.88
Latency to first novel object visit, s	15	25.46	12	25.32	9.31	0.99
Habituation towards the novel object, s/min	15	−1.60	12	−0.69	1.25	0.59
Sample object visit time, s	14	28.27	12	22.45	6.45	0.50
Number of sample object visits	15	4.77	12	4.62	0.56	0.84
Mean sample object visit time, s	15	6.18	12	5.51	1.34	0.71
Latency to first sample object visit, s	14	24.08	12	14.25	7.15	0.31
Habituation towards the sample object, s/min	14	−2.68	12	−1.78	0.73	0.35
Total object visit time, s	15	82.52	12	70.35	13.51	0.47
Mean object visit time, s	15	7.10	12	6.11	1.22	0.55

Table 4. *Cont.*

Measure	Diet: Control *n*	Control Mean	Sialyllactose *n*	Sialyllactose Mean	Pooled SEM	*p*-Value [2]
Number of object visits	15	13.13	12	11.42	1.34	0.31
Latency to first object visit, s	15	9.48	12	13.50	4.97	0.55
Habituation towards both objects, s/min	15	−4.32	12	−1.76	1.39	0.19
Total distance moved, m	15	2.43	11	2.11	0.19	0.11
Time spent in the center of the arena, %	15	58.76	12	56.73	6.95	0.80

[1] Abbreviations: NOR, novel object recognition; SEM, standard error of the mean; [2] *p*-Values derived from mixed model ANOVA.

3.4. Activity Analysis

Validation of the automated scoring method (i.e., computer-assisted analysis of actigraphy data) against the manual scoring of home-cage video was performed. A chi-square test for equality of two proportions showed that automated and manual scoring methods were not different ($p = 0.065$), with the automated scoring being only 7% more likely to score an epoch as "sleep" and less likely to score an epoch as "awake". Therefore, with the validation of the automated actigraphy data scoring method complete, all sleep/wake activity reported herein was generated using the automated software-based method. In general, there was no significant main effect of diet or interaction effect of diet by cycle for total activity or percent time asleep (all $p \geq 0.56$, Table 5). While intuitive, total activity counts and time asleep were both influenced by cycle (i.e., day vs. night; both $p < 0.01$).

Table 5. Effect of dietary sialyllactose supplementation on diurnal activity of pigs [1].

Measure	Diet [2]: Control, Day *n*	Control, Day Mean	Control, Night *n*	Control, Night Mean	Sialyllactose, Day *n*	Sialyllactose, Day Mean	Sialyllactose, Night *n*	Sialyllactose, Night Mean	Pooled SEM	*p*-Value [3] Diet	*p*-Value Cycle	*p*-Value Interaction
Total activity count	65	1.6×10^5	70	6.9×10^4	67	1.7×10^5	72	6.9×10^4	7.0×10^3	0.64	<0.01	0.56
Time asleep, %	65	67.47	70	84.90	71	67.43	72	85.63	0.97	0.61	<0.01	0.58

[1] Abbreviations: SEM, standard error of the mean; %, percent; [2] Data from 12 pigs per diet over a six-day period; [3] *p*-Value derived from repeated measures mixed model ANOVA.

4. Discussion

Siallylactose is one of several sources of SA, and comparisons of mature human and porcine milk demonstrate that the SA content of human milk is much greater than that of porcine milk. Mature human milk provides approximately 500 mg SA/L milk [21], porcine milk contains approximately 10 mg SA/L milk [22], and infant formula falls between 65–290 mg SA/L milk [23] (for a thorough review of SA content of milk and other food products, see Röhrig et al. [24]). In this study, a dose of 380 mg SL/L was tested as a previous study reported that this dose was most effective at eliciting changes in SA content and diffusivity in the brain [18]. This dose is well below the SL dose that was shown by Jacobi et al. [17] to enrich corpus callosum and hippocampal SA content [17], but is within the range found in mature human milk [19]. Here, the impact of dietary SL on growth, recognition memory, exploratory behavior, and diurnal activity was investigated, but no impact of diet was observed for any measure.

Pigs fed an SL-supplemented diet did not display altered sleep behavior, whereas a past report demonstrated that SL attenuated disruptions to sleep architecture after exposure to an acute inescapable stress [15]. An important distinction from past research is that diurnal activity was measured in a minimally stressful environment, whereas SL may provide a neuroprotective effect that is only observed in the context of a more extreme stressor. Additionally, Chichlowski et al. [15] used electroencephalography (EEG), allowing the experimenters to more accurately quantify the timing, stage, and quality of sleep. Although both treatment groups in our study had similar activity during the day and night, differences in the quality of sleep may have been observed if assessments were made using EEG.

While different doses and/or longer duration of SL administration may have produced a cognitive benefit, it is possible that supplemental SA (via SL) was not required in the behavioral paradigm under which the pigs were assessed. Active learning increases the expression of mRNA for the enzyme critical for regulating SA biosynthesis (UDP-N-acetylglucoasamine-2-epimerase/*N*-acetylmannosamine kinase, GNE) by 2- to 3-fold in the hippocampus and liver of pigs [25]. As the NOR task makes use of spontaneous behavior rather than operant conditioning the cognitive load required to learn a rule was not present, and there may not have been a physiological demand for increased SA utilization in the brain. Our data show that dietary SL supplementation did not provide a cognitive benefit as assessed by NOR, which conflicts with previous work that showed young pigs exhibit cognitive benefits from dietary SA supplementation when using behavioral tasks dependent on operant conditioning [12,13]. Moreover, these results may reflect the presence of prebiotics in both the control and experimental diet. We previously reported that pigs fed milk replacers containing the prebiotics PDX and GOS demonstrated increased exploratory behavior and improved recognition memory using the same behavioral paradigm (i.e., the NOR task with a delay of 48 h) [9]. Together with evidence that piglets are capable of performing the NOR task at younger ages using shorter delays [20], we believe the difficulty of the task was appropriate. Rather, the potential cognitive benefits from SL may have been masked by the inclusion of PDX and GOS in each diet.

To our knowledge, few studies have evaluated the ability of dietary SL to affect behavior and cognition. Tarr and colleagues [14] found that dietary SL attenuated stressor induced anxiety-like behaviors in rats and preliminary data suggests that SL may prevent stress-induced alterations in sleep architecture [15]. However, another report in rats demonstrated that feeding SL only produced a non-significant trend towards improved cognition on spatial tasks [16]. The majority of data suggesting dietary SL may be beneficial for cognitive development come indirectly from studies that investigated other SA-containing ingredients such as gangliosides [10,11,26], cGMP [12], and lactoferrin [13]. Each of these ingredients vary in structure and function, but are common in that they contain SA. Gangliosides are sialylated glycosphingolipids highly concentrated in the brain [6], cGMP is an SA-enriched peptide released during the formation of cheese from the protein kappa-casein [27], and lactoferrin is an iron binding glycoprotein enriched in SA with various functions related to iron metabolism [28].

Gangliosides contribute 75% of conjugated SA in the brain where they play a critical role in functions such as synaptic transmission, plasticity, neurogenesis, synaptogenesis, cell proliferation, and cell differentiation [6]. Exogenous, but not dietary, gangliosides and SA appear to be effective at promoting cognition in adult or aging models [29–33] and deficit (i.e., drug-induced amnesia, cortical lesions, malnourishment) models [34–36]. The impact on young, normal animals is mixed, but ganglioside and SA administration have shown both positive and neutral effects on cognition [31,37]. These studies provided preliminary evidence that exogenous SA improves cognition; however, there is less evidence that dietary gangliosides improve cognition in normative models (i.e., gangliosides are provided at physiological concentrations via the diet to healthy animals during typical development).

Male and female pigs fed formula containing a mix of 0.8% or 2.5% phospholipids and gangliosides displayed fewer errors in a spatial T-maze test compared with controls and had larger brain weights. Furthermore, volumes of several brain regions including the internal capsule, putamen, and thalamus appeared sensitive to supplementation [11]. As has been discussed for SA, the cognitive effects of dietary ganglioside supplementation appear dependent on dosage and behavioral task employed. Rats provided complex milk lipid in doses of 1.0% but not 0.2% exhibited greater behavioral performance in the novel object recognition and Morris water maze, but no improvement in operant conditioning tasks [10]. A subsequent report from the same group demonstrated that even lower doses of 0.05% and 0.01% had no effect on operant learning, and spatial or recognition memory [38]. In a separate study, dietary gangliosides fed to children with cerebral palsy for 3 months elicited improved muscle tension, limb function, language ability, and intelligence [26]. Due to the use of a developmentally-appropriate preclinical model for the human infant, this study provides strong evidence that gangliosides contribute to not only cognition but also motor function and development. Taken together these data suggest that, provided the correct dosage, gangliosides fed alone or as part of a complex milk lipid may have the capacity to promote cognitive development.

Young pigs supplemented with SA via cGMP from PND 3–35 displayed dose-dependent increases in performance in the radial arm maze, with those provided the most cGMP completing the difficult version of the task with the fewest mistakes. All groups fed cGMP had enriched protein-bound, but not ganglioside-bound, SA in the frontal cortex. Additionally, pigs fed the highest amount of cGMP had increased levels of *ST8SIAIV*, a polysialyltransferase important in SA metabolism. After a correlational analysis, it was revealed that sialyltransferase activity in the frontal cortex correlated inversely with number of mistakes on the behavioral task, with pigs exhibiting lower sialyltransferase activity making more mistakes. Despite this correlation, there were no dietary effects on sialyltransferase activity, suggesting sialyltransferase activity may not be involved in the mechanism by which performance was improved. In a later study by the same group, pigs supplemented with lactoferrin from PND 3–38 were found to have increased performance on the radial maze. More pigs in the treatment group were able to complete both easy and difficult versions of the task, with the pigs provided lactoferrin making fewer mistakes on the difficult version [13]. Gene microarray data in hippocampal tissue revealed that pigs fed lactoferrin had upregulated expression of genes in the brain-derived neurotrophic factor (BDNF) neurotrophic signaling pathway, affecting genes related to organization of the cytoplasm, cytoskeleton, growth of neurites, and anxiety [13]. The finding that the provision of dietary lactoferrin influenced the expression of genes related to anxiety suggested that this protein may decrease anxiety, which aligns with the previously discussed results from Tarr et al. [14], wherein mice provided SL demonstrated attenuated anxiety when introduced to a social stressor.

Overall, few studies have evaluated the impact of SL on cognition and behavior. However, there is evidence that SA-containing ingredients positively influence cognitive performance, but making cross-sectional comparisons is confounded by the use of several different SA-enriched ingredients. While containing SA, SL, gangliosides, cGMP, and lactoferrin differ vastly in structure and function, contributing to the variation between study results.

Although our intervention coincided with a significant portion of brain growth in the pig, our investigation may have been limited by the duration of the trial, which may not have allowed sufficient time for SL to confer cognitive benefits. As discussed, the novel object recognition task may not reflect a context wherein supplemental SA is beneficial, and comparisons between spontaneous and operant behavior may elucidate the conditions that lead to increased neural requirements for SA. While clinically translatable, the use of actigraphy instead of EEG did not allow the examination of neural activity during sleep and the quantification of sleep stages, thus our measures were only a gross representation of sleep activity. Lastly, although the goal of this study was to evaluate the efficacy of 380 mg SL/L at supporting cognitive development, we cannot exclude the possibility that a higher supplementation dose or longer supplementation period may have elicited cognitive benefits.

5. Conclusions

While there are several reports that SA-containing ingredients may influence cognitive development, we found no evidence that bovine-derived dietary SL provided at 380 mg SL/L was effective at altering recognition memory or sleep-related activity.

Acknowledgments: The authors would like to thank Kristen Karkiewicz for her assistance with animal rearing. The authors acknowledge the efforts of Mead Johnson Nutrition employees Shireen Doultani and Julieta Ortiz for assistance in formulating and manufacturing the diets. The authors would also like to thank Monique LeBourgeois for her assistance with adapting actigraphy to the pig model and the Mead Johnson Nutrition Medical Affairs Department for donating the actigraphy devices.

Author Contributions: All authors contributed to design of the study. S.A.F. performed study execution. S.A.F. and R.N.D. contributed to statistical analyses. All authors contributed to interpretation and manuscript preparation.

References

1. Ballard, O.; Morrow, A.L. Human milk composition: Nutrients and bioactive factors. *Pediatr. Clin. N. Am.* **2013**, *60*, 49–74. [CrossRef] [PubMed]
2. Horta, B.L.; de Mola, C.L.; Victora, C.G. Breastfeeding and intelligence: A systematic review and meta-analysis. *Acta Paediatr. Int. J. Paediatr.* **2015**, *104*, 14–19. [CrossRef] [PubMed]
3. Girard, L.-C.; Doyle, O.; Tremblay, R.E. Breastfeeding, Cognitive and Noncognitive Development in Early Childhood: A Population Study. *Pediatrics* **2017**, *139*, e20161848. [CrossRef] [PubMed]
4. Hoffman, D.R.; Boettcher, J.A.; Diersen-Schade, D.A. Toward optimizing vision and cognition in term infants by dietary docosahexaenoic and arachidonic acid supplementation: A review of randomized controlled trials. *Prostaglandins Leukot. Essent. Fat. Acids* **2009**, *81*, 151–158. [CrossRef] [PubMed]
5. Zeisel, S.H. Nutritional Importance of Choline for Brain Development. *J. Am. Coll. Nutr.* **2004**, *23*, 621S–626S. [CrossRef] [PubMed]
6. Palmano, K.; Rowan, A.; Guillermo, R.; Guan, J.; McJarrow, P. The role of gangliosides in neurodevelopment. *Nutrients* **2015**, *7*, 3891–3913. [CrossRef] [PubMed]
7. Morrow, A.L.; Ruiz-Palacios, G.M.; Jiang, X.; Newburg, D.S. Human-milk glycans that inhibit pathogen binding protect breast-feeding infants against infectious diarrhea. *J. Nutr.* **2005**, *135*, 1304–1307. [CrossRef] [PubMed]
8. Bode, L. Human milk oligosaccharides: Every baby needs a sugar mama. *Glycobiology* **2012**, *22*, 1147–1162. [CrossRef] [PubMed]
9. Fleming, S.A.; Monaikul, S.; Patsavas, A.J.; Waworuntu, R.V.; Berg, B.M.; Dilger, R.N. Dietary polydextrose and galactooligosaccharide increase exploratory behavior, improve recognition memory, and alter neurochemistry in the young pig. *Nutr. Neurosci.* **2017**, 1–14. [CrossRef] [PubMed]
10. Vickers, M.H.; Guan, J.; Gustavsson, M.; Krägeloh, C.U.; Breier, B.H.; Davison, M.; Fong, B.; Norris, C.; McJarrow, P.; Hodgkinson, S.C. Supplementation with a mixture of complex lipids derived from milk to growing rats results in improvements in parameters related to growth and cognition. *Nutr. Res.* **2009**, *29*, 426–435. [CrossRef] [PubMed]
11. Liu, H.; Radlowski, E.E.C.; Conrad, M.M.S.; Li, Y.; Dilger, R.N.; Johnson, R.W. Early supplementation of phospholipids and gangliosides affects brain and cognitive development in neonatal piglets. *J. Nutr.* **2014**, *144*, 1–7. [CrossRef] [PubMed]
12. Wang, B.; Yu, B.; Karim, M.; Hu, H.; Sun, Y.; McGreevy, P.; Petocz, P.; Held, S.; Brand-Miller, J. Dietary sialic acid supplementation improves learning and memory in piglets. *Am. J. Clin. Nutr.* **2007**, *85*, 561–569. [CrossRef] [PubMed]
13. Chen, Y.; Zheng, Z.; Zhu, X.; Shi, Y.; Tian, D.; Zhao, F.; Liu, N.; Hüppi, P.S.; Troy, F.A.; Wang, B. Lactoferrin Promotes Early Neurodevelopment and Cognition in Postnatal Piglets by Upregulating the BDNF Signaling Pathway and Polysialylation. *Mol. Neurobiol.* **2015**, *52*, 256–269. [CrossRef] [PubMed]
14. Tarr, A.J.; Galley, J.D.; Fisher, S.E.; Chichlowski, M.; Berg, B.M.; Bailey, M.T. The prebiotics 3′Sialyllactose and 6′Sialyllactose diminish stressor-induced anxiety-like behavior and colonic microbiota alterations: Evidence for effects on the gut-brain axis. *Brain Behav. Immun.* **2015**, *50*, 166–177. [CrossRef] [PubMed]
15. Chichlowski, M.; Morairty, S.; Berg, B.M. Early life diet alters sleep architecture following an acute stress: The potential role of milk oligosaccharides. *FASEB J.* **2017**, *31*, 636.
16. Sakai, F.; Ikeuchi, Y.; Urashima, T.; Fujihara, M.; Ohtsuki, K.; Yanahira, S. Effects of Feeding Sialyllactose and Galactosylated *N*-Acetylneuraminic Acid on Swimming Learning Ability and Brain Lipid Composition in Adult Rats. *J. Appl. Glycosci.* **2006**, *53*, 249–254. [CrossRef]
17. Jacobi, S.K.; Yatsunenko, T.; Li, D.; Dasgupta, S.; Yu, R.K.; Berg, B.M.; Chichlowski, M.; Odle, J. Dietary Isomers of Sialyllactose Increase Ganglioside Sialic Acid Concentrations in the Corpus Callosum and Cerebellum and Modulate the Colonic Microbiota of Formula-Fed Piglets. *J. Nutr.* **2016**, *146*, 200–208. [PubMed]
18. Mudd, A.A.T.; Fleming, S.S.A.; Labhart, B.; Chichlowski, M.; Berg, B.B.M.; Donovan, S.S.M.; Dilger, R.R.N.

Dietary Sialyllactose Influences Sialic Acid Concentrations in the Prefrontal Cortex and Magnetic Resonance Imaging Measures in Corpus Callosum of Young Pigs. *Nutrients* **2017**, *9*, 1297. [CrossRef] [PubMed]

19. Bruggencate, S.J.T.; Bovee-Oudenhoven, I.M.; Feitsma, A.L.; van Hoffen, E.; Schoterman, M.H. Functional role and mechanisms of sialyllactose and other sialylated milk oligosaccharides. *Nutr. Rev.* **2014**, *72*, 377–389. [CrossRef] [PubMed]
20. Fleming, S.A.; Dilger, R.N. Young pigs exhibit differential exploratory behavior during novelty preference tasks in response to age, sex, and delay. *Behav. Brain Res.* **2017**, *321*, 50–60. [CrossRef] [PubMed]
21. Martín-Sosa, S.; Martín, M.-J.; García-Pardo, L.A.; Hueso, P. Distribution of sialic acids in the milk of spanish mothers of full term infants during lactation. *J. Pediatr. Gastroenterol. Nutr.* **2004**, *39*, 499–503. [CrossRef] [PubMed]
22. Mudd, A.T.; Salcedo, J.; Alexander, L.S.; Johnson, S.K.; Getty, C.M.; Chichlowski, M.; Berg, B.M.; Barile, D.; Dilger, R.N. Porcine Milk Oligosaccharides and Sialic Acid Concentrations Vary throughout Lactation. *Front. Nutr.* **2016**, *3*. [CrossRef] [PubMed]
23. Spichtig, V.; Michaud, J.; Austin, S. Determination of sialic acids in milks and milk-based products. *Anal. Biochem.* **2010**, *405*, 28–40. [PubMed]
24. Röhrig, C.H.; Choi, S.S.H.; Baldwin, N. The nutritional role of free sialic acid, a human milk monosaccharide, and its application as a functional food ingredient. *Crit. Rev. Food Sci. Nutr.* **2017**, *57*, 1017–1038. [CrossRef] [PubMed]
25. Wang, B.; Hu, H.; Yu, B.; Troy, F.A. Molecular characterization of pig UDP-*N*-acetylglucosamine-2-epimerase/*N*-acetylmannosamine kinase (Gne) gene: Effect of dietary sialic acid supplementation on gene expression in piglets. *Curr. Top. Nutr. Res.* **2007**, *5*, 165–175.
26. Xu, X.; Zhu, T. Effect of ganglioside in repairing the neurological function of Chinese children with cerebral palsy. *Chin. J. Clin. Rehabil.* **2005**, *9*, 122–123.
27. Neelima; Sharma, R.; Rajput, Y.S.; Mann, B. Chemical and functional properties of glycomacropeptide (GMP) and its role in the detection of cheese whey adulteration in milk: A review. *Dairy Sci. Technol.* **2013**, *93*, 21–43. [CrossRef] [PubMed]
28. Levay, P.F.; Viljoen, M. Lactoferrin: A general review. *Haematologica* **1995**, *80*, 252–267. [PubMed]
29. Fagioli, S.; Rossi-Arnaud, C.; Castellano, C. Dose-dependent effect of GM1 ganglioside during development on inhibitory avoidance behaviour in mice: Influence of the period of administration. *Psychopharmacology (Berl.)* **1992**, *109*, 457–460. [CrossRef] [PubMed]
30. Silva, R.H.; Bellot, R.G.; Vital, M.A.; Frussa-Filho, R. Effects of long-term ganglioside GM1 administration on a new discriminative avoidance test in normal adult mice. *Psychopharmacology (Berl.)* **1997**, *129*, 322–328. [PubMed]
31. Fong, T.G.; Neff, N.H.; Hadjiconstantinou, M. GM1 ganglioside improves spatial learning and memory of aged rats. *Behav. Brain Res.* **1997**, *85*, 203–211. [CrossRef]
32. Silva, R.H.; Bergamo, M.; Frussa-Filho, R. Effects of neonatal ganglioside GM1 administration on memory in adult and old rats. *Pharmacol. Toxicol.* **2000**, *87*, 120–125. [CrossRef]
33. Popov, N.; Toffano, G.; Riechert, U.; Matthies, H. Effects of intraventricularly applied gangliosides and *N*-acetylneuraminic acid on acquisition and retention performance of a brightness discrimination task in rats. *Pharmacol. Biochem. Behav.* **1989**, *34*, 209–212. [CrossRef]
34. Silva, R.H.; Felicio, L.F.; Frussa-Filho, R. Ganglioside GM1 attenuates scopolamine-induced amnesia in rats and mice. *Psychopharmacology (Berl.)* **1999**, *141*, 111–117. [CrossRef] [PubMed]
35. Glasier, M.M.; Janis, L.S.; Goncalves, M.I.; Stein, D.G. GM1 produces attenuation of short-term memory deficits in Hebb-Williams maze performance after unilateral entorhinal cortex lesions. *Physiol. Behav.* **1999**, *66*, 441–446. [CrossRef]
36. Morgan, B.L.; Winick, M. Effects of administration of N-acetylneuraminic acid (NANA) on brain NANA content and behavior. *J. Nutr.* **1980**, *110*, 416–424. [CrossRef] [PubMed]
37. Wainwright, P.E.; Lomanowska, A.M.; McCutcheon, D.; Park, E.J.; Clandinin, M.T.; Ramanujam, K.S. Postnatal dietary supplementation with either gangliosides or choline: Effects on spatial short-term memory in artificially-reared rats. *Nutr. Neurosci.* **2007**, *10*, 67–77. [CrossRef] [PubMed]
38. Gustavsson, M.; Hodgkinson, S.C.; Fong, B.; Norris, C.; Guan, J.; Krageloh, C.U.; Breier, B.H.; Davison, M.; McJarrow, P.; Vickers, M.H. Maternal supplementation with a complex milk lipid mixture during pregnancy and lactation alters neonatal brain lipid composition but lacks effect on cognitive function in rats. *Nutr. Res.* **2010**, *30*, 279–289. [CrossRef] [PubMed]

3

Serine Phosphorylation of IRS1 Correlates with Aβ-Unrelated Memory Deficits and Elevation in Aβ Level Prior to the Onset of Memory Decline in AD

Wei Wang [1,†], Daisuke Tanokashira [1,†], Yusuke Fukui [1], Megumi Maruyama [1], Chiemi Kuroiwa [1], Takashi Saito [2,3], Takaomi C. Saido [2] and Akiko Taguchi [1,*]

1 Department of Integrative Aging Neuroscience, National Center for Geriatrics and Gerontology, Obu, Aichi 474-8511, Japan
2 Laboratory for Proteolytic Neuroscience, RIKEN Center for Brain Science, Wako, Saitama 351-0106, Japan
3 Department of Neurocognitive Science, Nagoya City University Graduate School of Medical Science, Nagoya, Aichi 467-8601, Japan
* Correspondence: taguchia@ncgg.go.jp
† These authors contributed equally.

Abstract: The biological effects of insulin signaling are regulated by the phosphorylation of insulin receptor substrate 1 (IRS1) at serine (Ser) residues. In the brain, phosphorylation of IRS1 at specific Ser sites increases in patients with Alzheimer's disease (AD) and its animal models. However, whether the activation of Ser sites on neural IRS1 is related to any type of memory decline remains unclear. Here, we show the modifications of IRS1 through its phosphorylation at etiology-specific Ser sites in various animal models of memory decline, such as diabetic, aged, and amyloid precursor protein (APP) knock-in $^{NL\text{-}G\text{-}F}$ (APPKI$^{NL\text{-}G\text{-}F}$) mice. Substantial phosphorylation of IRS1 at specific Ser sites occurs in type 2 diabetes- or age-related memory deficits independently of amyloid-β (Aβ). Furthermore, we present the first evidence that, in APPKI$^{NL\text{-}G\text{-}F}$ mice showing Aβ42 elevation, the increased phosphorylation of IRS1 at multiple Ser sites occurs without memory impairment. Our findings suggest that the phosphorylation of IRS1 at specific Ser sites is a potential marker of Aβ-unrelated memory deficits caused by type 2 diabetes and aging; however, in Aβ-related memory decline, the modifications of IRS1 may be a marker of early detection of Aβ42 elevation prior to the onset of memory decline in AD.

Keywords: IRS1; serine phosphorylation; hippocampus; diabetes; aging; Alzheimer's disease; memory decline; Aβ; AMPK; energy depletion

---

1. Introduction

Insulin signaling mediated by insulin receptor substrates 1 and 2 (IRS1 and IRS2) is involved in the regulation of growth, glucose homeostasis, energy metabolism, and lifespan [1–4]. The biological effects of insulin signaling are regulated by the modulation of IRS proteins through serine (Ser) and threonine (Thr) phosphorylation [5,6]. Notably, IRS1 is known to be abundantly phosphorylated at Ser and Thr residues regardless of insulin or IGF1 stimulation [5,7]. In vitro studies have demonstrated the relationship between IRS1 Ser/Thr phosphorylation and canonical downstream signaling components, including Akt/protein kinase B, glycogen synthase kinase 3 beta (GSK3β), and ribosomal protein S6 kinase (S6K) [5]. Under physiological and pathological conditions, Ser/Thr phosphorylation of IRS1 is potentially mediated by multiple kinases, including AMP-activated protein kinase (AMPK), conventional and novel protein kinase C (PKC), and c-Jun N-terminal kinases (JNKs), in response to intracellular energy status, nutritional conditions, and inflammatory stimulation [5,6,8].

Among the numerous Ser residues on IRS1, a few sites, including human(h)Ser312/mouse(m)Ser307, hSer616/mSer612, hSer636/mSer632, hSer639/mSer635, and hSer1101/mSer1097, have been studied because a limited number of phosphospecific antibodies were previously commercially available.

Nonetheless, hSer312/mSer307 has been widely investigated and implicated in insulin resistance under metabolic stress conditions and in inflammatory conditions such as obesity, hyperinsulinemia, and dyslipidemia [5,9,10]. However, IRS1 mSer307 knock-in mice display insulin resistance rather than increased insulin sensitivity, suggesting that IRS1 mSer307 is a positive regulatory site and is essential for normal insulin signaling [11]. IRS1 mSer612 and mSer632/635 have been cited as negative regulatory sites for IRS1 signaling through tyrosine phosphorylation [5], and mSer1097, regarded as a potential mammalian target of rapamycin (mTOR) /S6K signaling pathway, is activated in the liver of model animals of obesity [12]. However, the roles of these sites remain largely unknown because they have been examined in different context.

In the central nervous system, studies on postmortem brain tissues of patients with Alzheimer's disease (AD) have revealed increased phosphorylation of IRS1 at hSer312/mSer307, hSer616/mSer612, hSer636/mSer632, and hSer639/mSer635 compared with that in non-AD control subjects [13–16]. The phosphorylation levels of IRS1 at hSer312/mSer307 and hSer616/mSer612 are considerably elevated in the brains of patients with AD [15]. In animal studies, multiple AD mouse models display increased phosphorylation of IRS1 at mSer307 and/or mSer632 or mSer612 [16–18]. However, whether the modifications of IRS1 via Ser phosphorylation are involved in memory decline in amyloid precursor protein (APP) knock-in (KI)$^{NL\text{-}G\text{-}F}$ (APPKI$^{NL\text{-}G\text{-}F}$) mice, a novel AD mouse model, remains unclear [19]. Meanwhile, animals with diet-induced obesity (DIO), a model of type 2 diabetes mellitus (T2DM), that were fed a 40% or 60% high-fat diet (HFD) during different periods displayed cognitive impairment accompanied by increased phosphorylation of neural IRS1 at different Ser residues (mSer1097, mSer307, or mSer612) at different ages [20–22]. Few studies have reported the relationship between streptozotocin (STZ)-induced type 1 diabetes-related cognitive impairment and phosphorylation of neural IRS1 at Ser sites. Similarly, in aged animals, the phosphorylation of IRS1 at mSer307 has been shown to increase in the cortex; however, whether this alteration is correlated with age-related decline in cognitive function has not been explored [23].

In the present study, we investigated whether the modification of hippocampal IRS1 by Ser phosphorylation is commonly associated with different types of memory decline in DIO, STZ, aged, and APPKI$^{NL\text{-}G\text{-}F}$ mice and whether it occurs before or after the onset of memory decline in APPKI$^{NL\text{-}G\text{-}F}$ mice. We demonstrate that the concomitant activation of specific Ser sites on hippocampal IRS1 with amyloid-β (Aβ)-unrelated memory decline occurs in DIO and aged mice, whereas STZ mice exhibit memory deficits independent of IRS1 activity. We further show that increased phosphorylation of hippocampal IRS1 at Ser sites is already observed in young APPKI$^{NL\text{-}G\text{-}F}$ mice showing normal memory function despite increased Aβ42 level. These data suggest that the activation of Ser residues on hippocampal IRS1 is associated with non-AD-related memory impairment in T2DM and aging and with Aβ42 level, which is related to the onset of cognitive decline in AD.

2. Materials and Methods

2.1. Animals

C57BL/6J male mice (4 weeks of age) supplied by Japan SLC, Inc. (Shizuoka, Japan) were used to establish type 1 and 2 diabetes mellitus (T1DM, T2DM) mice and their respective control mice. Generation of high-fat-diet (HFD)-induced type 2 diabetes mice (DIO mice) was carried out as previously described [20]. Briefly, C57BL/6J mice were assigned to control wild-type (WT) mice] and HFD (DIO mice) groups, and were fed a normal diet (CE-2; CLEA Japan Inc., Tokyo, Japan) or a HFD (D12492, 60% kcal from fat; Research Diets, Inc., New Brunswick, NJ, USA) for 32 weeks, respectively. To generate Streptozotocin (STZ)-induced type 1 diabetes mice (STZ mice), eight-week-old C57BL/6J mice were intraperitoneally administered with 150 mg/kg STZ (Wako Pure Chemical Industries, Ltd.,

Osaka, Japan) dissolved in sodium citrate (pH 4.5) after overnight fasting, and control mice were injected with the sodium citrate buffer alone. Young and aged WT male mice, which were all pure C57BL/6J strains, were purchased from Charles River Inc., Kanagawa, Japan, or/and bred within our animal facility. APPKI^{NL-G-F} (Swedish (NL), Arctic (G), and Beyreuther/Iberian (F) mutations) homozygous mice were obtained from Dr. Saido at the Laboratory for Proteolytic Neuroscience, RIKEN Brain Science Institute, Saitama, Japan [19]. Age-matched WT mice of a similar strain (C57BL/6J) were used in the control experiments. All experiments were performed using DIO, STZ, and young and middle-aged APPKI^{NL-G-F} mice, and their respective age-matched control mice (DIO mice: 34–36 weeks, WT mice: 34–36 weeks; STZ mice: 10 weeks, WT mice: 10 weeks; young APPKI^{NL-G-F} mice: 12 weeks, WT mice: 12 weeks; middle-aged APPKI^{NL-G-F} mice: 34–36 weeks, WT mice: 34–36 weeks; young WT mice: 8–13 weeks, aged WT mice: 84 weeks). All mice were housed in a standard 12 h light–dark cycle with free access to water and food (room temperature: 25 ± 2 °C). Animal experiments were performed in compliance with the guidelines and with the approval of the ethics committee in Animal Care and Use of the National Center for Geriatrics and Gerontology in Obu, Aichi, Japan (Approval ID: 31-5).

2.2. Western Blotting

The protocol of western blotting used has been previously described [20]. In brief, hippocampal tissue was isolated on ice and homogenized in lysis buffer with a pellet mixer. The aliquot of hippocampal lysates was boiled for 5 min in Laemmli sodium dodecyl sulfate (SDS) sample buffer [60 mm Tris-Cl (pH 6.8), 2% sodium dodecyl sulfate, 10% glycerol, 4% β-mercaptoethanol, and 0.01% bromophenol blue]. A total of 10 µg of each SDS protein sample was loaded per lane, separated by 7.5% sodium dodecyl sulfate polyacrylamide gel electrophoresis (SDS-PAGE), and transferred to polyvinylidene difluoride membranes. Membranes were blocked using 4% Block Ace (Yukijirushi Ltd., Sapporo, Japan), incubated with the indicated primary antibodies, followed by incubation with horseradish peroxidase-conjugated secondary antibodies. Primary antibodies were rabbit anti-phospho-IRS1 [mouse Ser307/human Ser312 (mSer307/hSer312), mouse Ser612/human Ser616 (mSer612/hSer616), mouse Ser632/Ser635/human Ser636/Ser639 (mSer632/Ser635/hSer636/Ser639), mouse Ser1097/human Ser1101 (mSer1097/hSer1101)] (1:500; Cell Signaling Technology(CST)), rabbit anti-IRS1 (1:1000; CST), rabbit anti-phospho-Akt (Ser473) (1:1000; CST), rabbit anti-Akt (1:1000; CST), rabbit anti-phospho-p70S6K (Thr389) (1:1000; CST), rabbit anti-p70S6K (1:1000; CST), rabbit anti-phospho-AMPK (Thr172) (1:1000; CST), rabbit anti-AMPK (1:1000; CST), rabbit anti-phospho-GSK3β (Ser9)(1:1000; CST), rabbit anti-GSK3β (Ser9) (1:1000; CST), rabbit anti-phospho-JNK (Thr183/Tyr185) (1:1000; CST), rabbit anti-JNK (1:1000; CST), rabbit anti-phospho-aPKCζ/λ(Thr410/Thr403) (1:1000; CST), rabbit anti-aPKCζ/λ(1:1000; CST), and rabbit anti-β-tubulin (1:1000; CST). Immunodetection was performed with horseradish peroxidase-conjugated secondary antibodies (1:2000; CST) and chemiluminescence detection reagent Chemi-Lumi one L (Nacalai tesque, Kyoto, Japan) or the ImmunoStar LD (Fujifilm Wako Pure Chemical Corporation Japan, Osaka, Japan). The images were scanned using the Amersham Imager 680 (GE Healthcare UK Ltd., Little Chalfont, Buckinghamshire HP7 9NA, England).

2.3. Water T Maze Test

Hippocampal-dependent spatial memory was tested using a water T maze [24,25] according to our previous report [20]. The maze consisted of a start box, a left arm, and a right arm, which was filled with water at 23 ± 1 °C up to 1 cm above the surface of the platform. Mice were allowed to swim to the right or left arm. This screening step was repeated three times at 15 s intervals. The platform was placed on the side that the mice reached less often. After the screening step, mice were allowed to explore the maze freely. If mice reached the platform, they were allowed to rest there for 5 s (correct choice). If not, the arm entry was closed with a board and they were forced to swim for 15 s as a deterrent (incorrect choice). This trial step was repeated five times at 4-min intervals. Mice were subjected to this trial step for five days. To evaluate the results of the trial, the percentage of correct responses per day was determined. After two days of rest, to test hippocampal and prefrontal cortex (PFC)-dependent working memory, the platform was moved to the opposite arm. Similarly, mice were allowed to explore the maze freely. The trial step was repeated 15 times at 4-min intervals in a day. To evaluate the results of the trial, the percentage of the correct responses were calculated after every three responses.

2.4. *Measurement of Metabolic Parameters*

Body weight and the blood glucose levels were recorded after 6 h of fasting. Blood glucose levels were measured using a portable glucose meter (ACCU-CHEK® Aviva; Roche DC Japan K.K.). The level of plasma insulin at 6 h fasting was determined using an insulin enzyme-linked immunosorbent assay kit (Morinaga, Yokohama, Japan).

2.5. *Enzyme-Linked Immunosorbent Assay (ELISA) Quantitation of Aβ*

In order to measure the Aβ levels in the hippocampus, hippocampal tissue was isolated on ice and homogenized in a lysis buffer (T-PER® Tissue Protein Extraction Reagent; Thermo Fisher Scientific, Waltham, MA, USA) containing a protease inhibitor cocktail (Nacalai Tesque, Kyoto, Japan) and a phosphatase inhibitor cocktail (Nacalai Tesque) with a pellet mixer. After incubation on ice for 15 min, the lysates were centrifuged at 14,200× *g* for 5 min at 4 °C and the supernatants were placed in a fresh tube. Protein concentration was determined using a Bicinchoninic acid (BCA) protein assay kit (Thermo Fisher Scientific, Waltham, MA, USA). The levels of T-PER-extractable Aβ were measured with the Human β Amyloid (1–40) enzyme-linked immunosorbent assay (ELISA) Kit Wako II (#298-64601; Fujifilm Wako Pure Chemical Corp., Osaka, Japan), the Human β Amyloid (1–42) ELISA Kit Wako, High Sensitivity (#296-64401, Fujifilm Wako Pure Chemical Corp.), the Human/Rat/Mouse β Amyloid (1–40) ELISA Kit Wako II (#294-64701; Fujifilm Wako Pure Chemical Corp., Osaka, Japan), and the Human/Rat/Mouse β Amyloid (1–42) ELISA Kit Wako, High Sensitivity (#292-64501, Fujifilm Wako Pure Chemical Corp.) in accordance with the manufacturers' instructions.

2.6. *Statistics*

All results are presented as mean ± standard error of the mean (SEM) in the text. Statistical analyses were performed using Prism7 for Mac OS X v.7.0d (GrapPad Software Inc., La Jolla, CA, USA). Data were statistically analyzed using Student's *t*-test and two-way analysis of variance (ANOVA). Significance is indicated as * $p < 0.05$ and ** $p < 0.01$.

3. Results

3.1. *Activation of Specific Ser Residues on Hippocampal Insulin Receptor Substrate 1 (IRS1) Is Associated with T2DM-Induced Memory Impairment*

We recently reported that T2DM-related cognitive declines in 45-week-old DIO mice fed a 60% HFD for 42 weeks were accompanied by an increased phosphorylation of hippocampal IRS1 at mSer1097 [20]. While mice fed a 60% HFD for 17 days and mice or rats fed a 40% HFD for 6–8 weeks exhibited memory impairment accompanied by increased phosphorylation at hSer616/mSer612 or hSer312/mSer307 [21,22], 12-week-old DIO mice fed a 60% HFD for 9 weeks exhibited normal memory function under our experimental conditions (Figure S1), suggesting that changes in neural IRS1 Ser residues are variable on a temporal scale in DIO mice. Therefore, we investigated the phosphorylation levels of hippocampal IRS1 at Ser sites and the activities of downstream factors involved in memory impairment in 35-week-old (middle-aged) DIO mice fed a 60% HFD for 32 weeks (Figure 1A,C). At 35 weeks of age, DIO mice displayed significant weight gain, hyperglycemia, and hyperinsulinemia (Figure 1B, Figure S2A), as observed at other time points [20–22,26].

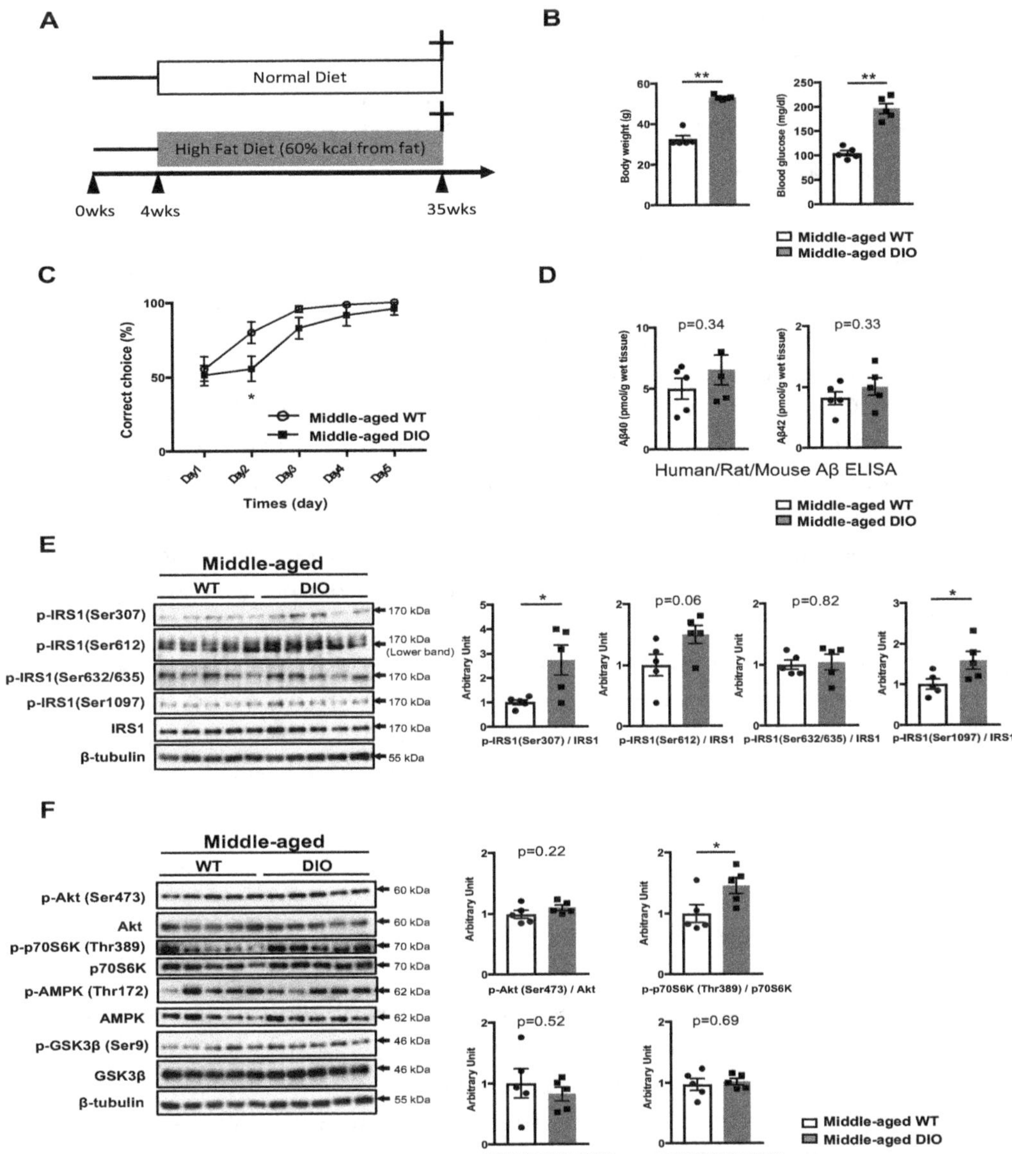

Figure 1. Changes in specific Ser sites on hippocampal insulin receptor substrate 1 (IRS1) in type 2 diabetes (T2DM)-induced memory impairment. (**A**) Schematic diagram of the experimental procedure. (**B**) Graphs of body weight and blood glucose level in wild-type (WT) and diet-induced obesity (DIO) mice (35 weeks of age, n = 5 mice per group). (**C**) Evaluation of learning memory function in middle-aged WT and DIO mice (n = 14 mice per group) using the water T-maze test. (**D**) Quantitative analysis of T-PER (Tissue Protein Extraction Reagent)-extractable Aβ40 and Aβ42 levels in the hippocampi of middle-aged WT and DIO mice using the human/rat/mouse β amyloid (1–40 and 1–42) enzyme-linked immunosorbent assay (ELISA) (35 weeks of age, n = 5 biologically independent samples per group). (E) Western blot analysis of phosphorylated insulin receptor substrates 1 mouse Ser307 [p-IRS1 (mSer307)], p-IRS1 (mSer612), p-IRS1 (mSer632/635), p-IRS1 (mSer1097), IRS1, and β-tubulin in the hippocampi of middle-aged WT and DIO mice (35 weeks of age, n = 5 biologically independent samples per group). Arrow indicates the p-IRS1 mSer612-corresponding band (lower band) in (**E**). Quantitative analysis of the phosphorylation of IRS1 at mSer307, mSer612, mSer632/635, and mSer1097 normalized to total protein. (**F**) Western blot analysis of phosphorylation levels of Akt Ser473, p70S6K Thr389, AMP-activated protein kinase (AMPK) Thr172, and glycogen synthase kinase 3 beta (GSK3β) Ser9 as well as total protein levels of Akt, p70 S6K, AMPK, GSK3β, and ß-tubulin in the hippocampi of middle-aged WT and DIO mice (35 weeks of age, n = 5 biologically independent samples per group). Quantitative analysis of the phosphorylation of Akt Ser473, p70S6K Thr389, AMPK Thr172, and GSK3β Ser9 normalized to the respective total protein contents. Results are presented as mean ± standard error of the mean (SEM), * $p < 0.05$; ** $p < 0.01$.

Furthermore, we examined whether memory impairment in middle-aged DIO mice is linked to increased levels of Aβ42, a pathological feature of AD. Biochemical analysis with specific kits (see Materials and Methods) demonstrated that, compared with age-matched wild-type (WT) mice, there was no change in Aβ40 and Aβ42 levels in the T-PER fractions obtained from the hippocampi of 35-week-old DIO mice (Figure 1D).

In contrast to DIO mice at 45 weeks of age, the phosphorylation of IRS1 at mSer307, which increases in insulin resistance, diabetes, and obesity [5], with phosphorylation at mSer1097 significantly increased in the hippocampus of DIO mice at 35 weeks of age, although there were no significant differences in phosphorylation at mSer612 and mSer632/635 between DIO and age-matched WT mice (Figure 1E, Figure S4A). Consistent with previous studies [27,28], the basal phosphorylation level of p70S6K slightly but significantly increased in the hippocampus of middle-aged DIO mice compared with that in the hippocampus of age-matched WT mice, whereas the basal phosphorylation of Akt and GSK3β and activation of AMPK and atypical protein kinase C ζ/λ (aPKC ζ/λ), downstream factors of insulin signaling, in the hippocampus were comparable between middle-aged WT and DIO mice (Figure 1F, Figures S3A, S4B and S5A). Additionally, the basal phosphorylation of JNK, an inflammation- and stress-related factor, remained unchanged in the hippocampus between the two groups (Figures S3A and S5A), although a relationship between the phosphorylation of IRS1 at mSer307 and activation of these factors in yeast cells, culture cells, and muscles has been reported [5]. These results indicate that T2DM-induced memory decline is provoked by an Aβ-independent mechanism and that the concomitant activation of IRS1 mSer307 and mSer1097 with p70S6K activation in the hippocampus is associated with memory deficits in 35-week-old DIO mice.

3.2. *Type 1 Diabetes Mellitus (T1DM)-Induced Memory Deficits Occur Independently of IRS1 Activity*

To investigate whether the alteration of IRS1 through Ser phosphorylation is associated with type 1 diabetes mellitus (T1DM)-induced memory deficits, we generated STZ-induced insulin-deficient T1DM mice. Two weeks after STZ injection, STZ mice exhibited weight loss, elevated blood glucose levels (>400 mg/dL), and low insulin levels (Figure 2A, Figure S2B). While there were no significant differences in hippocampus-dependent spatial memory between WT and STZ mice, STZ mice displayed hippocampus- and prefrontal cortex-related memory decline (Figure 2B), consistent with the findings reported in previous studies [29–32]. However, STZ-induced T1DM had no effect on Aβ40 and Aβ42 levels in the T-PER fractions of the hippocampus (Figure 2C).

Subsequently, we examined the impact of STZ-induced T1DM on the phosphorylation of IRS1 at Ser residues and downstream components in the hippocampus. In STZ mice that had already developed memory impairment, the phosphorylation levels of hippocampal IRS1 at Ser residues in STZ mice were comparable to those in WT mice (Figure 2D, Figure S4C). Although the activation of p70S6K and the monotonous activities of Akt, AMPK, aPKC ζ/λ, and JNK were observed in STZ mice as well as in middle-aged DIO mice regardless of the presence or absence of Ser phosphorylation on hippocampal IRS1, the phosphorylation of GSK3β at Ser9 significantly increased in the hippocampus of STZ mice (Figure 2E, Figure S3B, S4D and S5B). These data indicate that T1DM-induced memory deficits accompanied by increased phosphorylation of GSK3β arises independently of the modification of IRS1 signaling via Ser phosphorylation and independently of Aβ elevation.

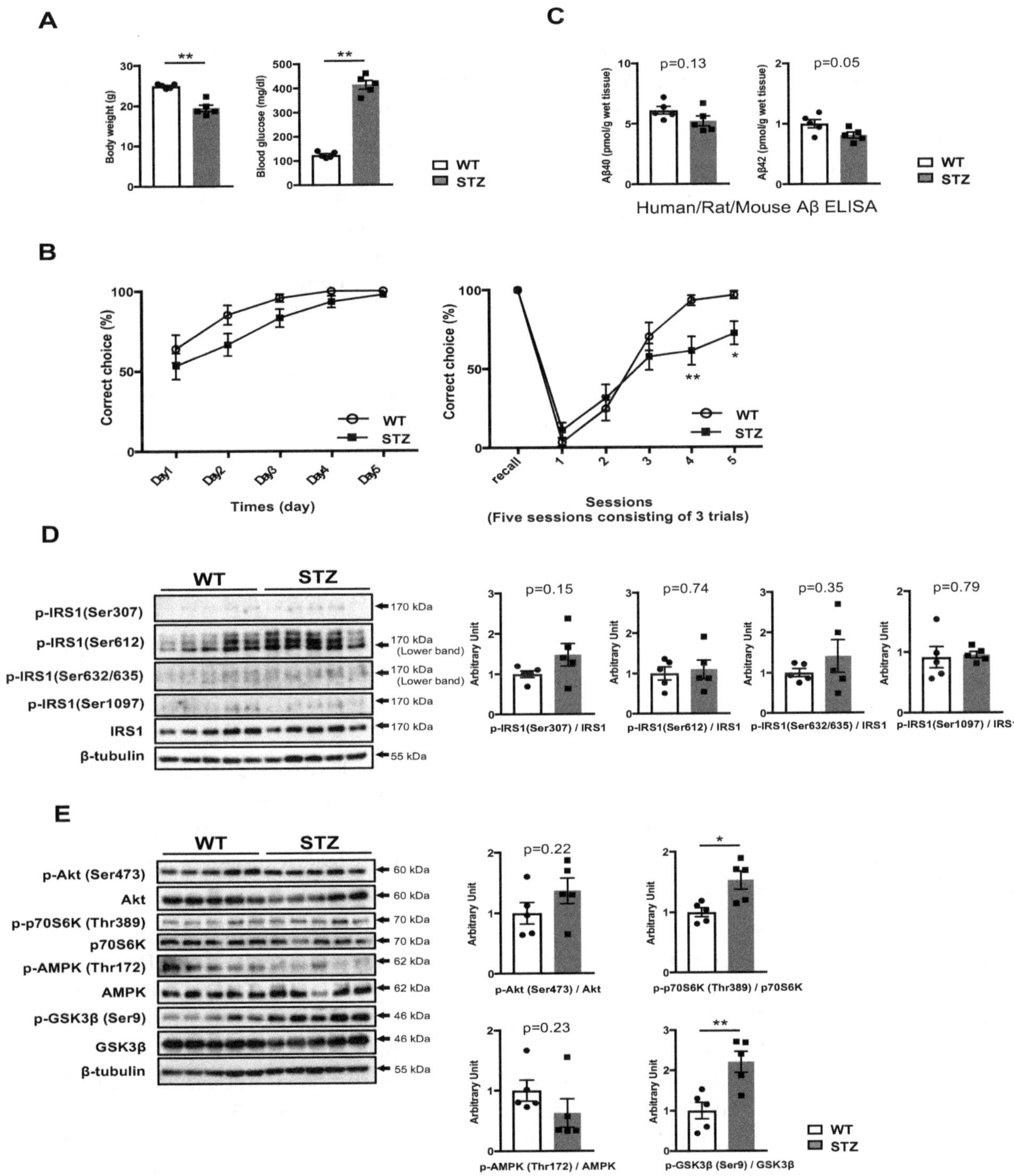

A
Body weight (g)
Blood glucose (mg/dl)
**
WT
STZ
C
p=0.13
p=0.05
Aβ40 (pmol/g wet tissue)
Aβ42 (pmol/g wet tissue)
Human/Rat/Mouse Aβ ELISA
WT
STZ
B
Correct choice (%)
Day1
Day2
Day3
Day4
Day5
Times (day)
WT
STZ
recall
Sessions
(Five sessions consisting of 3 trials)
D
WT
STZ
p-IRS1(Ser307)
p-IRS1(Ser612)
p-IRS1(Ser632/635)
p-IRS1(Ser1097)
IRS1
β-tubulin
170 kDa
170 kDa (Lower band)
55 kDa
p=0.15
p=0.74
p=0.35
p=0.79
Arbitrary Unit
p-IRS1(Ser307) / IRS1
p-IRS1(Ser612) / IRS1
p-IRS1(Ser632/635) / IRS1
p-IRS1(Ser1097) / IRS1
E
WT
STZ
p-Akt (Ser473)
Akt
p-p70S6K (Thr389)
p70S6K
p-AMPK (Thr172)
AMPK
p-GSK3β (Ser9)
GSK3β
β-tubulin
60 kDa
70 kDa
62 kDa
46 kDa
55 kDa
p=0.22
p=0.23
Arbitrary Unit
p-Akt (Ser473) / Akt
p-p70S6K (Thr389) / p70S6K
p-AMPK (Thr172) / AMPK
p-GSK3β (Ser9) / GSK3β
WT
STZ

Figure 2. No alteration of IRS1 Ser phosphorylation in the hippocampus of T1DM mouse models. (**A**) Graphs of body weight and blood glucose level in wild-type (WT) and streptozotocin (STZ)-induced insulin-deficient type 1 diabetes (T1DM) model mice (10 weeks of age, n = 5 mice per group). (**B**) Evaluation of hippocampus-dependent learning and memory function and hippocampus/prefrontal cortex associated working memory function in WT (10 weeks of age, n = 19 mice per group) and STZ mice (10 weeks of age, n = 18 mice per group) using the water T-maze test and reverse water T-maze test. (**C**) Quantitative analysis of T-PER-extractable Aβ40 and Aβ42 levels in the hippocampi of WT and STZ mice using the human/rat/mouse β amyloid (1–40 and 1–42) ELISA (10 weeks of age, n = 5 biologically independent samples per group). (**D**) In WT and STZ-induced type 1 diabetes mice (10 weeks of age, n = 5 biologically independent samples per group), western blot analysis of phosphorylated insulin receptor substrates 1 mouse Ser307 [p-IRS1 (mSer307)], p-IRS1 (mSer612), p-IRS1 (mSer632/635), p-IRS1 (mSer1097), IRS1, and ß-tubulin was performed. Quantitative analysis of the phosphorylation of IRS1 at mSer307, mSer612, mSer632/635, and mSer1097 normalized to total protein. (**E**) Western blot analysis of phosphorylation levels of Akt Ser473, p70S6K Thr389, AMPK Thr172, and GSK3β Ser9 as well as total protein levels of Akt, p70S6K, AMPK, GSK3β, ß-tubulin in WT and STZ mice (10 weeks of age, n = 5 biologically independent samples per group). Arrows indicate the p-IRS1 mSer612-corresponding band (lower band) and the p-IRS1 mSer632/635-corresponding band (lower band) in (**D**). Quantitative analysis of the phosphorylation of Akt Ser473, p70 S6K Thr389, AMPK Thr172, and GSK3β Ser9 normalized to the respective total protein contents. Results are presented as mean ± SEM, * $p < 0.05$; ** $p < 0.01$.

3.3. Phosphorylation of IRS1 at Age-Specific Ser Residues with the Activation of Downstream Kinases Is Linked to Age-Related Memory Deficits

Although memory decline associated with physiological aging can occur naturally, in contrast to pathogenic memory deficits, whether the onset processes of age-related memory impairment are related to the mechanisms underlying pathogenic memory deficits in T2DM and AD remains unclear.

We examined the modification of IRS1 at Ser residues and the activity of downstream factors in the hippocampi of 21-month-old mice (aged mice). Aged mice displayed memory impairments without an increase in blood glucose and plasma insulin levels, despite an increase in body weight (Figure 3A,B, Figure S2C). Meanwhile, the Aβ40 and Aβ42 levels in the T-PER fractions of the hippocampus were comparable between young and aged WT mice (Figure 3C).

In common with DIO mice, the activation of mSer307, but not of mSer1097, on IRS1 accompanied by p70S6K activation and unchanged AMPK was observed with increased phosphorylation of IRS1 at mSer612 and mSer632/635 in the hippocampi of aged mice (Figure 3D, Figure S4E). Nonetheless, unlike in DIO mice, the basal phosphorylation levels of Akt and GSK3β prominently increased in the hippocampus of aged mice (Figure 3E, Figure S4F); however, the basal activities of aPKC ζ/λ, and JNKs remained unchanged, similar to those in DIO mice (Figure S3C and S5C). These results suggest that aging causes the concomitant phosphorylation of hippocampal IRS1 at mSer307, mSer612, and mSer632/635 with the activation of canonical downstream kinases, which may be associated with Aβ-unrelated physiological decline in memory function.

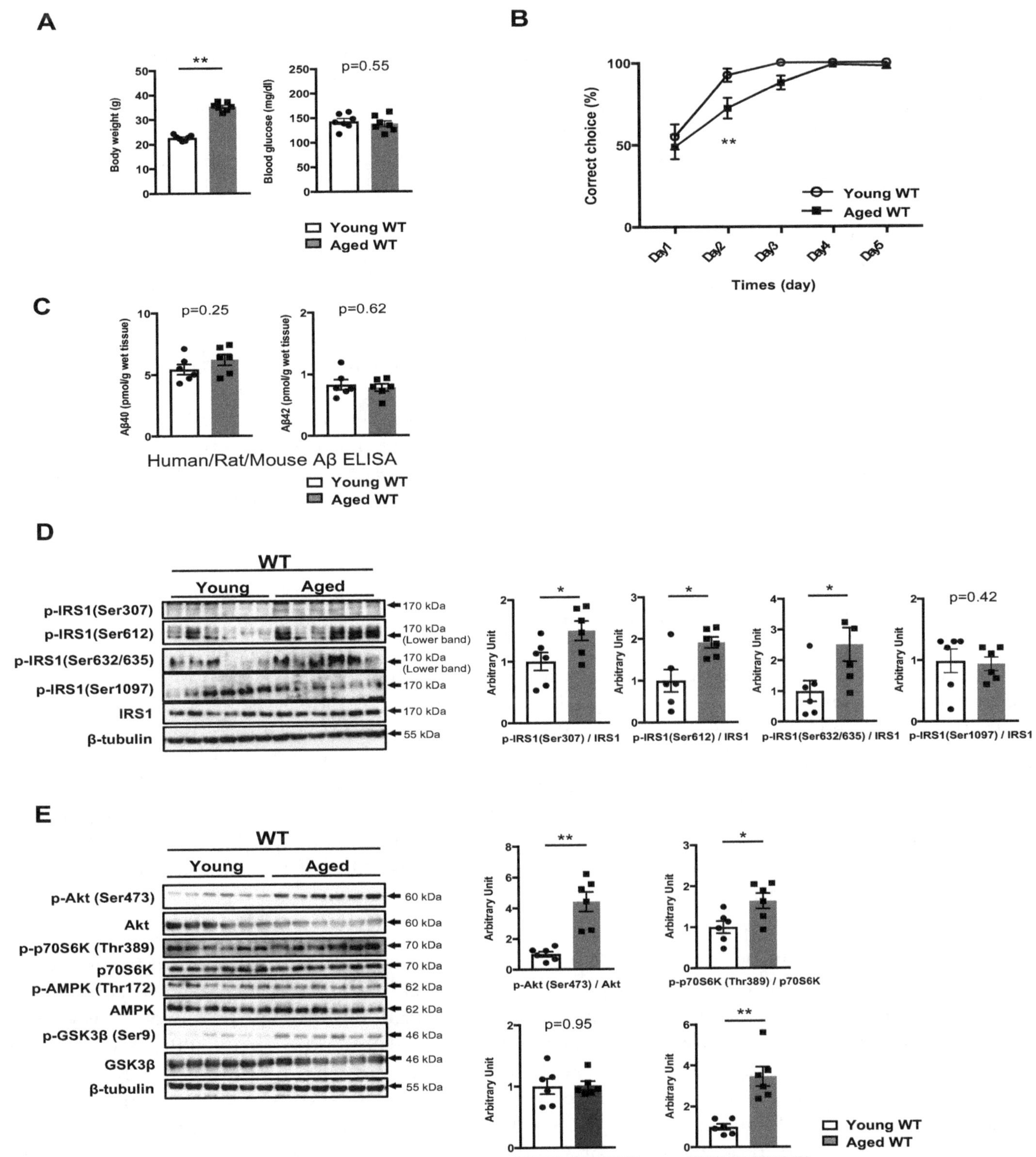
A
Body weight (g)
**
Blood glucose (mg/dl)
p=0.55
Young WT
Aged WT
B
Correct choice (%)
**
Young WT
Aged WT
Day1
Day2
Day3
Day4
Day5
Times (day)
C
Aβ40 (pmol/g wet tissue)
p=0.25
Aβ42 (pmol/g wet tissue)
p=0.62
Human/Rat/Mouse Aβ ELISA
Young WT
Aged WT
D
WT
Young
Aged
p-IRS1(Ser307)
p-IRS1(Ser612)
p-IRS1(Ser632/635)
p-IRS1(Ser1097)
IRS1
β-tubulin
170 kDa
170 kDa (Lower band)
170 kDa (Lower band)
170 kDa
170 kDa
55 kDa
Arbitrary Unit
p-IRS1(Ser307) / IRS1
p-IRS1(Ser612) / IRS1
p-IRS1(Ser632/635) / IRS1
p-IRS1(Ser1097) / IRS1
p=0.42
E
WT
Young
Aged
p-Akt (Ser473)
Akt
p-p70S6K (Thr389)
p70S6K
p-AMPK (Thr172)
AMPK
p-GSK3β (Ser9)
GSK3β
β-tubulin
60 kDa
60 kDa
70 kDa
70 kDa
62 kDa
62 kDa
46 kDa
46 kDa
55 kDa
Arbitrary Unit
p-Akt (Ser473) / Akt
p-p70S6K (Thr389) / p70S6K
p-AMPK (Thr172) / AMPK
p=0.95
p-GSK3β (Ser9) / GSK3β
Young WT
Aged WT

Figure 3. Age-related memory deficits accompanied by increased phosphorylation of IRS1 Ser sites in the hippocampus. (**A**) The graphs of body weight and blood glucose levels in young (12 weeks of age, n = 7 mice per group) and aged (84 weeks of age, n = 7 mice per group) wild-type (WT) mice. (**B**) Evaluation of learning memory functions in young WT mice (n = 16 mice per group) and aged WT mice (n = 18 mice per group) using the water T-maze test. (**C**) Quantitative analysis of T-PER-extractable Aβ40 and Aβ42 levels in the hippocampi of young (12 weeks of age, n = 6 biologically independent samples) and aged (84 weeks of age, n = 6 biologically independent samples) WT mice using the human/rat/mouse β amyloid (1–40 and 1–42) ELISA. (**D**) Western blot analysis of phosphorylated insulin receptor substrates 1 mouse Ser307 [p-IRS1 (mSer307)], p-IRS1 (mSer612), p-IRS1 (mSer632/635), p-IRS1 (mSer1097), IRS1, and ß-tubulin in the hippocampi of young WT mice (12 weeks of age, n = 6 biologically independent samples) and aged WT mice (84 weeks of age, n = 6 biologically independent samples). Quantitative analysis of the phosphorylation of IRS1 at mSer307, mSer612, mSer632/635, and mSer1097 normalized to total protein. (**E**) Western blot analysis of phosphorylation levels of Akt Ser473, p70S6K Thr389, AMPK Thr172, and GSK3β Ser9 as well as total protein levels of Akt, p70S6K, AMPK, GSK3β, and ß-tubulin in the hippocampi of young WT mice (12 weeks of age, n = 6 biologically independent samples) and aged WT mice (84 weeks of age, n = 6 biologically independent samples). Arrows indicate the p-IRS1 mSer612-corresponding band (lower band) and the p-IRS1 mSer632/635-corresponding band (lower band) in (**D**). Quantitative analysis of the phosphorylation of Akt Ser473, p70S6K Thr389, AMPK Thr172, and GSK3β Ser9 normalized to the respective total protein contents. Results are presented as mean ± SEM, * $p < 0.05$; ** $p < 0.01$.

3.4. Increased Phosphorylation of Hippocampal IRS1 at Ser Residues in Young Amyloid Precursor Protein (APP) Knock-In (APP KI$^{NL\text{-}G\text{-}F}$) Mice Occurs Prior to the Onset of Memory Decline

To investigate whether AD-related activation of Ser residues on neural IRS1 emerges before or after the onset of memory decline, we employed a novel AD mouse model, APPKI$^{NL\text{-}G\text{-}F}$ mice carrying a humanized Aβ sequence and three AD mutations, i.e., Swedish, Beyreuther/Iberian, and Arctic mutations, in the endogenous *App* gene [19]. First, we measured body weight and glucose metabolism in 12-week-old (young) APPKI$^{NL\text{-}G\text{-}F}$ mice. There were no differences in terms of body weight, blood glucose level, and plasma insulin concentration between WT and APPKI$^{NL\text{-}G\text{-}F}$ mice at 12 weeks of age (Figure 4A, Figure S2B). Next, we confirmed memory function as well as Aβ40 and Aβ42 levels in the hippocampi of young APPKI$^{NL\text{-}G\text{-}F}$ mice. At 12 weeks of age, APPKI$^{NL\text{-}G\text{-}F}$ mice exhibited normal memory function (Figure 4B).

Using monoclonal antibody (BNT77/BC05)-based sandwich ELISA for human/rat/mouse Aβ42, we successfully confirmed that T-PER-extractable Aβ42 level had already increased in young APP KI$^{NL\text{-}G\text{-}F}$ mice (Figure 4C, right). A conspicuous increase in T-PER-extractable Aβ42 level in these mice was detected by human Aβ42 sandwich ELISA using monoclonal antibodies (BAN50/BC05) (Figure 4D, right). However, T-PER-extractable Aβ42 levels in both ELISA were comparable to the range of Tris-buffered saline (TBS)-extractable Aβ42 level in the brain and cortex of APPKI$^{NL\text{-}G\text{-}F}$ mice reported by Saito et al. (2019) and Saito et al. (2014). Similarly, human/rat/mouse Aβ40 and human Aβ40 sandwich ELISA revealed the same range for Aβ40 level in the T-PER fractions of the hippocampi of young APPKI$^{NL\text{-}G\text{-}F}$ mice (black bar on the left in Figure 4C,D and Figure 5C,D). Meanwhile, regardless of age, human/rat/mouse Aβ40 or human Aβ40 sandwich ELISA showed almost the same levels (white bar on the left in Figures 1D, 2C, 3C, 4C and 5C) or range (white bar on the left in Figures 4D and 5D) of T-PER-extractable Aβ40 in WT mice, respectively.

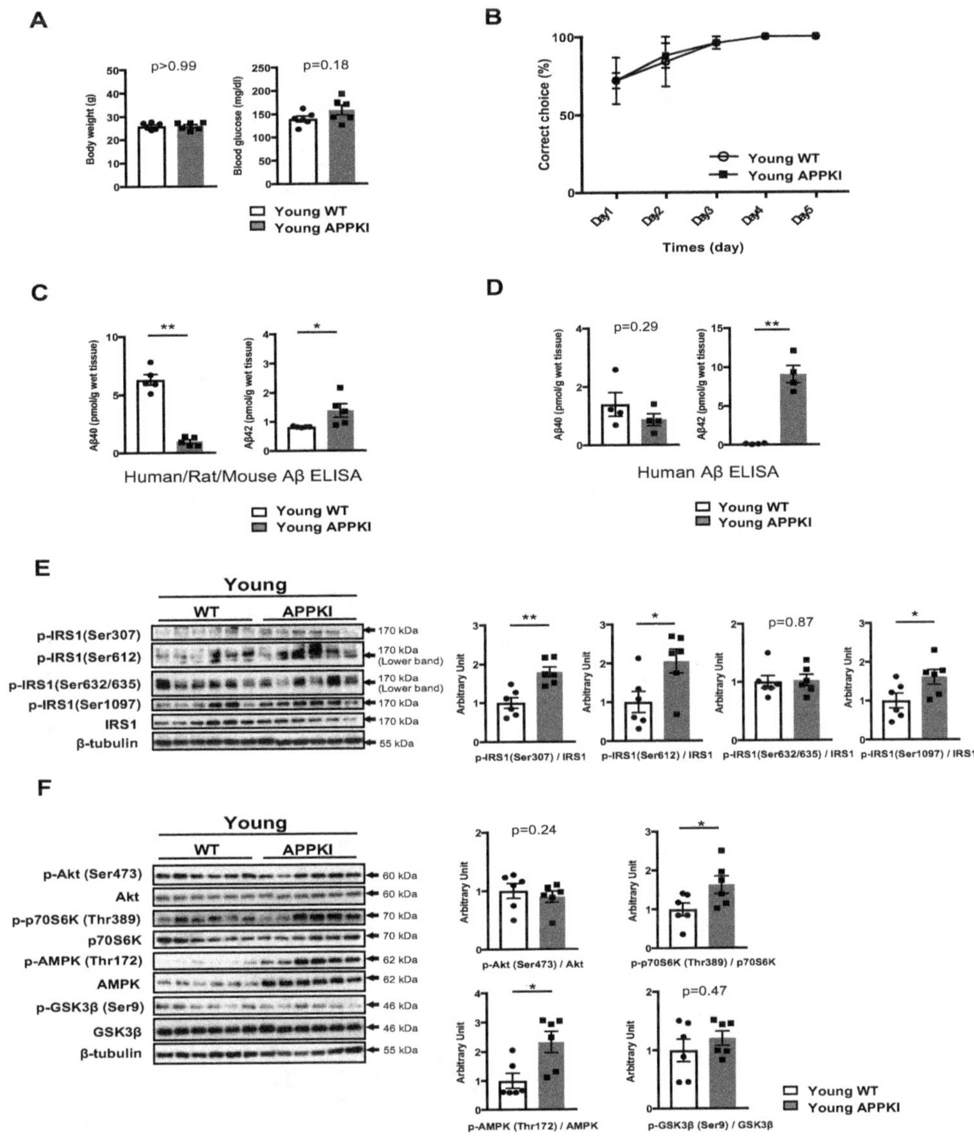

Figure 4. Activation of multiple Ser residues on hippocampal IRS1 unrelated to memory decline in young amyloid precursor protein (APP) knock-in (APPKI$^{NL\text{-}G\text{-}F}$) mice. (**A**) The graphs of body weight and blood glucose levels in young wild-type (WT) and APPKI$^{NL\text{-}G\text{-}F}$ mice (12 weeks of age, n = 6 mice per group). (**B**) Evaluation of learning memory function in young WT (n = 5 mice per group) and APP KI$^{NL\text{-}G\text{-}F}$ mice (n = 5 mice per group) using the water T-maze test. (**C**) Quantitative analysis of T-PER-extractable Aβ40 and Aβ42 levels in the hippocampi of young WT and APPKI$^{NL\text{-}G\text{-}F}$ mice using the human/rat/mouse β amyloid (1–40 and 1–42) ELISA (12 weeks of age, n = 5 biologically independent samples per group). (**D**) Quantitative analysis of T-PER-extractable Aβ40 and Aβ42 levels in the hippocampi of young WT and APPKI$^{NL\text{-}G\text{-}F}$ mice using the human β amyloid (1–40 and 1–42) ELISA (12 weeks of age, n = 5 biologically independent samples per group). (**E**) Western blot analysis of phosphorylated insulin receptor substrates 1 mouse Ser307 [p-IRS1 (mSer307)], p-IRS1 (mSer612), p-IRS1 (mSer632/635), p-IRS1 (mSer1097), IRS1, and ß-tubulin in the hippocampi of young WT and APP KI$^{NL\text{-}G\text{-}F}$ mice (12 weeks of age, n = 6 biologically independent samples per group). Arrows indicate the p-IRS1 mSer612-corresponding band (lower band) and p-IRS1 mSer632/635-corresponding band (lower band) in (**E**). Quantitative analysis of the phosphorylation of IRS1 at mSer307, mSer612, mSer632/635, and mSer1097 normalized to the respective total protein contents. (**F**) Western blot analysis of phosphorylation levels of Akt Ser473, p70S6K Thr389, AMPK Thr172, and GSK3β Ser9 as well as total protein levels of Akt, p70S6K, AMPK, GSK3β, and ß-tubulin in the hippocampi of young WT and APPKI$^{NL\text{-}G\text{-}F}$ mice (12 weeks of age, n = 6 biologically independent samples per group). Quantitative analysis of phosphorylation of Akt Ser473, p70S6K Thr389, AMPK Thr172, and GSK3β Ser9 normalized to the respective total protein contents. Results are presented as mean ± SEM, * $p < 0.05$; ** $p < 0.01$.

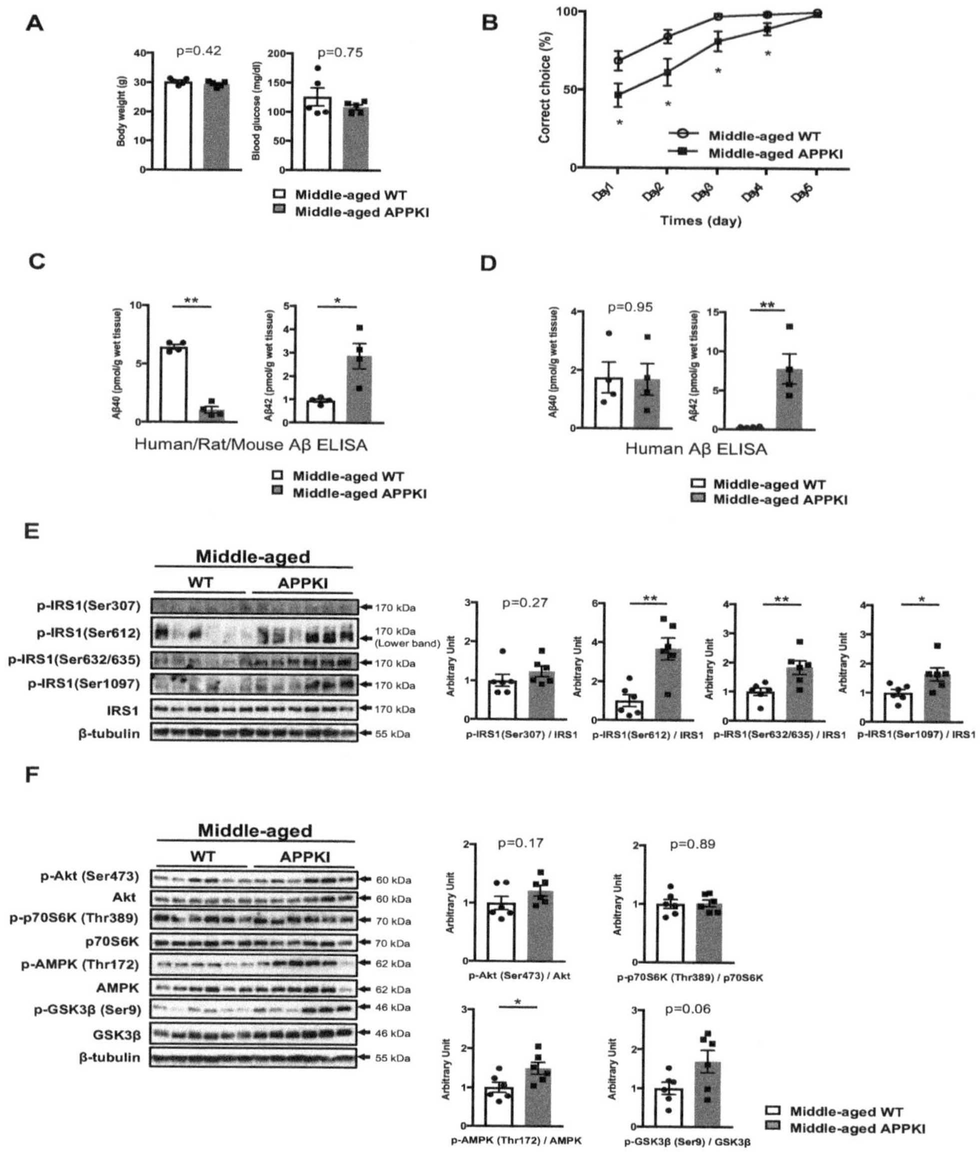

Figure 5. Memory decline accompanied by sustained phosphorylation of IRS1 Ser residues in the hippocampus of middle-aged APPKI$^{NL\text{-}G\text{-}F}$ mice. (**A**) The graphs of body weight and blood glucose levels in middle-aged wild-type (WT) and APPKI$^{NL\text{-}G\text{-}F}$ mice (34–36 weeks of age, n = 5 mice per group). (**B**) Evaluation of learning memory function in middle-aged WT (n = 14) and APPKI$^{NL\text{-}G\text{-}F}$ mice (n = 15 mice per group) using the water T-maze test. (**C**) Quantitative analysis of T-PER-extractable Aβ40 and Aβ42 levels in the hippocampi of middle-aged WT and APPKI$^{NL\text{-}G\text{-}F}$ mice using the human/rat/mouse β amyloid (1–40 and 1–42) ELISA (34–36 weeks of age, n = 4 biologically independent samples per group). (**D**) Quantitative analysis of T-PER-extractable Aβ40 and Aβ42 levels in the hippocampi of middle-aged WT and APPKI$^{NL\text{-}G\text{-}F}$ mice using the human β amyloid (1–40 and 1–42) ELISA (34–36 weeks of age, n = 4 biologically independent samples per group). (**E**) Western blot analysis of phosphorylated insulin receptor substrates 1 mouse Ser307 [p-IRS1 (mSer307)], p-IRS1 (mSer612), p-IRS1 (mSer632/635), p-IRS1 (mSer1097), IRS1, and ß-tubulin in the hippocampi of middle-aged WT and APPKI$^{NL\text{-}G\text{-}F}$ mice (34–36 weeks of age, n = 6 biologically independent samples per group). Arrow indicates the p-IRS1 mSer612 -corresponding band (lower band) in (**E**). Quantitative analysis of the phosphorylation of IRS1 at mSer307, mSer612, mSer632/635, and mSer1097 normalized to total protein. (**F**) Western blot analysis of phosphorylation levels of Akt Ser473, p70S6K Thr389, AMPK Thr172, and GSK3β Ser9 as well as total protein levels of Akt, p70S6K, AMPK, GSK3β, and ß-tubulin in the hippocampi of middle-aged WT and APPKI$^{NL\text{-}G\text{-}F}$ mice (34–36 weeks of age, n = 6 biologically independent samples per group). Quantitative analysis of the phosphorylation of Akt Ser473, p70S6K Thr389, AMPK Thr172, and GSK3β Ser9 normalized to the respective total protein contents. Results are presented as mean ± SEM, * $p < 0.05$; ** $p < 0.01$.

Subsequently, we investigated the phosphorylation levels of hippocampal IRS1 at Ser residues in young APPKI^{NL-G-F} mice. Importantly, the phosphorylation of hippocampal IRS1 at mSer307, mSer612, and mSer1097, but not at mSer632/635, significantly increased in 12-week-old APPKI^{NL-G-F} mice (Figure 4E, Figure S4G) displaying normal memory function (Figure 4B). In parallel to these increases, a concomitant elevation in the basal phosphorylation of AMPK, a metabolic energy sensor, with p70S6K activation and a slight decrease in basal JNK phosphorylation were observed in these mice, along with monotonous Akt, GSK3β, and aPKC ζ/λ activity (Figure 4F, Figure S3D, S4H and S5D). Thus, in young APPKI^{NL-G-F} mice exhibiting normal memory function, the increased phosphorylation of hippocampal IRS1 at multiple Ser sites accompanied by AMPK-related low energy conditions had already occurred in the presence of increased Aβ42 level, suggesting that the elevation of Aβ42 level and/or AMPK activation provokes the activation of Ser sites on IRS1 in brains of patients with AD prior to the onset of memory decline.

3.5. Memory Decline in Middle-Aged APPKI^{NL-G-F} Mice Is Accompanied by the Activation of Specific Ser Sites on IRS1 and Energy Depletion

Next, we examined age-related alterations in the patterns of phosphorylation of IRS1 at Ser sites and its downstream components in the hippocampi of middle-aged APPKI^{NL-G-F} mice at 34–36 weeks of age. Consistently, body weight, blood glucose level, and plasma insulin concentration were comparable between middle-aged WT and APPKI^{NL-G-F} mice (Figure 5A, Figure S2A).

Although the onset of memory deficits was reported by 6 months in APPKI^{NL-G-F} mice [19], 6-month-old APPKI^{NL-G-F} mice did not display memory decline under our experimental conditions (data not shown). However, the water T-maze test demonstrated that middle-aged APPKI^{NL-G-F} mice exhibited memory decline after 34 weeks under our experimental conditions (Figure 5B). Meanwhile, both human/rat/mouse Aβ42 and human Aβ42 sandwich ELISA demonstrated increased levels of T-PER-extractable Aβ42 in the hippocampi of middle-aged APPKI^{NL-G-F} mice (right in Figure 5C, D) and young APPKI^{NL-G-F} mice, which were comparable to TBS-extractable Aβ42 levels in the brain and cortex of APPKI^{NL-G-F} mice [33].

While an age-related increase in the phosphorylation of IRS1 at mSer612 and mSer632/635 accompanied by sustained phosphorylation of IRS1 at T2DM-related mSer1097 site and of AMPK was observed in the hippocampi of middle-aged APPKI^{NL-G-F} mice showing memory decline (Figure 5E, Figure S4I, Table S1), there were no significant differences in phosphorylation levels at mSer307 site and of p70S6K between middle-aged WT and APPKI^{NL-G-F} mice (Figure 5E,F) owing to the age-related elevation of these factors (Figure 3D,E). Regardless of age, the activity of downstream components, such as Akt, GSK3β, aPKC ζ/λ, and JNKs, remained almost unchanged in the hippocampi of APPKI^{NL-G-F} mice (Figure 5F, Figure S3E, S4J and S5E). Our data suggest that the increased phosphorylation of hippocampal IRS1 at multiple Ser residues and persistent AMPK activation that corresponds to energy depletion accompanied by age-related elevation of Aβ42 levels are associated with the onset of memory decline in these mice.

4. Discussion

The present study demonstrates that memory decline in T1DM and T2DM in middle age occurs in an Aβ-independent manner, which is consistent with the findings of previous studies [34–36]. Similarly, age-related memory impairments arise with no alteration in Aβ levels.

In middle-aged DIO and aged mice, Aβ-unrelated memory deficits are accompanied by increased basal phosphorylation of hippocampal IRS1 at specific Ser residues, whereas Aβ-unrelated memory impairments develop in STZ mice without the modification of IRS1. Although p70S6K activation accompanied by unchanged AMPK activity in the hippocampus is mutually observed with Aβ-unrelated memory deficits in middle-aged DIO, STZ, and aged mice regardless of the presence or absence of the phosphorylation of IRS1 at Ser residues, different alterations in other downstream components were observed in these mouse models. Furthermore, we found that, in APPKI^{NL-G-F} mice, a concomitant increase in the basal phosphorylation of hippocampal IRS1 at multiple Ser sites with the activation of AMPK and elevation of Aβ42 level had already arisen at a young age, before the onset of memory decline, and that memory decline in middle age was accompanied by the persistence of these changes with age-related increase in the phosphorylation of IRS1 at specific Ser sites and in Aβ42 level.

HFD and genetically obese animals exhibit increased phosphorylation at mSer307 and p70S6K-induced phosphorylation at mSer1097 in peripheral tissues [37,38]. In the central nervous system, the involvement of non-activated AMPK with/without phosphorylation of IRS1 at mSer307 accompanied by p70S6K activation or different combinations of alterations in Akt and GSK3β activity (i.e., increased or decreased phosphorylation) in cognitive impairment in 40–45% HFD-fed and STZ mice has been reported [21,22,27,28,32,34,39,40], whereas the monotonous levels of phosphorylation of IRS1 at Ser sites and of downstream kinases including Akt, AMPK, GSK3β, and p70S6K are observed in 45% HFD-induced cognitive deficits [41]. Consistent with these results, memory decline in middle-aged DIO mice is accompanied by a concomitant increase in the basal phosphorylation of IRS1 at mSer307 and mSer1097 with p70S6K activation and monotonous activity of Akt, GSK3β, and AMPK in the hippocampus. On the other hand, in aged mice, the concomitant activation of Akt and GSK3β with an increase in the basal phosphorylation of hippocampal IRS1 at mSer307, mSer612, and mSer632/635 with p70S6K activation is observed, which is consistent with previous studies showing that the increased phosphorylation of mSer632/635 or mSer1097 on IRS1 is associated with p70S6K [5,37,38]. Given that the activation of mSer612 on IRS1 may negatively correlate with intracellular signaling and that the activation of Ser632/635 on IRS1 may occur independently of Akt [5], it is likely that, in aged mice, the increased phosphorylation of IRS1 at mSer307, mSer612, and mSer632/635 with the activation of multiple downstream factors other than AMPK may arise through reciprocal feedback regulation.

Additionally, HFD- and STZ-induced diabetes increases the phosphorylation of JNK accompanied by the activation of mSer307 on IRS1 in the brain [21,32]. The activity of JNK is elevated in aged mice and transgenic mouse models of AD, although the involvement of phosphorylation of IRS1 at Ser sites in the altered activation of JNK has not been reported [16,42]. Furthermore, the activation of aPKC ζ/λ is associated with the phosphorylation of IRS1 at Ser sites, including mSer1097 [5,20]. However, in all types of mouse models of memory impairment in the present study, the basal phosphorylation levels of JNK and aPKC ζ/λ consistently remained unchanged under our experimental conditions. These discrepancies may be due to the differences in observation time, animal species, and HFD or STZ protocols, such as age, duration of exposure, diet fat content, and drug dosages. Taken together, these results suggest that the reciprocal effects of the phosphorylation of IRS1 at T2DM- or age-related Ser sites and downstream components via feedback loops that may lead to the common alterations in the activity of p70S6K and AMPK are involved in Aβ-unrelated memory decline; however, the modification of IRS1 through Ser sites is not required for the onset of memory deficits in STZ-induced T1DM mice.

Although a link between the phosphorylation of neural IRS1 at mSer307, mSer612, and mSer632/635 and brain insulin resistance has been proposed [14,16,43], brain insulin resistance is not yet defined, and the phosphorylation of IRS1 at Ser sites emerges in insulin-dependent and insulin-independent manners [5,6]. Given that diabetes- and obesity-induced memory impairments were accompanied by the phosphorylation of IRS1 at mSer307 [5], we found that young APPKI$^{NL\text{-}G\text{-}F}$ mice showing normal metabolism and memory function displayed increased phosphorylation of hippocampal IRS1 at three Ser residues including mSer307, mSer612, and mSer1097, in which the Aβ42 level had already increased before the onset of memory decline. Consistent with previous studies [13–16], the increased phosphorylation at mSer612 and mSer 632/635 and persistent activation of mSer1097 are observed in the hippocampus of middle-aged APPKI$^{NL\text{-}G\text{-}F}$ mice exhibiting memory decline with age-associated increase in the Aβ42 level.

Interestingly, in both young and middle-aged APPKI$^{NL\text{-}G\text{-}F}$ mice, the concomitant phosphorylation of hippocampal IRS1 at mSer612 and mSer1097 with the activation of AMPK is constantly observed regardless of the presence or absence of the activation of mSer307 or mSer 632/635, suggesting that persistent phosphorylation of mSer612 and mSer1097 accompanied by AMPK activation may contribute to memory dysfunction in AD.

Reportedly, the Arctic mutation in $APPKI^{NL\text{-}G\text{-}F}$ mice reduces immunoreactivity in ELISA because the location of this mutation on the Aβ sequences is overlapped with the binding region of monoclonal antibody to Aβ used in human/rat/mouse Aβ sandwich ELISA [19]; however, T-PER-extractable Aβ40 and Aβ42 levels were successfully determined by human/rat/mouse Aβ sandwich ELISA using BNT77 (binds to the location of the Arctic mutation) and human Aβ sandwich ELISA using BAN50 (does not bind to the location of the Arctic mutation). We confirmed that the elevation of Aβ42 level is evident in young $APPKI^{NL\text{-}G\text{-}F}$ mice and that the Aβ42 level increased in middle-aged $APPKI^{NL\text{-}G\text{-}F}$ mice. Owing to the elevation of Aβ42 level in the hippocampi of $APPKI^{NL\text{-}G\text{-}F}$ mice from a young age, it is likely that the increased phosphorylation of IRS1 at Ser sites is associated with Aβ42 level but not with memory decline. Consistent with this finding, a previous study showed that the phosphorylation of IRS1 at mSer307/hSer312 and mSer612/hSer616 increased in cultured hippocampal neurons exposed to Aβ oligomers prepared from synthetic Aβ1–42 peptide and in the AβO-injected hippocampi of non-human primates [16]. Interestingly, the increased basal phosphorylation of hippocampal IRS1 at multiple Ser sites in $APPKI^{NL\text{-}G\text{-}F}$ mice is accompanied by AMPK activation regardless of the presence or absence of memory decline. Consistent with our findings, recent studies suggest that AMPK activation is implicated in brain aging and development of neurodegenerative diseases, including AD [44,45]. These results suggest that the elevation of Aβ42 accompanied by AMPK activation induced by energy depletion that occurs from a young age before the onset of memory decline is associated with increased phosphorylation of hippocampal IRS1 at multiple Ser sites and that sustained activation of these factors contributes to the onset of memory decline in middle-aged $APPKI^{NL\text{-}G\text{-}F}$ mice.

In summary, whether the modification of IRS1 through its phosphorylation at Ser sites in the hippocampus has a pathogenic or an adaptive function remains unknown because the phosphorylation of hippocampal IRS1 at mSer307, mSer612, and mSer1097 increased when metformin improves memory deficits in middle-aged DIO mice [20,46]. Studies using mutant mice with IRS1 Ser residues in the brain will help us to understand the roles of Ser sites in memory function and to identify unrecognized downstream pathways.

5. Conclusions

Our findings indicate that the phosphorylation of IRS1 at disease-specific Ser residues in the hippocampus may be a potential marker of Aβ-unrelated memory impairments induced by T2DM and aging. Alternatively, in Aβ-related memory decline in AD, the modification of IRS1 via its phosphorylation at multiple Ser sites accompanied by the activation of AMPK, a sensor of energy metabolism, may be a marker of the response to an early detection of elevated Aβ42 level before the onset of memory decline in AD.

Author Contributions: W.W., D.T., Y.F., M.M., and C.K. researched data. W.W. and D.T. analyzed data. W.W., D.T., and Y.F. wrote the manuscript. T.S. and T.C.S. provided the APPKI mice and interpreted the data. A.T. designed experiments, analyzed data, and wrote and edited the manuscript. All authors read and approved the final manuscript.

Acknowledgments: We thank Kohei Tomita (Laboratory of Experimental Animal, National Center for Geriatrics and Gerontology) for animal care and M. Sawaura and K. Tabata for providing aged wild-type mice (Charles river, Japan).

References

1. Lin, X.; Taguchi, A.; Park, S.; Kushner, J.A.; Li, F.; Li, Y.; White, M.F. Dysregulation of insulin receptor substrate 2 in beta cells and brain causes obesity and diabetes. *J. Clin. Invest.* **2004**, *114*, 908–916. [CrossRef] [PubMed]
2. Dong, X.; Park, S.; Lin, X.; Copps, K.; Yi, X.; White, M.F. Irs1 and Irs2 signaling is essential for hepatic glucose homeostasis and systemic growth. *J. Clin. Invest.* **2006**, *116*, 101–114. [CrossRef] [PubMed]

3. Taguchi, A.; Wartschow, L.M.; White, M.F. Brain IRS2 signaling coordinates life span and nutrient homeostasis. *Science* **2007**, *317*, 369–372. [CrossRef] [PubMed]
4. Long, Y.C.; Cheng, Z.; Copps, K.D.; White, M.F. Insulin receptor substrates Irs1 and Irs2 coordinate skeletal muscle growth and metabolism via the Akt and AMPK pathways. *Mol. Cell. Biol.* **2011**, *31*, 430–441. [CrossRef] [PubMed]
5. Copps, K.D.; White, M.F. Regulation of insulin sensitivity by serine/threonine phosphorylation of insulin receptor substrate proteins IRS1 and IRS2. *Diabetologia* **2012**, *55*, 2565–2582. [CrossRef] [PubMed]
6. Hancer, N.J.; Qiu, W.; Cherella, C.; Li, Y.; Copps, K.D.; White, M.F. Insulin and metabolic stress stimulate multisite serine/threonine phosphorylation of insulin receptor substrate 1 and inhibit tyrosine phosphorylation. *J. Biol. Chem.* **2014**, *289*, 12467–12484. [CrossRef]
7. White, M.F.; Maron, R.; Kahn, C.R. Insulin rapidly stimulates tyrosine phosphorylation of a Mr-185,000 protein in intact cells. *Nature* **1985**, *318*, 183–186. [CrossRef]
8. Samuel, V.T.; Shulman, G.I. Mechanisms for insulin resistance: Common threads and missing links. *Cell* **2012**, *148*, 852–871. [CrossRef]
9. Jiang, G.; Dallas-Yang, Q.; Biswas, S.; Li, Z.; Zhang, B.B. Rosiglitazone, an agonist of peroxisome-proliferator-activated receptor gamma (PPARgamma), decreases inhibitory serine phosphorylation of IRS1 in vitro and in vivo. *Biochem. J.* **2004**, *377 Pt 2*, 339–346. [CrossRef]
10. Morino, K.; Petersen, K.F.; Dufour, S.; Befroy, D.; Frattini, J.; Shatzkes, N.; Neschen, S.; White, M.F.; Bilz, S.; Sono, S.; et al. Reduced mitochondrial density and increased IRS-1 serine phosphorylation in muscle of insulin-resistant offspring of type 2 diabetic parents. *J. Clin. Invest.* **2005**, *115*, 3587–3593. [CrossRef]
11. Copps, K.D.; Hancer, N.J.; Opare-Ado, L.; Qiu, W.; Walsh, C.; White, M.F. Irs1 serine 307 promotes insulin sensitivity in mice. *Cell Metab.* **2010**, *11*, 84–92. [CrossRef] [PubMed]
12. Tremblay, F.; Brule, S.; Hee Um, S.; Li, Y.; Masuda, K.; Roden, M.; Sun, X.J.; Krebs, M.; Polakiewicz, R.D.; Thomas, G.; et al. Identification of IRS-1 Ser-1101 as a target of S6K1 in nutrient- and obesity-induced insulin resistance. *Proc. Nat. Acad. Sci. USA* **2007**, *104*, 14056–14061. [CrossRef] [PubMed]
13. Moloney, A.M.; Griffin, R.J.; Timmons, S.; O'Connor, R.; Ravid, R.; O'Neill, C. Defects in IGF-1 receptor, insulin receptor and IRS-1/2 in Alzheimer's disease indicate possible resistance to IGF-1 and insulin signalling. *Neurobiol. Aging* **2010**, *31*, 224–243. [CrossRef] [PubMed]
14. Talbot, K.; Wang, H.Y.; Kazi, H.; Han, L.Y.; Bakshi, K.P.; Stucky, A.; Fuino, R.L.; Kawaguchi, K.R.; Samoyedny, A.J.; Wilson, R.S.; et al. Demonstrated brain insulin resistance in Alzheimer's disease patients is associated with IGF-1 resistance, IRS-1 dysregulation, and cognitive decline. *J. Clin. Invest.* **2012**, *122*, 1316–1338. [CrossRef] [PubMed]
15. Yarchoan, M.; Toledo, J.B.; Lee, E.B.; Arvanitakis, Z.; Kazi, H.; Han, L.Y.; Louneva, N.; Lee, V.M.; Kim, S.F.; Trojanowski, J.Q.; et al. Abnormal serine phosphorylation of insulin receptor substrate 1 is associated with tau pathology in Alzheimer's disease and tauopathies. *Acta Neuropathol.* **2014**, *128*, 679–689. [CrossRef] [PubMed]
16. Bomfim, T.R.; Forny-Germano, L.; Sathler, L.B.; Brito-Moreira, J.; Houzel, J.C.; Decker, H.; Silverman, M.A.; Kazi, H.; Melo, H.M.; McClean, P.L.; et al. An anti-diabetes agent protects the mouse brain from defective insulin signaling caused by Alzheimer's disease- associated Abeta oligomers. *J. Clin. Invest.* **2012**, *122*, 1339–1353. [CrossRef] [PubMed]
17. Lourenco, M.V.; Clarke, J.R.; Frozza, R.L.; Bomfim, T.R.; Forny-Germano, L.; Batista, A.F.; Sathler, L.B.; Brito-Moreira, J.; Amaral, O.B.; Silva, C.A.; et al. TNF-alpha mediates PKR-dependent memory impairment and brain IRS-1 inhibition induced by Alzheimer's beta-amyloid oligomers in mice and monkeys. *Cell Metab.* **2013**, *18*, 831–843. [CrossRef]
18. Ma, Q.L.; Yang, F.; Rosario, E.R.; Ubeda, O.J.; Beech, W.; Gant, D.J.; Chen, P.P.; Hudspeth, B.; Chen, C.; Zhao, Y.; et al. Beta-amyloid oligomers induce phosphorylation of tau and inactivation of insulin receptor substrate via c-Jun N-terminal kinase signaling: Suppression by omega-3 fatty acids and curcumin. *J. Neurosci. Off. J. Soc. Neurosci.* **2009**, *29*, 9078–9089. [CrossRef]
19. Saito, T.; Matsuba, Y.; Mihira, N.; Takano, J.; Nilsson, P.; Itohara, S.; Iwata, N.; Saido, T.C. Single App knock-in mouse models of Alzheimer's disease. *Nat. Neurosci.* **2014**, *17*, 661–663. [CrossRef]
20. Tanokashira, D.; Kurata, E.; Fukuokaya, W.; Kawabe, K.; Kashiwada, M.; Takeuchi, H.; Nakazato, M.; Taguchi, A. Metformin treatment ameliorates diabetes-associated decline in hippocampal neurogenesis and memory via phosphorylation of insulin receptor substrate 1. *FEBS Open Bio* **2018**, *8*, 1104–1118. [CrossRef]

21. Liang, L.; Chen, J.; Zhan, L.; Lu, X.; Sun, X.; Sui, H.; Zheng, L.; Xiang, H.; Zhang, F. Endoplasmic reticulum stress impairs insulin receptor signaling in the brains of obese rats. *PloS ONE* **2015**, *10*, e0126384. [CrossRef] [PubMed]
22. Arnold, S.E.; Lucki, I.; Brookshire, B.R.; Carlson, G.C.; Browne, C.A.; Kazi, H.; Bang, S.; Choi, B.R.; Chen, Y.; McMullen, M.F.; et al. High fat diet produces brain insulin resistance, synaptodendritic abnormalities and altered behavior in mice. *Neurobiol. Dis.* **2014**, *67*, 79–87. [CrossRef] [PubMed]
23. Jiang, T.; Yin, F.; Yao, J.; Brinton, R.D.; Cadenas, E. Lipoic acid restores age-associated impairment of brain energy metabolism through the modulation of Akt/JNK signaling and PGC1alpha transcriptional pathway. *Aging Cell* **2013**, *12*, 1021–1031. [CrossRef] [PubMed]
24. Makinodan, M.; Rosen, K.M.; Ito, S.; Corfas, G. A critical period for social experience-dependent oligodendrocyte maturation and myelination. *Science* **2012**, *337*, 1357–1360. [CrossRef] [PubMed]
25. Tsai, P.T.; Hull, C.; Chu, Y.; Greene-Colozzi, E.; Sadowski, A.R.; Leech, J.M.; Steinberg, J.; Crawley, J.N.; Regehr, W.G.; Sahin, M. Autistic-like behaviour and cerebellar dysfunction in Purkinje cell Tsc1 mutant mice. *Nature* **2012**, *488*, 647–651. [CrossRef] [PubMed]
26. Morrison, C.D.; Pistell, P.J.; Ingram, D.K.; Johnson, W.D.; Liu, Y.; Fernandez-Kim, S.O.; White, C.L.; Purpera, M.N.; Uranga, R.M.; Bruce-Keller, A.J.; et al. High fat diet increases hippocampal oxidative stress and cognitive impairment in aged mice: Implications for decreased Nrf2 signaling. *J. Neurochem.* **2010**, *114*, 1581–1589. [CrossRef]
27. Yang, Y.; Fang, H.; Xu, G.; Zhen, Y.; Zhang, Y.; Tian, J.; Zhang, D.; Zhang, G.; Xu, J. Liraglutide improves cognitive impairment via the AMPK and PI3K/Akt signaling pathways in type 2 diabetic rats. *Mol. Med. Rep.* **2018**, *18*, 2449–2457. [CrossRef]
28. Zhu, B.; Li, Y.; Xiang, L.; Zhang, J.; Wang, L.; Guo, B.; Liang, M.; Chen, L.; Xiang, L.; Dong, J.; et al. Alogliptin improves survival and health of mice on a high-fat diet. *Aging Cell* **2019**, *18*, e12883. [CrossRef]
29. Flood, J.F.; Mooradian, A.D.; Morley, J.E. Characteristics of learning and memory in streptozocin-induced diabetic mice. *Diabetes* **1990**, *39*, 1391–1398. [CrossRef]
30. Nakano, M.; Nagaishi, K.; Konari, N.; Saito, Y.; Chikenji, T.; Mizue, Y.; Fujimiya, M. Bone marrow-derived mesenchymal stem cells improve diabetes-induced cognitive impairment by exosome transfer into damaged neurons and astrocytes. *Sci. Rep.* **2016**, *6*, 24805. [CrossRef]
31. Wang, J.; Wang, L.; Zhou, J.; Qin, A.; Chen, Z. The protective effect of formononetin on cognitive impairment in streptozotocin (STZ)-induced diabetic mice. *Biomed. Pharmacother. Biomed. Pharmacother.* **2018**, *106*, 1250–1257. [CrossRef]
32. Chen, Q.; Mo, R.; Wu, N.; Zou, X.; Shi, C.; Gong, J.; Li, J.; Fang, K.; Wang, D.; Yang, D.; et al. Berberine ameliorates diabetes-associated cognitive decline through modulation of aberrant inflammation response and insulin signaling pathway in DM rats. *Front. Pharmacol.* **2017**, *8*, 334. [CrossRef]
33. Saito, T.; Mihira, N.; Matsuba, Y.; Sasaguri, H.; Hashimoto, S.; Narasimhan, S.; Zhang, B.; Murayama, S.; Higuchi, M.; Lee, V.M.Y.; et al. Humanization of the entire murine Mapt gene provides a murine model of pathological human tau propagation. *J. Biol. Chem.* **2019**. [CrossRef]
34. Minami, Y.; Sonoda, N.; Hayashida, E.; Makimura, H.; Ide, M.; Ikeda, N.; Ohgidani, M.; Kato, T.A.; Seki, Y.; Maeda, Y.; et al. p66Shc signaling mediates diabetes-related cognitive decline. *Sci. Rep.* **2018**, *8*, 3213. [CrossRef]
35. Fukazawa, R.; Hanyu, H.; Sato, T.; Shimizu, S.; Koyama, S.; Kanetaka, H.; Sakurai, H.; Iwamoto, T. Subgroups of Alzheimer's disease associated with diabetes mellitus based on brain imaging. *Dement. Geriatr. Cogn. Disord.* **2013**, *35*, 280–290. [CrossRef]
36. Fukasawa, R.; Hanyu, H.; Shimizu, S.; Kanetaka, H.; Sakurai, H.; Ishii, K. Identification of diabetes-related dementia: Longitudinal perfusion SPECT and amyloid PET studies. *J. Neurol. Sci.* **2015**, *349*, 45–51. [CrossRef]
37. Shah, O.J.; Hunter, T. Turnover of the active fraction of IRS1 involves raptor-mTOR- and S6K1-dependent serine phosphorylation in cell culture models of tuberous sclerosis. *Mol. Cell. Biol.* **2006**, *26*, 6425–6434. [CrossRef]
38. Zhang, J.; Gao, Z.; Yin, J.; Quon, M.J.; Ye, J. S6K directly phosphorylates IRS-1 on Ser-270 to promote insulin resistance in response to TNF-(alpha) signaling through IKK2. *J. Biol. Chem.* **2008**, *283*, 35375–35382. [CrossRef]

39. Wu, J.; Zhou, S.L.; Pi, L.H.; Shi, X.J.; Ma, L.R.; Chen, Z.; Qu, M.L.; Li, X.; Nie, S.D.; Liao, D.F.; et al. High glucose induces formation of tau hyperphosphorylation via Cav-1-mTOR pathway: A potential molecular mechanism for diabetes-induced cognitive dysfunction. *Oncotarget* **2017**, *8*, 40843–40856. [CrossRef]
40. Kang, S.; Kim, C.H.; Jung, H.; Kim, E.; Song, H.T.; Lee, J.E. Agmatine ameliorates type 2 diabetes induced-Alzheimer's disease-like alterations in high-fat diet-fed mice via reactivation of blunted insulin signalling. *Neuropharmacology* **2017**, *113 Pt A*, 467–479. [CrossRef]
41. McNeilly, A.D.; Williamson, R.; Balfour, D.J.; Stewart, C.A.; Sutherland, C. A high-fat-diet-induced cognitive deficit in rats that is not prevented by improving insulin sensitivity with metformin. *Diabetologia* **2012**, *55*, 3061–3070. [CrossRef]
42. O'Donnell, E.; Vereker, E.; Lynch, M.A. Age-related impairment in LTP is accompanied by enhanced activity of stress-activated protein kinases: Analysis of underlying mechanisms. *Eur. J. Neurosci.* **2000**, *12*, 345–352. [CrossRef]
43. Craft, S. Alzheimer disease: Insulin resistance and AD—Extending the translational path. *Nat. Rev. Neurol.* **2012**, *8*, 360–362. [CrossRef]
44. Liu, Y.J.; Chern, Y. AMPK-mediated regulation of neuronal metabolism and function in brain diseases. *J. Neurogenet.* **2015**, *29*, 50–58. [CrossRef]
45. Wang, X.; Zimmermann, H.R.; Ma, T. Therapeutic potential of AMP-activated protein kinase in alzheimer's disease. *J. Alzheimer's Dis. JAD* **2019**, *68*, 33–38. [CrossRef]
46. Tanokashira, D.; Fukuokaya, W.; Taguchi, A. Involvement of insulin receptor substrates in cognitive impairment and Alzheimer's disease. *Neural Regen. Res.* **2019**, *14*, 1330–1334.

4

Tryptophan-Tyrosine Dipeptide, the Core Sequence of β-Lactolin, Improves Memory by Modulating the Dopamine System

Yasuhisa Ano [1,*], Tatsuhiro Ayabe [1], Rena Ohya [1], Keiji Kondo [1], Shiho Kitaoka [2,3] and Tomoyuki Furuyashiki [2,3]

1 Research Laboratories for Health Science & Food Technologies, Kirin Company Ltd, Kanazawa-ku, Yokohama-shi, Kanagawa 236-0004, Japan; Tatsuhiro_Ayabe@kirin.co.jp (T.A.); Rena_Ohya@kirin.co.jp (R.O.); kondok@kirin.co.jp (K.K.)

2 Division of Pharmacology, Kobe University Graduate School of Medicine, Kobe 650-0017, Japan; skitaoka@med.kobe-u.ac.jp (S.K.); tfuruya@med.kobe-u.ac.jp (T.F.)

3 AMED-CREST, Chiyoda-ku 100-0004, Tokyo, Japan

* Correspondence: Yasuhisa_Ano@kirin.co.jp

Abstract: Tryptophan-tyrosine (WY)-related peptides including the β-lactopeptide of the glycine-threonine-tryptophan-tyrosine peptide, β-lactolin, improve spatial memory. However, whether and how the WY dipeptide as the core sequence in WY-related peptides improves memory functions has not been investigated. This study assessed the pharmacological effects of the WY dipeptide on memory impairment to elucidate the mechanisms. Here, we showed that oral administration of dipeptides of WY, tryptophan-methionine (WM), tryptophan-valine, tryptophan-leucine, and tryptophan-phenylalanine improved spontaneous alternation of the Y-maze test in scopolamine-induced amnesic mice. In contrast, tyrosine-tryptophan, methionine-tryptophan, tryptophan, tyrosine, and methionine had no effect. These results indicated that the conformation of dipeptides with N-terminal tryptophan is required for their memory improving effects. WY dipeptide inhibited the monoamine oxidase B activity in vitro and increased dopamine levels in the hippocampus and frontal cortex, whereas tryptophan did not cause these effects. In addition, the treatment with SCH-23390, a dopamine D1-like receptor antagonist, and the knockdown of the hippocampal dopamine D1 receptor partially attenuated the memory improvement induced by the WY dipeptide. Importantly, WY dipeptide improved the spontaneous alternations of the Y-maze test in aged mice. These results suggest that the WY dipeptide restores memory impairments by augmenting dopaminergic activity. The development of supplements rich in these peptides might help to prevent age-related cognitive decline.

Keywords: dipeptide; dopamine; hippocampus; memory; monoamine oxidase B

1. Introduction

The rapid growth of aging populations worldwide is associated with an increased incidence of cognitive decline and dementia that become a growing burden not only on patients and their families but also on national healthcare systems. Due to the lack of effective dementia therapies, increasing attention is given to preventive approaches. Recent epidemiological studies suggest that the consumption of certain dairy products reduces the risk of cognitive decline in the elderly and may prevent Alzheimer's disease [1].

Crichton et al. [2] reported that individuals who consumed low-fat dairy products, including yogurt and cheese, once a week had a higher cognitive function than those who did not. A survey-based study of self-reported health information showed that the consumption of low-fat dairy products was associated with increased memory recall, increased social functioning, and decreased stress [3,4]. Ozawa et al. [3,4] surveyed more than 1000 Japanese subjects who were living in the community, aged 60–79 years, and free from dementia to investigate their dietary patterns and any potential association with a reduced risk of dementia symptoms. The authors concluded that including milk or fermented dairy products in the diet reduces the risk of dementia in the general Japanese population. In a clinical trial, Ogata et al. [5] investigated the association between the intake of dairy products and short-term memory and found that the intake of dairy products is highly associated with improved short-term memory. It has also been demonstrated that the intake of dairy products fermented with *Penicillium candidum*, i.e., Camembert cheese, had preventive effects on Alzheimer's disease pathology in a mouse model [6].

We have previously identified tryptophan-tyrosine (WY)-related peptides, including the β-lactopeptide of glycine-threonine-tryptophan-tyrosine (GTWY) peptide, β-lactolin, derived from β-lactoglobulin in an enzymatic whey protein digest [7]. The β-lactolin was smoothly absorbed into the body and delivered to the brain where it was associated with a dopamine level increase, resulting in improved spatial and object memory [7]. In addition, we demonstrated that whey peptides rich in WY-related peptides improved memory and attention in a clinical trial [8]. These reports suggested that WY-related peptides improve cognitive function. However, whether and how the WY dipeptide, the core sequence of WY-related peptides, improves cognitive function has not been investigated. The gap in our knowledge about the pharmacological effects of the WY dipeptide on memory impairment hinders the assessment of the underlying mechanism of the effect of whey peptide preparations rich in WY-related peptides on cognitive performance in clinical trials.

In the present study, we examined the effects of tryptophan-containing dipeptides, including the WY dipeptide, on memory impairment and their mechanisms.

2. Materials and Methods

2.1. Materials

The dipeptides WY, tyrosine-tryptophan (YW), tryptophan-methionine (WM), methionine-tryptophan (MW), tryptophan-valine (WV), tryptophan-leucine (WL), and tryptophan-phenylalanine (WF) (purity > 98%) were purchased from NARD Chemicals, Ltd. (Amagasaki, Japan). Tryptophan, tyrosine, (−)-scopolamine hydrobromide trihydrate, and R(+)-SCH-23390 hydrochloride were purchased from Sigma Aldrich Co. (St. Louis, MO, USA).

2.2. Animals

Crl:CD1 (ICR) male mice, 6 weeks old, and C57BL/6J male mice, 7 months and 22 months old (Charles River Japan, Tokyo, Japan), were maintained at Kirin Company Ltd. Mice were maintained at room temperature (23 ± 1 °C) under a constant 12-h light/dark cycle (light period from 8:00 am to 8:00 pm) and were fed a standard rodent diet (CE-2 (Clea Japan, Tokyo, Japan)). Behavioral pharmacological tests were performed in a sound-isolated room with the same temperature and light/dark cycles. All efforts were made to minimize suffering. For euthanasia, mice were placed into a chamber filled with vapor of isoflurane (Wako, Osaka, Japan). All experiments were approved by the Animal Experiment Committee of Kirin Company Ltd and conducted in strict accordance with their guidelines in 2016.

2.3. Spontaneous Alteration Test

A spontaneous alternation test was conducted in accordance with our previous report [7]. The Y-maze is a three-arm maze with equal angles between all arms (25 cm long × 5 cm wide × 20 cm high). The maze walls were constructed from dark black, polyvinyl plastic. Each mouse was initially placed in one arm, and the sequence and number of arm entries were counted for 8 minutes. The alternation score (%) for each mouse was defined as the ratio of the actual number of alternations to the possible number (defined as the total number of arm entries minus two) multiplied by 100 as follows: % Alternation = ((Number of alternations) / (Total arm entries − 2)) × 100.

To evaluate the effects of the samples on scopolamine-induced memory impairment, 6-week-old Crl:CD1 male mice were orally administered distilled water with or without peptides to be tested 1 h before evaluation. Forty minutes after the oral administration, memory impairment was induced by the intraperitoneal administration of 0.85 mg/kg scopolamine dissolved in saline. One hour after the oral administration, mice were subjected to the Y-maze test. In some experiments, mice were administered 0.85 mg/kg scopolamine and 0.05 mg/kg SCH-23390 (dopamine D1 antagonist) intraperitoneally at 40 min after the oral administration of 0 or 1 mg/kg WY peptide and subjected to the Y-maze test at 1 h after the oral administration. There were 10 mice per group.

In other experiments, C57BL/6J mice were orally administered a daily dose of 0 or 1 mg/kg WY peptide for 14 days. One hour after the last administration, mice were subjected to a Y-maze trial.

2.4. Monoamine Analysis

To evaluate the levels of dopamine and its metabolites (DOPAC and HVA) in the brain, tissue was homogenized in 0.2 M perchloric acid (PCA, Wako, Tokyo, Japan) containing 100 μM EDTA·2Na (Sigma-Aldrich, St. Louis, MO, USA). After centrifugation, the supernatant was analyzed by high-performance liquid chromatography (HPLC) using an EICOMPAK SC-5ODS column and PREPAK column (Eicom, Kyoto, Japan) with an electrochemical detection (ECD) unit. The mobile phase consisted of 83% 0.1 M acetic acid in citric acid buffer (pH 3.5), 17% methanol (Wako), 190 mg/ml of sodium 1-octanesulfonate sodium (Wako), and 5 mg/mL EDTA·2Na. For ECD, the applied voltage was 750 mV vs. an Ag/AgCl reference electrode.

2.5. Monoamine Oxidase (MAO) Activity Assay

MAO-B activity was measured using the MAO assay kit (Cell Biolabs, San Diego, CA, USA) according to the manufacturer's instructions. Human MAO-B (50 μg/mL; Sigma-Aldrich) was incubated with 1 mM WY dipeptide or 1 mM tryptophan for 30 min. The substrates for MAO-B were added and the amount of hydrogen peroxide in the reaction was measured.

2.6. Injection of Adeno-Associated Viruses (AAV) to the Hippocampus

The adeno-associated virus (AAV) injection method used to knock down the dopamine D1 receptor and the following behavioral evaluation were performed as described in our previous study [9,10]. The AAV construct that expresses artificial microRNA (miRNA) targeting the dopamine D1 receptor with an emerald green fluorescent protein (EmGFP) under the control of the elongation factor (EF)1α promoter only in the presence of Cre recombinase (AAV10-EF1α-double-floxed inverted (DIO)-EmGFP-D1miRNA), an AAV construct that expresses control miRNA in the same arrangement (AAV10-EF1α-DIO-EmGFP-control), and an AAV construct that expresses Cre recombinase under the CMV promoter (AAV10-CMV-Cre) were produced as previously described [9]. After anesthetized with sodium pentobarbital, 8-week-old Crl:CD1 male mice were injected with 0.5 μL of the AAV solution (1.0×10^{12} genomics copies/mL) per site, applied at two sites in the hippocampal regions of both hemispheres (four sites per mouse; from bregma: posterior, −3.5 mm; lateral, ± 3 mm; ventral, −3.8 mm and −1.8 mm) according to the atlas of Paxinos and Franklin [11] and using a PV-830 Pneumatic PicoPump (World Precision Instruments, Sarasota, FL, USA). Mice were allowed to recover for 4 weeks and then used for the Y-maze test.

2.7. Statistical Analysis

All values are expressed as means ± standard error of the mean (SEM). Data was analyzed by one-way analysis of variance (ANOVA), followed by Tukey–Kramer test, Dunnett's test, or Student's *t*-test as described in the figure legends. All statistical analyses were performed using the Ekuseru–Toukei 2012 software program (Social Survey Research Information, Tokyo, Japan). A *p*-value < 0.05 was considered statistically significant.

3. Results

3.1. Tryptophan-Containing Dipeptides Improved Memory Impairment in Amnesic Mice

To evaluate the effects of the WY, WM, WV, WL, and WF dipeptides, which are known to be derived from milk proteins, on spatial memory, amnesia was induced by treatment with scopolamine, a muscarinic antagonist, according to a previous study [7]. The spontaneous alternation test using the Y-maze is well-established as a behavioral evaluation method for examining short-term spatial memory performance. A single dose of 1 mg/kg WY, WM, WV, WL, or WF dipeptide significantly increased the spontaneous alternation (Figure 1A–E, respectively). Further, the administration of 0.3 mg/kg WY or WM dipeptide already increased the alternation, which showed higher improvement than that of WV, WL, or WF (Figure 1A and B). The number of arm entries was not changed among the groups (data not shown). These results indicated that the administration of certain dipeptides with N-terminal tryptophan improved short-term spatial memory in amnestic mice.

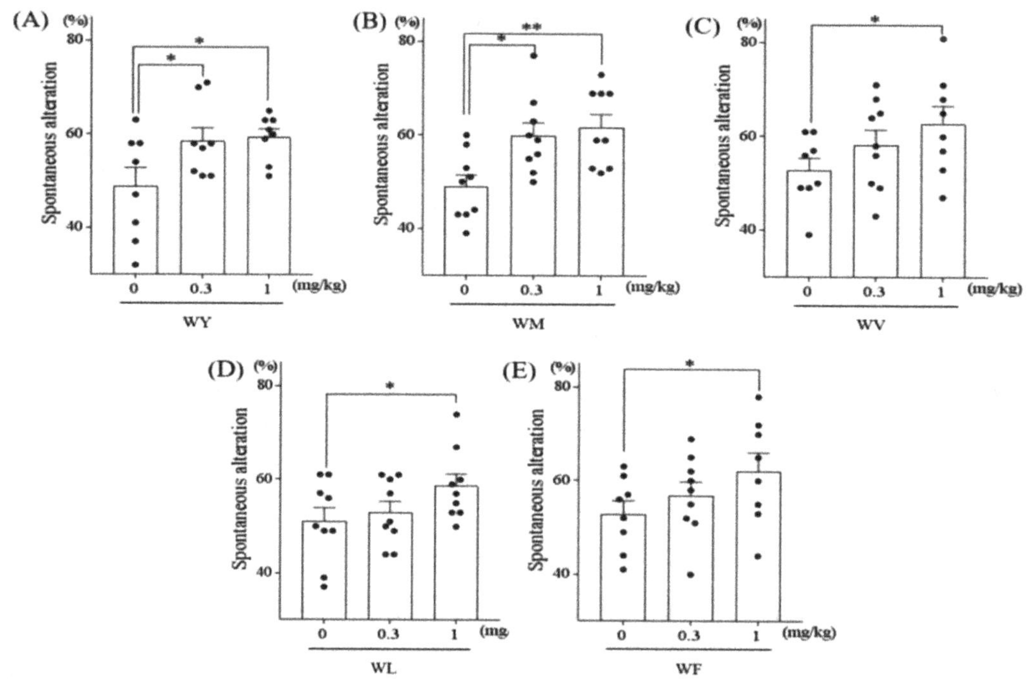

Figure 1. The effects of dipeptides (**A**) WY, (**B**) WM, (**C**) WV, (**D**) WL, and (**E**) WF on spatial memory in amnesic mice. Six-week-old Crl:CD1 male mice were orally administered 0, 0.3, or 1 mg/kg of dipeptide (WV, WM, WV, WL, and WF) and, 40 min later, injected intraperitoneally with 0.85 mg/kg of scopolamine. At 1 h after oral administration, each mouse was allowed to explore the Y-maze for 8 min. Spontaneous alternations were also measured. Data represent the mean ± SEM of 10 mice per group. The p values shown were calculated using the Dunnett's test. *$p < 0.05$ and **$p < 0.01$.

3.2. Dipeptides Containing Tryptophan at the N-Terminus But Not at the C-Terminus Improved Memory Impairment

Next, to evaluate the effect of the tryptophan position within the dipeptides, we assessed the effect of tryptophan, tyrosine, and the dipeptides WY and YW on spatial memory in the spontaneous alternation test. A single administration of 1 mg/kg WY dipeptide, but not tryptophan, tyrosine, or YW dipeptide, increased the spontaneous alternation (Figure 2A). We also tested the effect of tryptophan, methionine, and the dipeptides WM and MW on spatial memory. A single administration of 1 mg/kg WM peptide, but not tryptophan, methionine, or MW dipeptide, also increased the alternation (Figure 2B). These results suggested that the conformation of dipeptides with an N-terminal tryptophan is required to improve the spatial memory in amnestic mice.

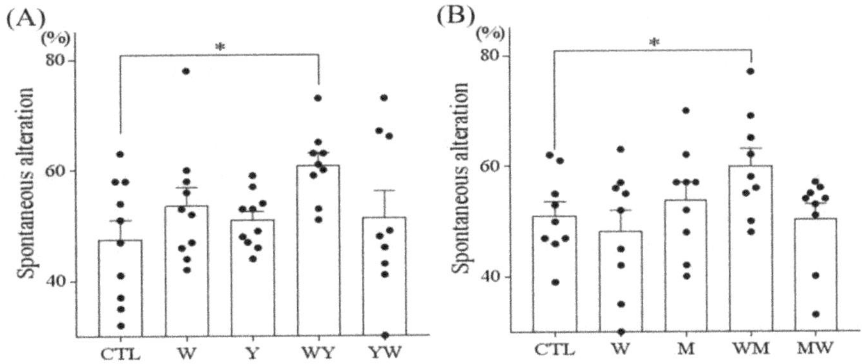

Figure 2. The effects of the dipeptides and single amino acids of (A) WY and (B) WM on spatial memory in amnesic mice. Six-week-old Crl:CD1 male mice were orally administered 0 or 1 mg/kg of dipeptide or single amino acid (WY, YW, WM, MW, tryptophan (W), tyrosine (Y), and methionine (M)) and, 40 min later, injected intraperitoneally with 0.85 mg/kg of scopolamine. At 1 h after oral administration, each mouse was allowed to explore the Y-maze for 8 min. Spontaneous alternations were also measured. Data represent the mean ± SEM of 10 mice per group. The p values shown were calculated using the Dunnett's test. * $p < 0.05$.

3.3. WY Peptide Increased Dopamine Levels in the Hippocampus and Frontal Cortex

Because we previously reported that the GTWY peptide inhibits MAO-B activity in vitro and in vivo and increases dopamine contents in the frontal cortex and hippocampus, we further evaluated the effect of the WY dipeptide on the catecholamine levels in the hippocampus and frontal cortex. In both the hippocampus and frontal cortex, a single administration of the WY dipeptide significantly increased the level of dopamine (Figure 3A–F). The levels of DOPAC and HVA appear to be slightly increased, though not statistically significant. Thus, the administration of WY dipeptide increased the level of dopamine in the brain without affecting the levels of its metabolites.

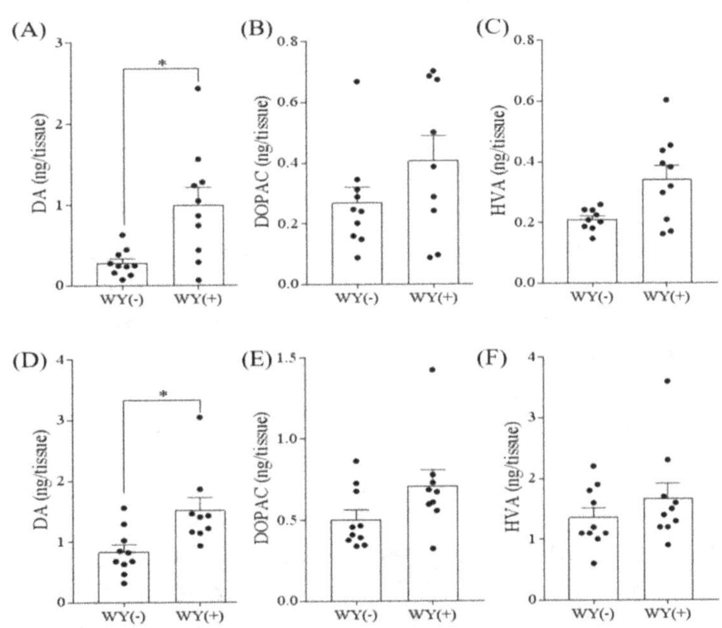

Figure 3. The levels of dopamine and its metabolites in the hippocampus and frontal cortex. Six-week-old Crl:CD1 male mice were orally administered 0 or 1 mg/kg of WY dipeptide. At 1 h after oral administration, the following monoamine levels were measured in the hippocampus (**A–C**) and frontal cortex (**D–F**) by HPLC: dopamine (DA) (**A, D**), 3,4-dihydroxyphenylacetic acid (DOPAC) (**B, E**), and homovanillic acid (HVA) (**C, F**). Data represent the mean ± SEM of 10 mice per group. The p values shown were calculated using the Student's t-test. * $p < 0.05$.

3.4. WY Peptide Inhibited the Activity of MAO

We evaluated the effect of WY dipeptide and tryptophan on MAO-B activity. Tyrosine and YW dipeptide were not tested in this assay because the compounds could not be dissolved in the assay buffer. Treatment with 1 mM WY dipeptide decreased MAO-B activity by 48 ± 1.95% compared to that of the control treatment. By contrast, treatment with 1 mM tryptophan did not inhibit MAO-B activity (Figure 4A). These results suggested that the WY dipeptide increased the dopamine content in the hippocampus by inhibiting MAO-B activity and that its chemical structure (Figure 4B) was important to inhibit the MAO-B activity.

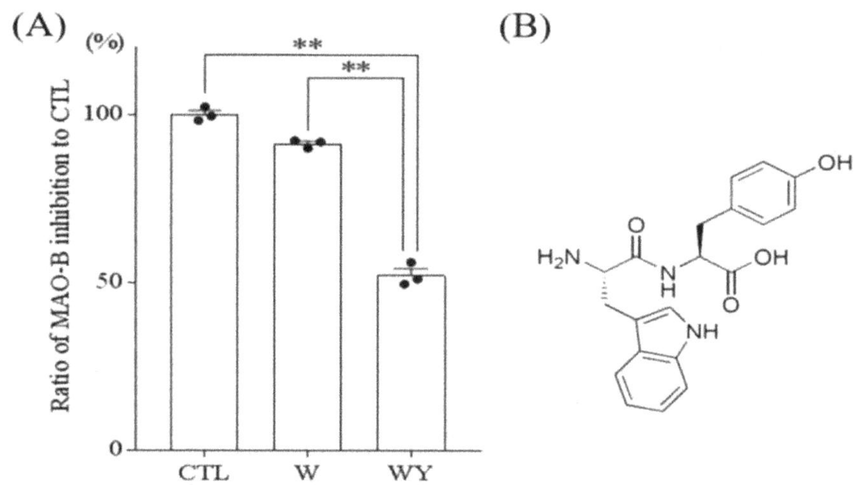

Figure 4. The inhibition of monoamine oxidase by the WY dipeptide and tryptophan and the chemical structure of the WY dipeptide. (**A**) The activity of monoamine oxidase B (MAO-B) was tested in the presence of 1 mM WY dipeptide or tryptophan (W). Data represent the mean ± SEM of triplicate per sample. The p values shown were calculated using the Dunnett's test. ** $p < 0.01$. (**B**) The chemical structure of the WY dipeptide.

3.5. Inhibition of the Dopamine D1 Receptor Attenuated the WY-Induced Memory Improvement

To investigate the link between dopamine and the memory-improving effect of the WY dipeptide, we examined the effect of SCH-23390, a dopamine D1-like receptor antagonist on the WY-dipeptide-induced memory improvement. Whereas WY-dipeptide increased spontaneous alteration in scopolamine-induced amnestic mice with prior treatment with saline (control group), SCH-23390 treatment abolished the memory improvement induced by the WY dipeptide (Figure 5A). These results indicated that the dopamine D1-like receptor was involved in the improvement of spatial memory induced by the WY dipeptide.

To further determine the involvement of the dopamine D1 receptor in the memory-improving effect of the WY dipeptide, the mRNA expression of the dopamine D1 receptor was knocked down in hippocampal neurons using the AAV system expressing artificial miRNA targeting this receptor according to our previous study [10]. While the WY dipeptide administration increased the spontaneous alternation in amnestic mice expressing control miRNA, this memory improvement was not significant with the dopamine D1 receptor knockdown in hippocampal neurons (Figure 5B). These results suggested that the dopamine D1 receptor in the hippocampus is involved in the memory improvement caused by the WY dipeptide at least in part.

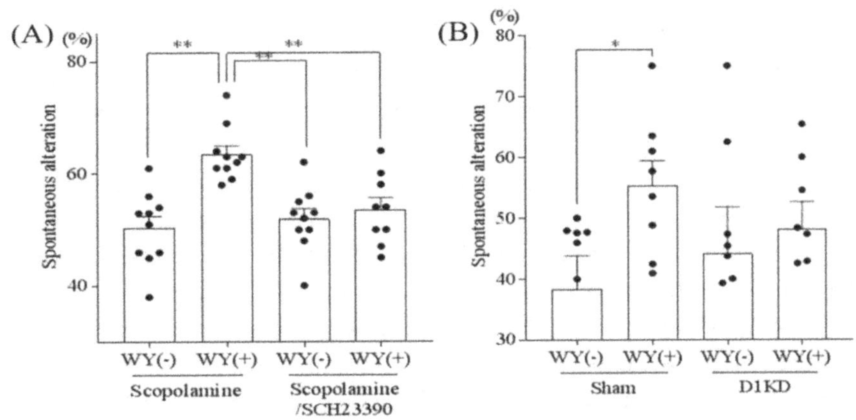

Figure 5. The dopamine receptor is involved in memory improvement linked to the WY dipeptide. (**A**) Six-week-old Crl:CD1 male mice were orally administered 0 or 1 mg/kg of WY dipeptide and, 40 min later, intraperitoneally injected with 0.85 mg/kg of scopolamine alone or scopolamine plus 0.05 mg/kg of SCH-23390. At 1 h after oral administration of the peptide, mice were allowed to explore the Y-maze for 8 min. Data represent the mean ± SEM of 10 mice per group. (**B**) Eight-week-old Crl:CD1 male mice were administered either a control microRNA or dopamine D_1 receptor microRNA containing AAV, which suppresses the dopamine D_1 receptor, to the hippocampus. Mice were orally administered 0 or 1 mg/kg of WY dipeptide and, 40 min later, intraperitoneally injected with 0.85 mg/kg of scopolamine. At 1 h after oral administration of the peptide, mice were allowed to explore the Y-maze for 8 min. Data represent the mean ± SEM of 7–8 mice per group. The p values were calculated using one-way ANOVA followed by the Tukey–Kramer test. ** $p < 0.01$ and * $p < 0.05$.

3.6. WY Peptide Improved Age-Related Memory Impairment

Our results showed that the WY dipeptide restored pharmacologically-induced memory impairment in mice. Therefore, we further examined whether the WY dipeptide would have a similar effect on memory impairment in aged mice. Aged (22 months) and young (7 months) C57BL/6J mice were orally administered WY dipeptide, and their performance in the spontaneous alternation test was evaluated. The proportion of spontaneous alternation was reduced in aged mice, compared with young mice, indicating age-related memory impairment. The administration of the WY dipeptide increased the proportion of spontaneous alteration in aged mice (Figure 6), indicating that WY dipeptide also restored memory impairment in aged mice.

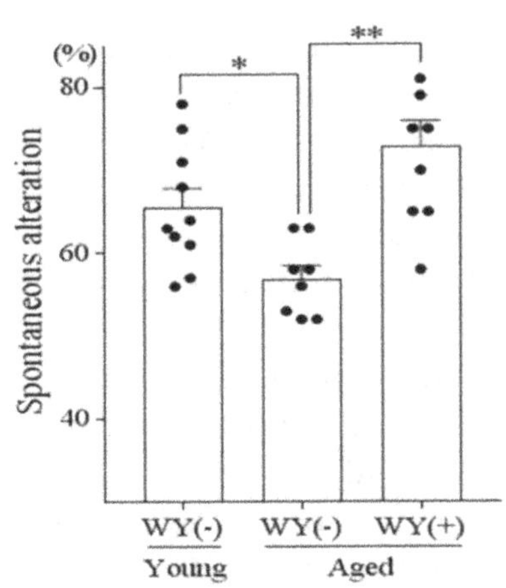

Figure 6. The effects of the WY peptide on aged mice: 7- and 22-month-old C57BL/6 mice were orally administered a daily dose 1 mg/kg of WY dipeptide for 14 days. At 1 h after oral administration of the peptide, mice were allowed to explore the Y-maze for 8 min. Data represent the mean ± SEM of 8–10 mice per group. The p values were calculated using one-way ANOVA followed by the Tukey–Kramer test. * $p < 0.05$ and ** $p < 0.01$.

4. Discussion

Epidemiological studies have reported that the consumption of fermented dairy products is beneficial for the prevention of cognitive decline in the elderly [1]. Our previous study demonstrated that WY-related peptides derived from enzymatic whey protein digests, such as the GTWY peptide β-lactolin, improve memory impairment in mice with pharmacologically-induced amnesia [7]. However, the underlying mechanism of the effects of the WY dipeptide core included in WY-related peptides on memory improvement is not well-understood. In the present study, we demonstrated that dipeptides with an N-terminal tryptophan, such as WY, WM, WV, WL, and WF improved memory impairment in scopolamine-induced amnesic mice. Especially, the WY dipeptide increased the dopamine levels in the hippocampus and frontal cortex, and the WY-induced memory improvement was attenuated by the blockade of the dopamine D1 receptor. Moreover, the WY dipeptide improved spatial memory impairment in aged mice. These results suggested that orally administered WY dipeptide improved spatial memory impairments in pharmacologically-induced amnestic mice and aged mice via modulating the dopamine system.

We showed that the WY dipeptide inhibited MAO-B activity and increased dopamine levels in the hippocampus and frontal cortex and improved spatial memory impairment in pharmacologically-induced amnestic mice and aged mice. Previous reports have indicated that dopamine is involved in hippocampus-dependent memory functions [12,13]. The dopamine neuronal network is related to an age-related decline in cognitive performance and executive function, and the dopamine precursor levodopa has been shown to improve the task-based learning rate and task performance in the elderly [14]. It has also been reported that MAO-B inhibitors improve cognitive function in rodents [15–17]. MAO-B is an enzyme for dopamine metabolism and thus decreases dopamine levels in the brain [18]. Therefore, MAO-B inhibitors have been used as drugs to induce dopamine levels [19]. It is suggested that some MAO-B inhibitors have a potential as therapeutic or preventive treatment for dementia including Alzheimer's disease [20,21]. We also showed that the administration of WY dipeptide increased total dopamine levels in the hippocampus and frontal cortex. These results suggest that WY dipeptide increase dopamine levels in the brain by inhibiting MAO-B activity. Those findings suggest that the WY dipeptide exerts its beneficial effect on the prevention of age-related cognitive decline by increasing dopaminergic activity in the brain.

In addition, we showed that dopamine D1 receptor is involved in the spatial memory improvement induced by the WY dipeptide. Dopamine exerts its functions via multiple receptor subtypes, D1-like (D1 and D5) and D2-like (D2, D3, and D4) receptors. In the present study, the treatment with D1-like receptor antagonist, SCH-23390 attenuated the improvement caused by the WY dipeptide in scopolamine-induced amnesic mice. It has been reported that activation of dopamine D1-like receptors enhances hippocampus-dependent memory functions [22–25]. Because the hippocampus is crucial for spatial memory as measured by the Y-maze test [26], we examined the involvement of the dopamine D1 receptor in the hippocampus in WY-dipeptide-induced memory improvement. Dopamine D1-like receptors are expressed in many brain areas including the hippocampus, but due to the lack of selective pharmacological drugs, most studies failed to discriminate dopamine receptor subtypes. Recently, the brain-region-specific knockdown of the dopamine D1 receptor subtype was achieved by injecting AAV vectors that express recombinant miRNA targeting this dopamine receptor subtype [9]. This technique made it possible to further examine a potential link between the spatial memory improvement by the WY dipeptide and the dopamine D1 receptors in the hippocampus. Dopamine D1 receptor knockdown in the hippocampus attenuated the improvement by the WY peptide, but it was a partial reduction. These data suggested that the dopamine D1 receptor in the hippocampus is involved in the WY-dipeptide-induced memory improvement for spatial information measured in the Y-maze test at least in part. The reason why the effect of the D1 receptor knockdown was partial remains unclear. It could be due to the partial knockdown of the dopamine D1 receptor in the hippocampus. This finding is consistent with previous reports suggesting that D1 receptor stimulation in the hippocampus augments spatial memory.

Alternatively, dopamine in the frontal cortex could be involved in the WY-dipeptide-induced memory improvement, since the WY dipeptide increased the dopamine levels in frontal cortex as well.

In the present study, we compared the effects of several dipeptides containing tryptophan and tryptophan as a single amino acid. We found that the administration of a single dose of dipeptides with an N-terminal tryptophan, WY, WM, WV, WL, and WF improved spatial memory in mice, whereas YW and MW dipeptides did not have this effect. These findings suggest that the dipeptide conformation with an N-terminal tryptophan is crucial for effectively improving the memory impairment after oral administration. It has been shown that dipeptides with an N-terminal tryptophan have a high affinity to peptide transporters, and among the dipeptide library, the WY dipeptide is one of the dipeptides with the highest affinities [27]. Thus, the conformation of dipeptides with an N-terminal tryptophan could be necessary for transporter-mediated absorption from the gut and delivery to the brain. On the other hand, based on our finding that the WY dipeptide, but not tryptophan as a single amino acid, inhibited MAO-B activity in vitro, the dipeptide conformation with an N-terminal tryptophan could be crucial for enhancing dopaminergic activity. Note that these two possibilities are not mutually exclusive but rather synergetic for the memory improving effect of the WY dipeptide.

5. Conclusions

In summary, the present study showed that the WY dipeptide improves pharmacologically-induced and age-related memory impairment in mice. Effective intake of the WY dipeptide and other dipeptides with N-terminal tryptophan via supplements or nutraceutical foods including certain whey peptide preparations might be beneficial for improving cognitive function in older age.

Author Contributions: Y.A., T.A., and R.O. conducted the experiments and analyzed the results. Y.A., S.K., and T.F. wrote the paper, and K.K. supervised this research.

References

1. Ano, Y.; Nakayama, H. Preventive effects of dairy products on dementia and the underlying mechanisms. *Int. J. Mol. Sci.* **2018**, *19*, 1927. [CrossRef] [PubMed]
2. Crichton, G.E.; Bryan, J.; Murphy, K.J.; Buckley, J. Review of dairy consumption and cognitive performance in adults: Findings and methodological issues. *Dement. Geriatr. Cogn. Disord.* **2010**, *30*, 352–361. [CrossRef] [PubMed]
3. Ozawa, M.; Ninomiya, T.; Ohara, T.; Doi, Y.; Uchida, K.; Shirota, T.; Yonemoto, K.; Kitazono, T.; Kiyohara, Y. Dietary patterns and risk of dementia in an elderly Japanese population: The Hisayama Study. *Am. J. Clin. Nutr.* **2013**, *97*, 1076–1082. [CrossRef] [PubMed]
4. Ozawa, M.; Ohara, T.; Ninomiya, T.; Hata, J.; Yoshida, D.; Mukai, N.; Nagata, M.; Uchida, K.; Shirota, T.; Kitazono, T.; et al. Milk and dairy consumption and risk of dementia in an elderly Japanese population: The Hisayama Study. *J. Am. Geriatr. Soc.* **2014**, *62*, 1224–1230. [CrossRef] [PubMed]
5. Ogata, S.; Tanaka, H.; Omura, K.; Honda, C.; Hayakawa, K. Association between intake of dairy products and short-term memory with and without adjustment for genetic and family environmental factors: A twin study. *Clin. Nutr. (Edinburgh, Scotland)* **2016**, *35*, 507–513. [CrossRef] [PubMed]
6. Ano, Y.; Ozawa, M.; Kutsukake, T.; Sugiyama, S.; Uchida, K.; Yoshida, A.; Nakayama, H. Preventive effects of a fermented dairy product against Alzheimer's disease and identification of a novel oleamide with enhanced microglial phagocytosis and anti-inflammatory activity. *PloS ONE* **2015**, *10*, e0118512. [CrossRef] [PubMed]
7. Ano, Y.; Ayabe, T.; Kutsukake, T.; Ohya, R.; Takaichi, Y.; Uchida, S.; Yamada, K.; Uchida, K.; Takashima, A.; Nakayama, H. Novel lactopeptides in fermented dairy products improve memory function and cognitive decline. *Neurobiol. Aging* **2018**, *72*, 23–31. [CrossRef]
8. Kita, M.; Obara, K.; Kondo, S.; Umeda, S.; Ano, Y. Effect of supplementation of a whey peptide rich in tryptophan-tyrosine-related peptides on cognitive performance in healthy adults: A randomized, double-blind, placebo-controlled study. *Nutrients* **2018**, *10*, 899. [CrossRef]
9. Shinohara, R.; Taniguchi, M.; Ehrlich, A.T.; Yokogawa, K.; Deguchi, Y.; Cherasse, Y.; Lazarus, M.; Urade, Y.; Ogawa, A.; Kitaoka, S.; et al. Dopamine D1 receptor subtype mediates acute stress-induced dendritic growth

in excitatory neurons of the medial prefrontal cortex and contributes to suppression of stress susceptibility in mice. *Mol. Psychiatr.* **2017**, *23*, 1717. [CrossRef]

10. Ano, Y.; Hoshi, A.; Ayabe, T.; Ohya, R.; Uchida, S.; Yamada, K.; Kondo, K.; Kitaoka, S.; Furuyashiki, T. Iso-alpha-acids, the bitter components of beer, improve hippocampus-dependent memory through vagus nerve activation. *FASEB J. Off. Publ. Fed. Am. Soc. Exp. Biol.* **2019**. [CrossRef]
11. Franklin, K.; Paxinos, G. *The Mouse Brain in Stereotaxic Coordinates, Compact*; Academic Press: San Diego, CA, USA, 2008.
12. McNamara, C.G.; Dupret, D. Two sources of dopamine for the hippocampus. *Trends Neurosci.* **2017**, *40*, 383–384. [CrossRef] [PubMed]
13. Takeuchi, T.; Duszkiewicz, A.J.; Sonneborn, A.; Spooner, P.A.; Yamasaki, M.; Watanabe, M.; Smith, C.C.; Fernandez, G.; Deisseroth, K.; Greene, R.W.; et al. Locus coeruleus and dopaminergic consolidation of everyday memory. *Nature* **2016**, *537*, 357–362. [CrossRef] [PubMed]
14. Chowdhury, R.; Guitart-Masip, M.; Lambert, C.; Dayan, P.; Huys, Q.; Duzel, E.; Dolan, R.J. Dopamine restores reward prediction errors in old age. *Nat. Neurosci.* **2013**, *16*, 648–653. [CrossRef] [PubMed]
15. Bar-Am, O.; Amit, T.; Kupershmidt, L.; Aluf, Y.; Mechlovich, D.; Kabha, H.; Danovitch, L.; Zurawski, V.R.; Youdim, M.B.; Weinreb, O. Neuroprotective and neurorestorative activities of a novel iron chelator-brain selective monoamine oxidase-A/monoamine oxidase-B inhibitor in animal models of Parkinson's disease and aging. *Neurobiol. Aging* **2015**, *36*, 1529–1542. [CrossRef] [PubMed]
16. Justo, L.A.; Duran, R.; Alfonso, M.; Fajardo, D.; Faro, L.R.F. Effects and mechanism of action of isatin, a MAO inhibitor, on in vivo striatal dopamine release. *Neurochem. Int.* **2016**, *99*, 147–157. [CrossRef] [PubMed]
17. Schulz, D.; Mirrione, M.M.; Henn, F.A. Cognitive aspects of congenital learned helplessness and its reversal by the monoamine oxidase (MAO)-B inhibitor deprenyl. *Neurobiol. Learn. Mem.* **2010**, *93*, 291–301. [CrossRef] [PubMed]
18. Gaweska, H.; Fitzpatrick, P.F. Structures and mechanism of the monoamine oxidase family. *Biomol. Concepts* **2011**, *2*, 365–377. [CrossRef]
19. Cai, Z. Monoamine oxidase inhibitors: Promising therapeutic agents for Alzheimer's disease (Review). *Mol. Med. Rep.* **2014**, *9*, 1533–1541. [CrossRef]
20. Wang, Y.; Sun, Y.; Guo, Y.; Wang, Z.; Huang, L.; Li, X. Dual functional cholinesterase and MAO inhibitors for the treatment of Alzheimer's disease: Synthesis, pharmacological analysis and molecular modeling of homoisoflavonoid derivatives. *J. Enzyme Inhib. Med. Chem.* **2016**, *31*, 389–397. [CrossRef]
21. Borroni, E.; Bohrmann, B.; Grueninger, F.; Prinssen, E.; Nave, S.; Loetscher, H.; Chinta, S.J.; Rajagopalan, S.; Rane, A.; Siddiqui, A.; et al. Sembragiline: A novel, selective monoamine oxidase type B inhibitor for the treatment of Alzheimer's disease. *J. Pharmacol. Exp. Ther.* **2017**, *362*, 413–423. [CrossRef]
22. Da Silva, W.C.; Kohler, C.C.; Radiske, A.; Cammarota, M. D1/D5 dopamine receptors modulate spatial memory formation. *Neurobiol. Learn. Mem.* **2012**, *97*, 271–275. [CrossRef] [PubMed]
23. De Bundel, D.; Femenia, T.; DuPont, C.M.; Konradsson-Geuken, A.; Feltmann, K.; Schilstrom, B.; Lindskog, M. Hippocampal and prefrontal dopamine D1/5 receptor involvement in the memory-enhancing effect of reboxetine. *Int. J. Neuropsychopharmacol.* **2013**, *16*, 2041–2051. [CrossRef] [PubMed]
24. Yuan Xiang, P.; Janc, O.; Grochowska, K.M.; Kreutz, M.R.; Reymann, K.G. Dopamine agonists rescue Abeta-induced LTP impairment by Src-family tyrosine kinases. *Neurobiol. Aging* **2016**, *40*, 98–102. [CrossRef] [PubMed]
25. Hao, J.R.; Sun, N.; Lei, L.; Li, X.Y.; Yao, B.; Sun, K.; Hu, R.; Zhang, X.; Shi, X.D.; Gao, C. L-Stepholidine rescues memory deficit and synaptic plasticity in models of Alzheimer's disease via activating dopamine D1 receptor/PKA signaling pathway. *Cell Death Dis.* **2015**, *6*, e1965. [CrossRef] [PubMed]
26. Pioli, E.Y.; Gaskill, B.N.; Gilmour, G.; Tricklebank, M.D.; Dix, S.L.; Bannerman, D.; Garner, J.P. An automated maze task for assessing hippocampus-sensitive memory in mice. *Behav. Brain Res.* **2014**, *261*, 249–257. [CrossRef] [PubMed]
27. Ito, K.; Hikida, A.; Kawai, S.; Lan, V.T.; Motoyama, T.; Kitagawa, S.; Yoshikawa, Y.; Kato, R.; Kawarasaki, Y. Analysing the substrate multispecificity of a proton-coupled oligopeptide transporter using a dipeptide library. *Nat. Commun.* **2013**, *4*, 2502. [CrossRef] [PubMed]

5

The Potential Influence of the Bacterial Microbiome on the Development and Progression of ADHD

Stephanie Bull-Larsen and M. Hasan Mohajeri *

Institute of Anatomy, Department of medicine, University of Zurich, Winterthurerstrasse 190, 8057 Zürich, Switzerland; stephanie.bull-larsen@uzh.ch

* Correspondence: mhasan.mohajeri@uzh.ch

Abstract: The latest research cumulates staggering information about the correlation between the microbiota-gut-brain axis and neurodevelopmental disorders. This review aims to shed light on the potential influence of the microbiome on the development of the most prevalent neurodevelopmental disease, attention-deficit-hyperactive disorder (ADHD). As the etiology and pathophysiology of ADHD are still unclear, finding viable biomarkers and effective treatment still represent a challenge. Therefore, we focused on factors that have been associated with a higher risk of developing ADHD, while simultaneously influencing the microbial composition. We reviewed the effect of a differing microbial makeup on neurotransmitter concentrations important in the pathophysiology of ADHD. Additionally, we deduced factors that correlate with a high prevalence of ADHD, while simultaneously affecting the gut microbiome, such as emergency c-sections, and premature birth as the former leads to a decrease of the gut microbial diversity and the latter causes neuroprotective *Lactobacillus* levels to be reduced. Also, we assessed nutritional influences, such as breastfeeding, ingestion of short-chain fatty acids (SCFAs) and polyunsaturated fatty acids (PUFAs) on the host's microbiome and development of ADHD. Finally, we discussed the potential significance of *Bifidobacterium* as a biomarker for ADHD, the importance of preventing premature birth as prophylaxis and nutrition as a prospective therapeutic measurement against ADHD.

Keywords: microbiome; microbiota-gut-brain axis; ADHD; attention-deficit-hyperactive-disorder

---

1. Introduction

The microbiota-gut-brain axis is a bidirectional communication pathway between the microbiota, gut and central nervous system (CNS). It has been estimated that over 10^{14} microorganisms, which include bacteria, archaea, and eukaryota, reside in the gastrointestinal tract (GI-tract) [1]. According to the latest study, this results in an approximately equal number of microbial compared to human cells in an individual [2]. The microorganisms residing in the GI-tract play an important role in protecting humans from potential GI pathogens [3], and also exert neuroactive properties which explains why this ecosystem does not only influence the gut, but also the brain. Research shows the great importance of a healthy microbial composition in the gut at an early stage in life (2–3 years of age), a period also characterized by intense neurodevelopment in humans. Several reports conclude that early gut dysbiosis can influence the neurodevelopment in the short run and may also lead to mental health issues later in life [4,5].

Research highlights this risk, as gut dysbiosis in child or adulthood has not only been associated with various diseases, such as irritable bowel syndrome [6] or obesity [7], but also with psychiatric disorders as, for example, depression [8], Parkinson's disease (PD) [9], schizophrenia [10], autism spectrum disorder (AS) [11], and lastly, attention-deficite-hyperactive-disorder (ADHD) [12].

ADHD is an early onset neurodevelopmental disease that, according to the fifth edition of Diagnostic and Statistical Manual (DSM-V), can be characterized into different representations:

Hyperactivity and/or impulsivity, inattentiveness or all combined [13]. The worldwide prevalence of ADHD in children under the age of 18 ranges from 5.3% [14] to 7.2% [15], making it the most frequent neurobehavioral diagnosis in children. Interestingly, varying prevalence levels are reported in different geographies, which are primarily due to different characteristics of methods employed for ADHD diagnosis rather than geographic variations [14]. Nonetheless, 30–60% of the children continue to show symptoms into adulthood and thus, 1–6% of the population develop adult ADHD [16]. This is predominantly represented by the inattentive type [17].

This literature review attempts to identify and discuss factors that may influence the microbiome, and thus, could be associated with the development or progression of ADHD. Thereby we concentrate solely on the influence of bacteria rather than archaea and eukaryota. Furthermore, we evaluate the biochemical changes in ADHD patients and to what extent these can be related to microbial alterations in the gut. Finally, we reconfirm known biomarkers and deduce possible new ones for the diagnosis of ADHD and conclude what factors worsen or alleviate the development and progression of ADHD as this might lead to potential intervention methods of the neurodevelopmental disorder.

2. Materials and Methods

The key research question of this literature review is: What factors may influence the microbiome and could be associated with the development and/or progression of ADHD? The databases Pubmed and Scopus were searched until the 1 July 2019 with the following MeSH and search terms: "Microbiome", "microbiota", "gut-brain axis", "microbiota-gut-brain-axis", "ADHD". Most of the research papers included in this review were published between 2010 and 2019.

As our primary focus was on bacteria, we excluded studies that concentrated on archaea and eukaryota. The incorporated studies had to fulfill all of the following inclusion criteria:

- Articles were directly related to the topic;
- ADHD patients were diagnosed by a medical expert;
- Publication in a peer-reviewed journal;
- Availability of the full-text publication;
- Studies were written in English.

A total of 208 citations were included in this article.

3. Evidence Linking Microbiota to ADHD

3.1. Microbiome

The influence of the microbiome on the ADHD pathophysiology is being intensively researched. The microbiota consists of the different microorganisms [18], and the microbiome describes the entire genome of the microbiota [18]. The primary functions of the microbiota include: (i) Protecting the host organism against pathogens by increasing the mucine production, and thus, stabilizing the gut-blood barrier; (ii) support of the immune system [19]; (iii) the production of vitamins [20]; and (iv) short-chain fatty acids (SCFAs), whereby the latter are products of microbial catabolism of indigestible carbohydrates [21]. Throughout the GI-tract, the composition and density of microbes changes, increasing from 10^2 cells per gram of content in the stomach to 10^8 cells per gram in the cecum [22]. Additionally, up to 1000 different bacterial species have been found to inhabit the GI-tract of humans [23]. Thereby the composition in species of the microbiome can be influenced by genetics [24], geography [25], disease, medication [26], and age [27].

The GI-microbiota goes through a physiological change from its prenatal period until the age of three [27]. For a long time, it has been thought that the intrauterine environment is sterile and that the first bacterial colonization of the newborn happens during delivery [28]. However, numerous studies have shown that bacteria exist in the placenta, amniotic fluid [29–31], and meconium [32] indicating that the unique microbial composition in utero may already influence the development of the microbiome of the fetus before birth. Research demonstrates that the microbiome of the placenta is low in richness and diversity and is predominantly colonized by the phyla Proteobacteria and Bacteroidetes. The former is mostly represented by the spp. *Escherichia coli* and *Neisseria lactamica*, while Bacteroidetes is dominated by *Bacteroides* spp. [31]. Other important phyla include Firmicutes, Fusobacteria and Tenericutes [31], whereby the latter includes genera, such as *Mycoplasma* and *Ureaplasma* [33].

The colonization of the gut in the postnatal period is sensitive to environmental factors. Nonetheless, the normal composition of the microbiome in a newborn is low in diversity and shows dominance in Proteobacteria and Actinobacteria [34]. More specifically, Proteobacteria shows its peak at birth, whereas Actinobacteria increases and dominates at the age of four months [35]. At this point, Proteobacteria is still mostly represented by *Escherichia coli* and Actinobacteria by the genus *Bifidobacterium longum* [35]. As seen in Figure 1, at the age of three and onwards, the microbiome stabilizes to four major phyla: Firmicutes, Bacteroidetes, Actinobacteria, and Proteobacteria, which normally cover more than 90% of the total bacterial population in a human body [36].

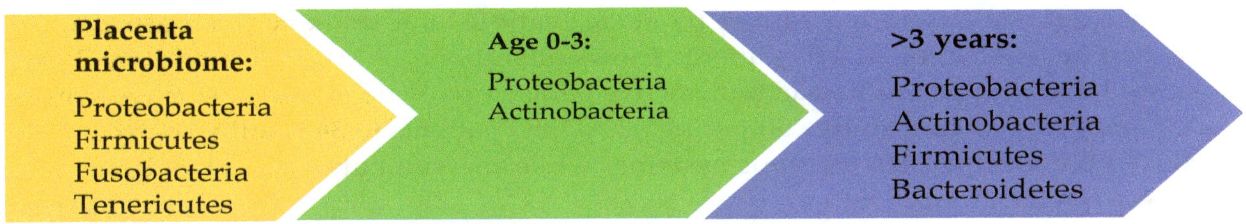

Figure 1. The most prevalent bacterial phyla in utero and in the GI-tract of humans. This figure represents the dynamic and development of the composition of the microbiome from fetuses in utero until the age of three years, at which point the microbiome gains its stability and consists of mostly four phyla: Proteobacteria, Actinobacteria, Firmicutes, and Bacteroides.

3.2. Gut-Brain Axis

The gut-brain axis describes the bidirectional communication between the microbes, enteric nervous system and the CNS [37]. So far, there are three known means of communication between these compartments: Neural, immune, and endocrine [4,38].

The neural pathway describes the hypothalamic-pituitary-adrenal axis (HPA axis), which is the most important efferent stress pathway. It is of great importance to understand to what extent the HPA axis plays a role in the pathogenesis of ADHD, as it influences pathways in the body that are often deviating in ADHD patients [39,40] as for example: Circadian rhythm [41], sleep [42], and emotions [43]. The stimulation of the HPA axis by stress or pro-inflammatory cytokines results in a release of corticotropin-releasing factor (CRF) from the hypothalamus, as well as adrenocorticotropic hormone (ACTH) from the pituitary gland, finally resulting in the secretion of cortisol from the suprarenal (adrenal) glands [38].

One study using 69 healthy children and 123 children with ADHD observed an increase in salivatory cortisol in ADHD patients after waking up in the morning [44]. The effect of stressors was studied in one paper showing that after being exposed to stress children with ADHD of combined type (high levels of hyperactivity and impulsivity) have decreased salivary cortisol levels in comparison to other ADHD patients [45]. In contrast, adult ADHD patients with an inattentive type showed higher levels of cortisol in comparison to the combined types, which showed normal levels of cortisol [46]. Finally, Lackschewitz et al. discovered that adults with ADHD who undergo a stress-inducing exam show a trend towards reduced cortisol levels [47]. These reports portray the association between altered cortisol levels and different types of ADHD. However, the heterogeneity of the results can be explained by various stressors on a differing target group all acting as confounders. Thus, only future studies using the same stressor, examining similar and large patient groups will allow drawing further reliable conclusions.

The neuroimmune communication pathway describes how intestinal microbes influence the function and maturation of immune cells in the CNS, whereby microglia cells play an important role [48]. These cells are activated, as well as produced, by pro-inflammatory cytokines, and are important regulators for autoimmunity, neuroinflammation, and neurogenesis [49]. Germ-free (GF) mice showed defects in microglia activation, which in turn lead to a deficient innate immune response when exposed to pathogenic bacteria [50]. The same study showed the immense effect the microbiome has on microglial cells, as introducing microbiota into GF mice resulted in restored microglial functions. Reversely, eradicating various bacteria in specific pathogen-free (SPF) mice resulted in microglial cells maturing less rapidly [50]. As neuroinflammation plays an important part in the pathophysiology of ADHD, the proper activation and maturation of microglia in ADHD patients have to be thoroughly investigated in order to determine if it has a pathogenic influence.

The enteric nervous system communicates with the brain mainly through the parasympathetic vagus nerve [51], and partially though the sympathetic spinal cord pathway [52]. Furthermore, the vagus nerve predominantly consists of afferent nerve fibers with a ratio of 9:1 to efferent fibers [53]. Even though a definite conclusion cannot be made, various studies have demonstrated that the autonomic nervous system of ADHD patients shows alterations. A study testing 19 children with ADHD showed that the patients had an underactive parasympathetic and an overactive sympathetic nervous system [54]. Another study comparing 32 ADHD patients to 34 healthy controls registered under-aroused parasympathetic nervous systems, while the sympathetic part did not show any difference between the groups [55].

It has become clear that all three ways of communication between the microbiome, gut, and CNS could play an important role in the pathophysiology of ADHD. The neural communication over the HPA axis shows abnormalities in ADHD patients. Additionally, studies detected that microbes influence the function of pro-inflammatory microglia, a key finding, as neuroinflammation in ADHD patients is commonly found. Finally, the autonomic nervous system shows aberrations as the main research results show an under-arousal of the parasympathetic nervous system.

3.3. *Etiology of ADHD and the Genetic and Environmental Influences*

As the exact pathophysiology of ADHD is still unclear, its causes are still being researched. Nevertheless, it has been established that there is an interplay between genes and the environment resulting in a complex etiology. Genetic predisposition plays an important part in the pathophysiology of ADHD as children from parents that have been diagnosed with ADHD have a 50% higher chance to be diagnosed with the same disorder [56]. Similarly, twin studies have shown a high heritability, as especially for inattentive and combined types an inheritance of 71–90% could be discovered [56,57]. On the other hand, one study showed, that 20–30% of the risk of developing ADHD is due to environmental factors [58]. These include perinatal maternal smoking, stress, mineral and micronutrient deficiencies and premature birth [59]. Additionally, research showed that 10–40% of the variance inheritance of ADHD could be caused due to the environment highlighting the interplay of genetic and environmental risk factors [60]. Due to these complex interactions, it is believed that ADHD can be manifested with highly heterogenous symptoms depending on the exact pathway and etiology involved [61].

Research shows that the dysfunction of monoaminergic neurotransmitters, including noradrenaline (NE), serotonin (5-HT) and dopamine (DA), plays an important role in the pathophysiology of ADHD [62].

3.3.1. Dopamine

DA is a catecholamine that acts both as a hormone and neurotransmitter (NT). It is a product of the essential amino acid L-phenylalanine, which must be provided in our diet. As seen in Figure 2, this is then turned into L-tyrosine, and finally into DA and NE [63].

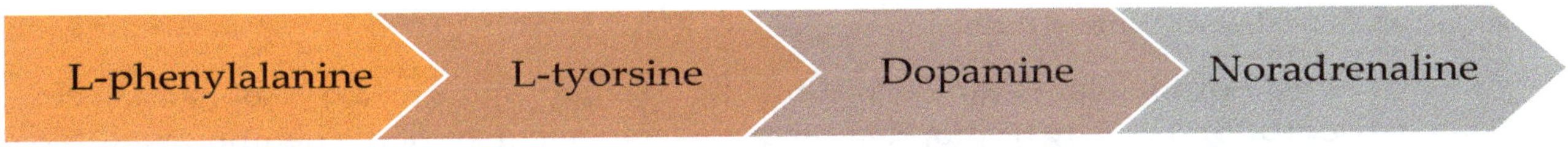

Figure 2. The synthesis pathway from L-phenylalanine to noradrenaline including all its intermediary products. Dopamine acts as an important metabolite for the emotional response and reward system [64].

The dopamine hypothesis links ADHD to alterations in dopamine metabolism. The hypothesis describes the increased expression of presynaptic dopamine transports (DAT) in ADHD patients leading to an increased dopamine transporter density (DTD), and finally results in a decreased level of the bioavailable NT [65]. The dopamine hypothesis gained attention due to the way methylphenidate (MPH) and amphetamines (AMP), the most commonly used pharmacotherapies to treat ADHD, interact with the DA and NE metabolism. MPH and AMP exert a stimulatory effect in ADHD as they inhibit the reuptake of NE and DA by blocking the metabolizing enzyme, monoamine oxidase (MAO), thereby increasing the concentration of the two monoamines in the synaptic cleft. One differentiates between MAO-A and MAO-B as the former is mostly expressed in the liver and GI-tract and the latter in blood platelets [66]. Nevertheless, both are manifested in the CNS and are able to break down DA [66]. Furthermore, amphetamines have the ability to release NTs from the presynaptic neuron, which additionally increases the monoaminergic concentration in the synapse [67].

Moreover, recent research shows that not only the metabolization, but also the production of DA plays an important role in the pathophysiology of ADHD. One of the influencers on the production of NTs seems to be the microbiome in the GI-tract [68]. Bacteria, such as the genus Bifidobacterium belonging to the phylum Actinobacteria potentially influence the levels of available DA in the body by encoding cyclohexadienyl dehydratase (CDT) [69]. This enzyme is important for the synthesis of the essential amino acid phenylalanine [69], which acts as a precursor of the amino acid tyrosine, which in turn is metabolized into DA and lastly to NE [70]. Aarts et al. found an increase in Bifidobacterium in ADHD patients, and thus, higher levels of CDT. By analyzing BOLD responses of the ventral striatal using fMRI measurements they deduced a negative correlation between the abundance of CDT and reward anticipation [69], a key symptom in ADHD [71], and target of DA [72]. Finally, this study concluded that high levels of phenylalanine might be a risk factor for abnormal dopamine signaling and could lead to a reduced reward response [69]. Although another study supports the findings by Aarts et al. [73], the correlation still appears to be inconsistent as two older studies found a decreased level of phenylalanine in ADHD patients [74,75], even if data of source [74] are not statistically significant. Finally, a more recent study found no correlation between phenylalanine levels and ADHD [76]. A summary of these finfings is given in Table 1.

Table 1. Various studies that tested phenylalanine levels in ADHD patients. ↑ represent the increase of phenylalanine found in ADHD patients and ↓ the decrease of the amino acid in comparison to healthy controls (HC). The symbol — describes that the study found no correlation between ADHD and phenylalanine levels. The accumulative data to date do not allow a definite correlation between a change in phenylalanine levels and ADHD. p levels less than 0.05 were considered statistically different.

Source	Levels of Phenylalanine in ADHD Patients	Sample Size (n)	Statistical Significance (p)
[69]	↑	96	$p < 0.001$
[73]	↑	79	$p < 0.001$
[74]	↓	44	$p < 0.1$
[75]	↓	48	$p < 0.05$
[76]	—	155	$p < 0.01$

3.3.2. Tryptophan and Serotonin

Upon intestinal absorption into the bloodstream, the essential amino acid tryptophan can cross the blood-brain barrier (BBB). Thereby tryptophan can act as the precursor of the neurotransmitter 5-HT, which plays an important part in the microbiome-gut-brain axis [77]. Although it is still unclear to what extent the microbiome influences the synthesis of 5-HT, it has been established that certain strains of bacteria, such as *Streptococcus* spp., *Enterococcus* spp., and *Escheria* spp. are capable of producing this NT [78]. Most of the 5-HT is produced and stored in gastrointestinal cells and affects peristalsis, nausea, satiety and abdominal pain [79]. Meanwhile, in the brain, it influences other NTs, such as DA, Cholin (CH) and GABA, which influence memory and mood [80].

Banerjee et al. showed that 5-HT may have an influence on hyperactive and impulsive symptoms in ADHD [81]. Another study implied lower levels of 5-HT in the CNS of ADHD patients due to a decreased transport capacity of its precursor, tryptophan, into the brain [82]. Finally, one study showed that inflammation in the intestine affects 5-HT signaling pathways due to a decreased function and expression of the serotonin selective reuptake transporter (SERT) resulting in an increased level of 5-HT in the body [79]. However, it is important to remember that serotonin is not able to cross the BBB, and thus, the 5-HT pools in the CNS and the periphery do not directly interact with each other.

To demonstrate the importance of microbes on the 5-HT system, one study concluded that GF male mice have a 1.3 fold increased level of 5-HT in their hippocampus. This is an important finding as certain therapeutic medications of ADHD, such as escitalopram and lithium increase serotonin levels in a similar amount [83]. Thus, the composition and the modulation of the gut microbiota might become an interesting, future therapeutic intervention strategy.

Although the studies do not allow us to make a precise conclusion in what way bacterial-produced 5-HT influences ADHD, they do make it clear that it is one of the several catecholamines that play an important role in the pathophysiology of ADHD.

3.3.3. Kynurenine Pathway

Although tryptophan is the key amino acid for the production of 5-HT, 90% of tryptophan is catabolized by the kynurenine pathway [84]. This process produces nicotinamide adenine dinucleotide (NAD) through the stimulation of inflammatory and glucocorticoid metabolites. The kynurenine pathway has received attention in regards to psychiatric diseases, such as depression and schizophrenia [80,85,86] as it uses most of the tryptophan, and thus, leaves a limiting amount of substrate for the synthesis of serotonin.

Intermediate products, such as kynurenine, kynurenic acid (KA), xanthurenic acid (XA) and quilonoic acid (QA) can influence the immune system and neurotransmission [87]. The three former metabolites have anti-inflammatory properties as KA inhibits the NMDA-gated ion channels [88], and XA interferes with the glutamatergic neurotransmission [89]. Also, these products decrease the amount of pro-inflammatory IFN gamma in comparison to the anti-inflammatory IL-10 [87]. In contrast, QA stimulates microglial cells and increases the ratio of IFN gamma/IL-10 [87], resulting in pro-inflammatory effects [90]. Although KA shows neuroprotective properties, human and animal studies show that high levels of KA are associated with cognitive abnormalities, such as attention and memory issues typically associated with psychiatric disease [91,92].

Studies regarding levels of tryptophan and metabolites of the kynurenine pathway show inconclusive results. A Norwegian study, using 133 adult ADHD patients and 133, did not find that the ADHD group had lower levels of tryptophan and neuroprotective KA and XA [86]. These data were confirmed by another study testing ADHD children, which exhibited lower KA and XA levels [93]. These researchers, however, recorded higher levels of tryptophan in ADHD subjects [93]. These data do suggest an association between low levels of KA and XA in ADHD, but as there are still too few studies on this topic, it is difficult to deduce a definitive connection between tryptophan, its metabolites, and ADHD.

The various steps of the kynurenine pathway are dependent on coenzymes, such as the activated form of vitamin B6, pyridoxal 5′-phosphate (PLP). One study found an inverse correlation between serum levels of vitamin B6 and ADHD including its symptom severity [94]. Similarly, Aarsland et al. also observed a decrease in vitamin B6 in their patient group. Other data suggested that vitamin B6 metabolism plays a key part in the pathophysiology of ADHD, as vitamin B6 dependent enzymes show severe abnormalities in the ADHD test group [95]. Thus, lower levels of intermediate metabolites could be related to a deficiency of enzyme substrate. This data supports the importance of optimal coverage of ADHD patients with vitamin B6. The microbiome could play a potentially important role, as bacteria in the large intestine produce this vitamin [96]. As the correlation between levels of vitamin B6 and ADHD are relatively new, future studies are warranted to asses to what extent the microbiome can influence vitamin B6 levels on a therapeutic level.

3.3.4. Gut Dysbiosis and Immunology

High variability in gut flora prevents the growth of pathogenic bacteria, and thus, stops gut dysbiosis [97]. The term dysbiosis describes a microbial imbalance in which there is a shift from protective to pathogenic microbes in the GI-tract [98]. This can lead to a growing GI-permeability which leads to an increase in migration of pathogenic microbes and translocation of their metabolites into the systemic circulation potentially resulting in systemic inflammation [99]. This can, in turn, decrease the permeability of the BBB, which can lead to inflammation of brain parenchyma [100]. Severe dysbiosis has been associated with chronic inflammatory intestinal disorders and psychiatric illnesses, such as schizophrenia, anxiety, depression [98], and ADHD [90,101]. A systematic review supports the latter findings concluding that patients with ADHD have increased levels of inflammatory cytokines [102]. Similarly, Verlaet et al. also detected increased levels of pro-inflammatory cytokines (IFN gamma and IL-6) in the serum of ADHD patients [101].

An imbalance of pro-inflammatory cytokines can also lead to allergic disease [103], and a positive correlation between ADHD and allergies has been shown in different cohorts [104–106]. Additionally, research has shown an association between an altered gut microbial composition and the tendency to suffer from the allergic disease [107].

An important pro-inflammatory cytokine is interleukin (IL-6). This has been inversely associated with the bacterium *Dialister* spp. [108]. *Dialister* spp. is shown to correlate with an altered temperament and impulsiveness in toddlers positively. These commonly found ADHD symptoms were measured using the Early Childhood Behavior Questionnaire (ECBQ), which measures extroversion, activity levels and feelings of high-intensity pleasure [109]. Furthermore, a review evaluating multiple studies concluded an increase in pro-inflammatory metabolites, such as IL-6 and IL-1 in patients with ADHD [110]. Nonetheless, one study showed that ADHD patients had significantly lower levels of *Dialister* spp. in comparison to healthy controls (HC), hinting towards decreased feelings of activity and lower levels of intense pleasure, and finally higher levels of IL-6 [111].

Although the association between *Dialister* spp. and feelings of pleasure are new findings; and it is important to note that pro-inflammatory interleukin levels are increased in ADHD patients. As high levels of pro-inflammatory interleukins can be linked to neurological inflammation that can lead to a decrease of cortical volume and altered behavior [110,112], reducing the activity of these pro-inflammatory cytokines could represent a vital prophylaxis strategy in ADHD management.

Patients with th2-mediated atopic disorders, such as eczema, asthma and allergic rhinitis have a 30–50% higher chance of developing ADHD [113]. Eczema is an inflammatory skin disease and is the most prevalent chronic condition in early childhood [114]. Children suffering from atopic dermatitis (eczema) have a 50% likelihood of developing asthma and allergic rhinitis, exhibiting airway inflammation and clear nasal discharge, respectively [115]. Th2-cytokines are important for eosinophilic recruitment and the production of IgE by B-lymphocytes. All of these processes are associated with allergies and inflammation of the skin (e.g., eczema) [116,117] as they activate the production of pro-inflammatory cytokines, such as IL-6, IL-1beta, TNF-alpha and IL-8 [103]. Studies have shown that these atopic diseases are associated with a low level of *Faecalbacteria* spp. In the gut [118]. This species is known to have anti-inflammatory effects on the organisms [119,120]. As explained above, patients with ADHD seem to exhibit higher levels of inflammatory markers which could potentially support the hypothesis that low levels of *Feacalbacteria* spp. Cause an increase of inflammation which affects the development of the brain, and finally the pathogenesis of ADHD.

4. Results

4.1. Obstetric Mode of Delivery: Vaginal Birth vs. Caesarean Section (C-Section)

As infants delivered by vaginal birth move through the birth canal, they get colonized by their mother's vaginal microbiota, and thus, adopted a resembling gut microbiome. In contrast, infants born via c-section are colonized by the microbiota of their mother's skin. Therefore, the delivery mode affects the composition of the gut microbiota in infants [121].

Results of various studies showed that in comparison to vaginally born infants, babies delivered by c-section had a decreased gut microbiota diversity including lower levels of *Bifidobacterium* spp. and Bacteroidetes, but increased levels *Clostridium difficile* [122] up until the age of two years [123].

Several research groups studied the correlation between c-section delivery and ADHD (see Table 2). An animal study showed a correlation between offspring born via c-section and altered dopamine metabolism throughout development [124]. It is important to note that these results might have been confounded by indication, which means that the altered dopamine response might be due to triggers that lead to a c-section [125]. In contrast to the above findings, two previous case-control studies found no significant correlation between c-sections and ADHD [126,127] in humans. A systematic review by Curran et al. initially showed a slight increase in the prevalence of ADHD in children born via c-section [128]. This correlation was challenged in their later study due to confounders, such as not differentiating between elective and emergency c-sections [129]. The only correlation that still seemed to be consistent was an increased prevalence of ADHD in children born via emergency c-sections. Confirmative data were obtained in a prospective cohort study using 671,592 Danish children. They found a significantly increased chance of children developing ADHD (Hazard Ratio 1.21) for intrapartum c-sections, but no effect when born by an elective c-section [130]. In contrast, the Millenium UK cohort study testing 13,141 children found no correlation between ADHD and mode of delivery despite differentiating between emergency, planned and induced c-sections [131].

Table 2. List of seven studies that tested the effects of c-section delivery on the development of ADHD. The table describes if the studies differentiated between the types of c-sections and their effects, and finally shows the sample size and statistical significance level of the individual studies. The symbol - represents that for these studies, this information could not be found as the studies were systematic reviews. The data shows that elective vs. emergency c-sections seem to have different effects on ADHD. *p* levels less than 0.05 were considered statistically different.

Source	Type of C-Section	Effect	Sample Size (n)	Statistical Significance (p)
[124]	No differentiation	Altered dopamine response	-	-
[126]	No differentiation	No effect	248	$p = 0.005$
[127]	No differentiation	No effect	12,991	$p < 0.05$
[128]	No differentiation	Positive correlation to ADHD	-	-
[129]	Elective vs. intrapartum	Only intrapartum c-sections showed a positive correlation to ADHD	1,722,548	$p < 0.05$
[130]	Elective vs. intrapartum	Only intrapartum c-sections showed a positive correlation to ADHD	671,592	$p < 0.05$
[131]	Elective vs. intrapartum	No effect	13,141	$p < 0.05$

The reasons for finding a positive correlation between intrapartum c-sections and ADHD development cannot unequivocally be explained as multiple confounders, such as unobserved familial factors, birth weight or gestational age also directly influence the mode of delivery and ADHD. However, there is a strong indication that the microbiota plays a subordinate role in this correlation as Axelsson et al. discovered that exposure of the newborn to ruptured vs. non-ruptured membranes prior to c-section did not influence the correlation between c-section and ADHD development [130].

To conclude, the accumulative data show that the mode of delivery affects the composition of the gut microbiota. However, a clear correlation between c-section delivery and a higher chance of developing ADHD cannot be found as results depend on various confounders and the type of c-section, whereby intrapartum c-sections show a positive correlation with the development of ADHD in comparison to elective c-sections.

4.2. Stress of the Mother

A prospective follow up study, and a Dutch population-based cohort study concluded a correlation between prenatal maternal stress exposure and an increase in ADHD in their offspring [132,133]. This data was confirmed by a Canadian study enrolling 203 pregnant women exposed to stress. Sixty-two of them were exposed to severe prenatal stress (experienced physical or sexual abuse, or death of a close relative) and delivered children with more severe ADHD symptoms in comparison to the 48 mothers who experienced moderate stress (financial or marital troubles) [134].

An animal study using quantitative PCR determined that maternal stress significantly decreased one of the most abundant taxa in the maternal vaginal flora, *Lactobacillus* spp. [135]. Consequently, *Lactobacillus* spp. was also significantly decreased in the distal colon of the offspring of stress exposed mothers. Additionally, a review focusing on the immunomodulatory effects of *Lactobacillus* spp. shows that stress reduces the abundance of this species independent of the host being pregnant or not [136]. *Lactobacillus* spp. is important for the synthesis of acetylcholine, while together with *Bifidobacteria* spp. it is contributing to the production of the main inhibitory neurotransmitter GABA [137]. Alterations in the GABAergic system have been associated with neurodevelopmental diseases, such as autism spectrum disorder and ADHD. This system is especially susceptible to alterations during development as GABAergic neurons originate from a different part of the neural tube than GABA's most important counterpart, the glutamatergic system. ADHD symptoms may be explained by the hypothesis that inhibitory functions of the cerebral cortex are reduced, leading to a reduction of filtering sensory influences, and finally having difficulties choosing the right behavioral reaction [138].

As described above, several studies have associated low levels of cerebral GABA concentrations with symptoms of ADHD [139–141]. Furthermore, a randomized controlled study showed that *Lactobacillus rhamnosus* also has a preventive effect as the administration of this bacterium in the first six months of life reduced the risk of ADHD and Asperger Syndrome (AS) [142]. The positive effects of this species may be due to the fact that *Lactobacillus rhamnosus* is, on the one hand, implicated in the development of tight junctions responsible for a strong gut barrier, and on the other hand, important for the immunoglobulin A and mucin production [143].

Various factors influence the development of ADHD, among which the neuroinhibitory neurotransmitter GABA seems to play a crucial role. However, to what extent low levels of *Lactobacillus* spp. and decreased concentrations of GABA are associated and how they precisely affect the development of ADHD remains unclear and has to be thoroughly investigated.

4.3. Preterm

Preterm babies that, thus, have gone through stressful situations similarly show lower levels of *Lactobacillus* spp. [144], and simultaneously have a significant increase in the prevalence of ADHD [58,145,146]. More specifically, Barrett et al. showed an increased abundance of *Proteobacteria* spp., while discovering undetectable levels of *Lactobacillus* spp. and *Bifidobacteria* spp. [144,147]. Chou et al. discovered that certain strains of *Lactobacillus* spp. show a protective trait towards the CNS. Preterm babies received strains of *Lactobacillus reuteri* and *Lactobacillus rhamnous* as probiotics for six weeks. This treatment resulted in a significantly reduced number of babies with neurological aberrations at one year of age in comparison to the group fed with *Lactobacillus acidophilus* and *Bifidobacterium infantis* [148].

It is widely known that preterm infants own an immature immune system as the innate and adaptive immune system has not developed fully. Due to their immature immune response and their usual extended hospital stay, infants are highly susceptible to nosocomial spread infections [149]. The increased number of infections may impair the neurodevelopment, and thus, might influence the development of the most common neurodevelopmental disorder ADHD. In addition to this, the weeks before term delivery (between 37 0/7 and 41 6/7) [150] represent an important stage in the neurodevelopment of the brain usually occurring in the protective womb of the mother [151,152]. Thus, preterm babies suffer from underdeveloped brain structures that in combination with postnatal complications, such as infections can lead to cell death of neurons, and finally lead to a decrease in the volume of specific areas of the brain [153].

As the prevalence of infection in premature newborns is high, the use of therapeutic antibiotics is similarly increased. Antibiotics have been associated with altering functions in the host's brain [154], while simultaneously, they are notoriously known for reducing the diversity of the microbiota [155]. Nevertheless, the direct effects of a lower microbiota diversity on the neurodevelopment have still not been thoroughly researched on, and thus, a concrete correlation cannot be made.

To summarize, a preterm baby is exposed to increased levels of stress, may have underdeveloped brain structures and owns an immature immune system. All of these result in a higher susceptibility to infections, and finally may lead to increased exposure to therapeutic antibiotics. These factors influence the neurodevelopment either directly through inflammatory processes during infections or indirectly by changing the composition of the gut microbiome.

4.4. Breastfeeding vs. Formula Feeding

Studies have associated breastfeeding with a lower prevalence of ADHD [156]. In contrast, formula-fed newborns showed a strong correlation with ADHD diagnosis [157–159]. The nutritious breast milk not only contains human milk oligosaccharides acting as prebiotics important for establishing a healthy gut microbiome, but also consists of vitamins and antibodies [160]. The latter being important in the first couple of months for the maturation of the innate immune system of the newborn [161]. Additionally, breast milk is marked to have a rich fat content due to its high levels of long-chain fatty acids, which are said to have protective effects on the CNS and the development of ADHD [162,163]. The gut microbiota of breastfed infants is less diverse in comparison to formula-fed infants [164]. Importantly, various groups utilizing differing methods for microbiome analysis, such as 16S sequencing or cytogenic FISH technique discovered that in both groups, the most prevalent genus is *Bifidobacterium* [122,164,165].

A systematic review by Guaraldi et al. showed that bottle-fed infants have a higher number of *Escherichia coli, Clostridium difficile, Bacteroides* spp. and *Lactobacilli* [166]. As seen in Table 3, research papers demonstrated that increased levels of *Lactobacillus acidophilus* [122], *Streptococcus, Veillonella parvula* [164], and *Clostridium coccoides* [165], were found in formula-fed infants. Although *Bifidobacterium* is the most prevalent genus found in both groups, breastfed infants show more than double of *Bifidobacteria* cells in comparison to formula-fed infants [164]. *Bifidobacterium infantis* has protective properties against pathogens as it supports the barrier function of the mucosa and concurrently has anti-inflammatory properties, thus, promotes a healthy immunological response [167,168].

Although the effect on the microbial composition could be the main cause of developing ADHD when being formula-fed, one has to consider the fact that other ingredients in the formula may also act as important influences. One study found that there were more cases of ADHD in formula-fed infants in 2007, than in December 2011. During the latter, the neurotoxic chemical Bisphenol A (BPA) was significantly reduced in formula cans and baby bottles in comparison to the former, suggesting that BPA might be the actual trigger of the correlation [169].

Table 3. Listing the different genera, predominantly found in formula-fed vs. breastfed infants. The arrow ↑ describes that this genus is increased in variously fed infants, while '-' represents that there is no significant change in this genus. One can clearly see that microbial diversity is increased in formula-fed in comparison to breastfed infants. p levels less than 0.05 were considered statistically different.

Genus	Formula-Fed	Sample Size (n)	Statistical Significance (p)	Breastfed	Sample Size (n)	Statistical Significance (p)
Bifidobacterium	↑ [122]	232	$p < 0.01$	↑ [122]	700	$p < 0.01$
	↑ [164]	6	$p < 0.05$	↑ [164]	6	$p < 0.05$
	↑ [165]	182	$p < 0.001$	↑ [165]	312	$p < 0.001$
Escherichia coli	↑ [122]	232	$p < 0.01$	-	700	$p < 0.01$
Bacteroides	↑ [122]	232	$p < 0.01$	-	700	$p < 0.01$
Lactobacillus	↑ [122]	232	$p < 0.01$	-	700	$p < 0.01$
Veillonella parvula	↑ [164]	6	$p < 0.05$	-	6	$p < 0.05$
Streptococcus	↑ [164]	6	$p < 0.05$	-	6	$p < 0.05$
Clostridium coccoides	↑ [165]	182	$p < 0.014$	-	312	$p < 0.014$

In summary, studies show that breastfeeding correlates negatively with the risk of developing ADHD, whereas formula-feeding increases this risk. Nevertheless, despite the highly nutritious content of breast milk, the gut microbiota of breastfed infants seems less diverse, but still contains the same or higher amount of protective components than formula-fed infants. Thus, alteration of the microbiome composition could potentially be a reason for the positive correlation between formula-feeding and the risk of developing ADHD.

4.5. Short Chain Fatty Acids

SCFAs are products of polysaccharides which could not be properly digested by the human digestive system, and thus, are broken down by microbial fermentation. Bacteria, such as *Bacteroides* spp. and *Clostridiae* spp., are two of the most important microbes for the production of SCFAs [21]. SCFAs represent not only a major energy source for microorganisms, but also show neuroactive and anti-inflammatory effects on the host [170,171]. A study by MacFabe et al. demonstrated that when SCFAs, such as propionic acid are intracebreoventriculary (ICV), administered to rodents, they show biochemical alterations similar to individuals who from autism [172]. Besides, the same authors found that high levels of the SCFA worsened symptoms of autistic individuals [172].

As ADHD, similar to autism, is a neurodevelopmental disease, it seems likely that SCFAs may affect the development of ADHD. Research shows that SCFAs influence the immune system, and as discussed earlier, this can influence the CNS [50]. An animal study using mice showed that the microbiome could influence the levels of the brain-derived neurotrophic factor (BDNF) via SCFA production [173]. The neurotrophin BDNF is important for neurogenesis and has a positive effect on the survival of neurons meaning that the microbiome can indirectly influence neural functions via SCFA's modulating effect on the BDNF production. The same study showed that GF mice whose BDNF levels had been decreased displayed problems with their working memory [173]. Confirmatory data were generated by Corominas-Roso et al. who showed in a human study that adults with ADHD have lower levels of BDNF compared to healthy controls [174]. Similarly, Akay et al. tested the effects of methylphenidate on BDNF levels on 50 drug-naïve ADHD boys and detected significantly increased BDNF levels in the serum and improved ADHD symptoms after eight weeks of methylphenidate treatment [175]. The same findings were found by an older study by Amiri et al. [176]. This is a direct confirmation of a potential link between the dopaminergic system, BDNF function, and ADHD. In contrast, another study enrolling 41 untreated ADHD and 107 control patients concluded that drug-naïve ADHD children had higher levels of BDNF in their plasma and that these levels are positively associated with the severity of inattentiveness [177].

Besides hypothesizing a compensatory mechanism in ADHD children, a potential reason for these differing results could be varying methodology as Akay et al. measured BDNF levels in the serum, known to have a higher BDNF concertation in comparison to the plasma [178].

In conclusion, SCFAs most probably affect the development of ADHD indirectly by influencing the production of BDNF.

4.6. Polyunsaturated Fatty Acids

Another regulator of BDNF seems to be omega-3 polyunsaturated fatty acids (PUFAs). PUFAs are long chains of carbon atoms characterized by a carboxyl group at one end and a methyl group at the other end. As they are unsaturated, they own one or more double bonds between the carbon atoms. Naturally, plant and fish oils, such as flaxseed or salmon have a high content of omega-3 PUFAs [179]. PUFAs play an important role in membrane fluidity, neuronal membranes, neurotransmission, and receptor function [180]. Furthermore, the omega-3 fatty acid, docosahexaenoic acid (DHA), is indispensable for cognition function throughout the lifespan [181]. Indeed, already intrauterine PUFA deficiencies lead to altered cognitive and attentive skills [182].

An animal study showed that omega-3 PUFAs did not only affect the levels of BDNF, but also of glial cell-derived neurotrophic factor (GDNF). The latter is especially important for the recovery of dopaminergic neurons in Parkinson's disease (PD) as it promotes the survival of the dopamine system in the nigrostriatum. Hence, GDNF is shown to be neuroprotective and supporting dopaminergic neurons in PD models, and thus, could potentially be utilized as a therapy against neurodegenerative diseases, especially PD [183,184]. Furthermore, another study found that lower levels of omega-3 fatty acids were associated with lower levels of BDNF in the frontal cortex of rats [185], a part of the brain where various psychiatric illnesses, such as bipolar disease can be manifested [186]. Additionally, omega-3 PUFAs show antimicrobial effects as they increase levels of *Enterobacteria* and *Bifidobacteria*, which both strengthen intestinal permeability, reducing the risk of inflammation [187]. Finally, omega-3 PUFAs have the ability to stimulate macrophages that inhibit the activation of the NLRP3 inflammasome, and thus, decrease levels of the previously mentioned pro-inflammatory IL-1beta [188]. Nevertheless, it is important to note that an excess of omega-6 PUFAs benefits the development of endotoxemia leading to low-grade systematic inflammation, explaining why a low ratio of omega-6/omega-3 PUFAs should be targeted [189,190].

Human studies have discovered a negative correlation between patients with ADHD and levels of PUFAs. An Italian study examined the levels of PUFAs in the blood of 51 ADHD and 22 non-ADHD patients. PUFA levels in the blood of ADHD patients were significantly lower and correlated with behavioral symptoms, but were not associated with cognitive skills [191]. Similarly, a systematic review concluded that in all randomized control trials (RCT) analyzed (7 RCTs, n = 534), omega-3 PUFA supplementation led to an improvement in clinical ADHD symptoms. Furthermore, in three out of the seven RCT's (n = 396), the omega-3 PUFA supplementation was associated with improvements in cognitive skills [192]. Due to these findings, questions of PUFAs being a potential therapeutic medication for ADHD patients seem to be warranted.

Moreover, a double-blind trial [193] assessed the effects of inducing the noradrenaline reuptake inhibitor (Atomoxetine) conventionally used to treat ADHD, to the patient and control group and PUFAs, such as eicosapentanoic acid (EPA) and DHA solely to the ADHD patients. The medication was given on a daily basis for four months to a total of 50 children. Although PUFAs improved ADHD symptoms, this experiment showed no clinically significant difference in the ADHD Conners Parent rating scale, questioning the overall therapeutic effect of PUFAs against ADHD, even if some beneficial effects are evident [193]. Supporting these results, a systematic review discussing results of 14 meta-analyses inducing PUFAs to ADHD children showed a very small effect size when parents and teachers rated children's behavior using the Conners scale [194].

Lastly, on a microbial level, an RCT showed that the intake of PUFAs does not seem to affect the alpha or beta diversity of the microbiota of the participants. Nevertheless, it did show a reversible increase in genera, such as *Bifidobacterium roseburia* and *Lactobaccilus* spp., all of which are important for the production of SCFAs and maintain an anti-inflammatory environment [195]. Similarly, a commentary discussing the importance of long-chain PUFAs as a mean to restore a healthy gut microbiome, deduced that PUFA ingestion may act as a protector from developing systemic inflammation and in the long term, chronic disease. It is, therefore, hypothesized that PUFA supplementation would not only be of therapeutic importance for ADHD, but also a prophylactic measurement against cancer as inflammation leads to immunosuppression and activates immune checkpoints resulting in an optimal tumor microenvironment [196].

Although the collected data show inconclusive results concerning the effect of PUFA supplementation as a therapeutic measurement for ADHD, the indirect effects of ingesting PUFAs and its impact on the microbiome may as well be crucial determinants that could modify the metabolism and consequently the behavioral and cognitive symptoms of ADHD.

4.7. Antibiotics

Although the development of antibiotics has made it possible to treat life-threatening infections, the use of antibiotics reduces the microbiota diversity in the GI-tract [197]. Consequently, the use of antibiotics may elevate the number of pathogenic bacteria, such as *Enterobacter, Klebsiella, Citrobacter, and Pseudomonas* and decrease anaerobic bacteria [197]. For example, a human study analyzing the short term parenteral-neonatal antibiotic usage showed that it reduced the number of protective *Bifidobacteria* in the first couple of months of life [198]. Supporting these results, Penders et al. not only found a decrease of *Bifidobacteria*, but also of *Bacteroides* when infants administered antibiotics [122].

Results concerning the correlation of early antibiotic use and later risk of developing ADHD seem to be incoherent. A Danish population-based cohort study did not find an association in sibling-stratified Cox model between antibiotic use in the first two years of life and the risk of developing ADHD [130]. Another study, however, using 871 European newborns examined the effects of early antibiotic treatment on cognitive functions with the help of IQ and reading tests, and on symptoms of ADHD using the mentioned Conners Rating Scale-Revised (CRS-R). Thereby they discovered that children who consumed antibiotics in the first year of life showed a reduced reading ability score, higher scores on the CRS-R, rated by parents, and increased symptoms of ADHD at the ages of 7–11 years. Nonetheless, this association was not made for babies and children that used antibiotics between the ages of 12 months and 3.5 years. This indicates that one of the vital factors for developing ADHD is the age in which the newborn consumes the antibiotics. It seems that during the first 12 months of life, important developments of the gut-brain axis take place, which when disrupted influence the neurodevelopment, and thus, the CNS in the long run [12]. These data, however, must be interpreted with caution, as this was not an RCT. Accordingly, direct causation between the antibiotic use and later seen ADHD cannot be correctly made [199].

4.8. Probiotics

By definition of the FAO/WHO probiotics are "live microorganisms which when administered in adequate amounts confer a health benefit on the host" [200]. Benefits of probiotics include reinforcing a more desirable environment in the gut, a healthy digestive system, and finally an adequate immune system [201]. Thereby probiotics help to sustain and produce healthy enzymes while eradicating potentially harmful pathogens [202,203]. Naturally occurring probiotic sources include lactic acid fermented vegetables, such as kimchi or fermented dairy products as, for example, yogurt [204].

The influence of probiotic strains on psychiatric diseases has been examined by multiple studies, concluding a positive effect on such illnesses and are, thus, described as "psychobiotics" [90]. An animal study using mice showed that probiotic ingestion of *Bifidobacterium longum* and *breve* led to a reduction of depression and anxiety symptoms [205].

The seminal study by Pärtty et al. researched the effects of probiotic use on the development of ADHD in children by randomly administering strains of *Lactobacillus rhamnosus* into 75 infants.

The infants were monitored at three weeks, 3, 6, 12, 18 and 24 months, and finally, at 13 years of age. The authors concluded that at the age of 13 years, ADHD was diagnosed in 6/35 (17.1%) children using the placebo, whereas no children had this disorder in the probiotic group. These results, even if encouraging, do not identify any specific composition of the microbiota to the neurodevelopmental disease, and thus, might mean that probiotics decrease ADHD in a different way rather than influencing the composition of the microbiome [142]. However, it is important to conclude that these findings potentially represent a method to reduce the risk of developing ADHD.

5. Discussion

This literature review demonstrates that the ADHD population has a different gut microbial composition in comparison to healthy controls as the phylum Actinobacteria is more and Firmicutes less abundant in ADHD patients. The genus *Bifidobacterium*, belonging to the phylum Actinobacteria, seems to play a significant role in the pathogenesis of ADHD and is recurrently influenced by several factors. *Bifidobacteria* do not only protect the barrier function in the gut and support a healthy immune response [168], but also influence the dopamine system by elevating the production of CDT which increases phenylalanine levels, and finally, results in higher levels of dopamine. This review showed that *Bifidobacterium* was decreased in offspring that were born (i) via c-section delivery ([122,123], (ii) as preterms [144,206], (iii) were breastfed [164] or (iv) were given antibiotics in the first months of life [122,198]. All of these factors are simultaneously associated with an increased risk of developing ADHD. Nevertheless, using *Bifidobacterium* as a potential biomarker for diagnosis of ADHD seems uncertain due to varying results regarding *Bifidobacterium* levels in ADHD patients. Although Pärtty et al. observed decreased levels of *Bifidobacterium* in 3 and 6-month-old ADHD patients [142], Aarts et al. detected slightly increased levels of the genus using a larger sample size and a more sensitive methodology [69]. Thus, for future research, well-designed studies, using a larger sample size, are needed to deduce a definite correlation between levels of *Bifidobacterium* and ADHD and the importance of this genus as a biomarker.

Additionally, this article concludes that the concertation of neuroprotective BDNF, indirectly influenced by the microbiome [173], plays a vital role in the pathogenesis of ADHD. The majority of reports showed a negative correlation between levels of BDNF and ADHD [173,174,207]. As the levels of SCFAs [173], and PUFAs [185] are positively correlated with BDNF, omega-3 fatty acids may prove to be of therapeutic importance. So far, various studies have shown that adding PUFAs to the diet only marginally decreases the symptoms of ADHD [193,194,208]. Future studies could assess the effects of various concentrations of PUFAs and age at which these were ingested on the symptom development of ADHD. BDNF shows properties important for neurogenesis in the critical stages of neurodevelopment. The production of SCFAs by the microbiome has been positively associated with levels of BDNF [173]. Therefore, increasing SCFAs through fiber-rich nutrition in combination with the appropriate gut microbial composition could also be a beneficial means for the treatment of ADHD symptoms.

It is widely known that c-section delivery causes the offspring's microbiome to be more similar to the mother's skin rather than her vaginal flora. However, it is still under debate to what extent this change impacts the development of ADHD. We decided to concentrate on the more recent papers, that used a large sample size and a precise methodology by differentiating between elective and emergency c-sections. These studies show that not every c-section increases the risk of developing ADHD, but only those that were done intrapartum [129,130]. Although this correlation is most probably not due to a differing microbial composition and rather due to various confounders, such as gestational age and birth weight [130], it is still important to note that emergency c-sections bear an intrinsic risk for the offspring developing ADHD.

Additionally, it has become increasingly clear to what extent prematurity plays a role in the development of ADHD. As the GI-tract and its colonization with bacteria are still underdeveloped, the microbiome shows lower levels of neuroprotective *Lactobacillus* [144]. Nonetheless, this decrease of the genus has not yet been directly associated with the development of ADHD. Much more important seems to be the combination of premature infants having underdeveloped brain structures and an immature immune system resulting in being more prone to neuronal cell death and infections that promote neuroinflammation, and finally influence the neurodevelopment. It is difficult to deduce the exact impact of microbial changes in preterms on the development of ADHD, as there are numerous confounders [153]. Thus, future studies should elucidate and concentrate on levels of pro-inflammatory cytokines in neonates and determine the extent to which underdeveloped brain structures influence the development of ADHD. Once these have been thoroughly understood, one can assess in what way the microbiome plays a role in the pathophysiology of prenates having a higher prevalence of ADHD. As the topic of this literature review is relatively new, only a limited number of studies examining the link between ADHD and the microbiota could be found. Hence, it was challenging to draw concrete conclusions from the scarce available data. A solid conclusion will require future investigations enrolling larger populations with defined pathologies to be able to analyze the study outcomes using robust statistical analysis. Finally, it is important that future trials use standardized methodologies for an unambiguous comparison of the outcomes and results. This literature review has made it clear that certain factors are associated with ADHD, while simultaneously changing the guts microbiome. Nevertheless, it remains yet to be determined to what extent the composition of the microbiome in the gut influences the development of ADHD.

6. Conclusions

To determine to what extent the microbiome plays a role in the pathophysiology of ADHD, further studies are needed. We discussed several triggers that have been associated with ADHD, how these correlate with an altered microbial composition, and thus, how various microbes might act as possible biomarkers for ADHD. Further research, on the microbial composition of ADHD patients using large, well-diagnosed cohorts is needed in order to find future conclusive biomarkers and therapeutic methods to treat ADHD.

Author Contributions: Conceptualization, S.B.-L. and M.H.M.; Methodology, S.B.-L. and M.H.M.; Validation, M.H.M.; Formal Analysis, S.B.-L., and M.H.M.; Investigation, S.B.-L., and M.H.M., Resources, S.B.-L. and M.H.M.; Data curation, S.B.-L.; Writing—Original Draft Preparation, S.B.-L.; Writing—Review and Editing, S.B.-L. and M.H.M.; Visualization, S.B.-L.; Supervision, M.H.M.; Project Administration, M.H.M. and S.B.-L.

Acknowledgments: We thank David Wolfer for helpful discussions and for critically reading this manuscript.

References

1. Thursby, E.; Juge, N. Introduction to the human gut microbiota. *Biochem. J.* **2017**, *474*, 1823–1836. [CrossRef] [PubMed]
2. Sender, R.; Fuchs, S.; Milo, R. Revised Estimates for the Number of Human and Bacteria Cells in the Body. *PLoS Biol.* **2016**, *14*, 1002533. [CrossRef] [PubMed]
3. Bäumler, A.J.; Sperandio, V. Interactions between the microbiota and pathogenic bacteria in the gut. *Nature* **2016**, *535*, 85–93. [CrossRef] [PubMed]
4. Mohajeri, M.H.; La Fata, G.; Steinert, R.E.; Weber, P. Relationship between the gut microbiome and brain function. *Nutr. Rev.* **2018**, *76*, 481–496. [CrossRef]
5. Mohajeri, M.H.; Brummer, R.J.M.; Rastall, R.A.; Weersma, R.K.; Harmsen, H.J.M.; Faas, M.; Eggersdorfer, M. The role of the microbiome for human health: From basic science to clinical applications. *Eur. J. Nutr.* **2018**, *57*, 1–14. [CrossRef]
6. Dinan, T.G.; Cryan, J.F. The Microbiome-Gut-Brain Axis in Health and Disease. *Gastroenterol. Clin. N. Am.* **2017**, *46*, 77–89. [CrossRef]
7. Cotillard, A.; ANR MicroObes consortium; Kennedy, S.P.; Kong, L.C.; Prifti, E.; Pons, N.; Le Chatelier, E.;

Almeida, M.; Quinquis, B.; Levenez, F.; et al. Dietary intervention impact on gut microbial gene richness. *Nature* **2013**, *500*, 585–588. [CrossRef]

8. Stower, H. Depression linked to the microbiome. *Nat. Med.* **2019**, *25*, 358. [CrossRef]
9. Gerhardt, S.; Mohajeri, M.H. Changes of Colonic Bacterial Composition in Parkinson's Disease and Other Neurodegenerative Diseases. *Nutrients* **2018**, *10*, 708. [CrossRef]
10. Dickerson, F.; Severance, E.; Yolken, R. The microbiome, immunity, and schizophrenia and bipolar disorder. *Brain Behav. Immun.* **2017**, *62*, 46–52. [CrossRef]
11. Srikantha, P.; Mohajeri, M.H. The Possible Role of the Microbiota-Gut-Brain-Axis in Autism Spectrum Disorder. *Int. J. Mol. Sci.* **2019**, *20*, 2115. [CrossRef] [PubMed]
12. Borre, Y.E.; O'Keeffe, G.W.; Clarke, G.; Stanton, C.; Dinan, T.G.; Cryan, J.F. Microbiota and neurodevelopmental windows: Implications for brain disorders. *Trends Mol. Med.* **2014**, *20*, 509–518. [CrossRef] [PubMed]
13. Association, A.P. *Diagnostic and Statistical Manual of Mental Disorders*; American Psychiatric Pub: Washington, DC, USA, 2013.
14. Polanczyk, G.; De Lima, M.S.; Horta, B.L.; Biederman, J.; Rohde, L.A. The Worldwide Prevalence of ADHD: A Systematic Review and Metaregression Analysis. *Am. J. Psychiatry* **2007**, *164*, 942–948. [CrossRef] [PubMed]
15. Thomas, R.; Sanders, S.; Doust, J.; Beller, E.; Glasziou, P. Prevalence of Attention-Deficit/Hyperactivity Disorder: A Systematic Review and Meta-analysis. *Pediatrics* **2015**, *135*, e994–e1001. [CrossRef]
16. Wender, P.H.; Wolf, L.E.; Wasserstein, J. Adults with ADHD. An overview. *Ann. N. Y. Acad. Sci.* **2001**, *931*, 1–16. [CrossRef]
17. Wilens, T.E.; Biederman, J.; Faraone, S.V.; Martelon, M.; Westerberg, D.; Spencer, T.J. Presenting ADHD symptoms, subtypes, and comorbid disorders in clinically referred adults with ADHD. *J. Clin. Psychiatry* **2009**, *70*, 1557–1562. [CrossRef]
18. Ding, H.T.; Taur, Y.; Walkup, J.T. Gut Microbiota and Autism: Key Concepts and Findings. *J. Autism. Dev. Disord.* **2017**, *47*, 480–489. [CrossRef]
19. Rescigno, M. Intestinal microbiota and its effects on the immune system. *Cell. Microbiol.* **2014**, *16*, 1004–1013. [CrossRef]
20. Bora, S.A.; Kennett, M.J.; Smith, P.B.; Patterson, A.D.; Cantorna, M.T. The Gut Microbiota Regulates Endocrine Vitamin D Metabolism through Fibroblast Growth Factor. *Front. Immunol.* **2018**, *9*, 408. [CrossRef]
21. Macfarlane, S.; Macfarlane, G.T. Regulation of short-chain fatty acid production. *Proc. Nutr. Soc.* **2003**, *62*, 67–72. [CrossRef]
22. Dethlefsen, L.; Eckburg, P.B.; Bik, E.M.; Relman, D.A. Assembly of the human intestinal microbiota. *Trends Ecol. Evol.* **2006**, *21*, 517–523. [CrossRef] [PubMed]
23. Douglas-Escobar, M.; Elliott, E.; Neu, J. Effect of Intestinal Microbial Ecology on the Developing Brain. *JAMA Pediatr.* **2013**, *167*, 374. [CrossRef] [PubMed]
24. Goodrich, J.K.; Davenport, E.R.; Waters, J.L.; Clark, A.G.; Ley, R.E. Cross-species comparisons of host genetic associations with the microbiome. *Science* **2016**, *352*, 532–535. [CrossRef] [PubMed]
25. Carmody, R.N.; Gerber, G.K.; Luevano, J.M.; Gatti, D.M.; Somes, L.; Svenson, K.L.; Turnbaugh, P.J. Diet dominates host genotype in shaping the murine gut microbiota. *Cell Host Microbe* **2015**, *17*, 72–84. [CrossRef]
26. Bik, E.M. The Hoops, Hopes, and Hypes of Human Microbiome Research. *Yale J. Boil. Med.* **2016**, *89*, 363–373.
27. Buie, T. Potential Etiologic Factors of Microbiome Disruption in Autism. *Clin. Ther.* **2015**, *37*, 976–983. [CrossRef]
28. Koenig, J.E.; Spor, A.; Scalfone, N.; Fricker, A.D.; Stombaugh, J.; Knight, R.; Angenent, L.T.; Ley, R.E. Succession of microbial consortia in the developing infant gut microbiome. *Proc. Natl. Acad. Sci. USA* **2011**, *108*, 4578–4585. [CrossRef]
29. Collado, M.C.; Rautava, S.; Aakko, J.; Isolauri, E.; Salminen, S. Human gut colonisation may be initiated in utero by distinct microbial communities in the placenta and amniotic fluid. *Sci. Rep.* **2016**, *6*, 23129. [CrossRef]
30. MacIntyre, D.A.; Chandiramani, M.; Lee, Y.S.; Kindinger, L.; Smith, A.; Angelopoulos, N.; Lehne, B.; Arulkumaran, S.; Brown, R.; Teoh, T.G.; et al. The vaginal microbiome during pregnancy and the postpartum period in a European population. *Sci. Rep.* **2015**, *5*, 8988. [CrossRef]
31. Aagaard, K.; Ma, J.; Antony, K.M.; Ganu, R.; Petrosino, J.; Versalovic, J. The Placenta Harbors a Unique Microbiome. *Sci. Transl. Med.* **2014**, *6*, 237ra65. [CrossRef]

32. Human Microbiome Jumpstart Reference Strains Consortium; Nelson, K.E.; Weinstock, G.M.; Highlander, S.K.; Worley, K.C.; Creasy, H.H.; Wortman, J.R.; Rusch, D.B.; Mitreva, M.; Sodergren, E.; et al. A catalog of reference genomes from the human microbiome. *Science* **2010**, *328*, 994–999. [CrossRef] [PubMed]
33. Brotman, R.M. Vaginal microbiome and sexually transmitted infections: An epidemiologic perspective. *J. Clin. Investig.* **2011**, *121*, 4610–4617. [CrossRef] [PubMed]
34. Dogra, S.; Sakwinska, O.; Soh, S.-E.; Ngom-Bru, C.; Brück, W.M.; Berger, B.; Brüssow, H.; Karnani, N.; Lee, Y.S.; Yap, F.; et al. Rate of establishing the gut microbiota in infancy has consequences for future health. *Gut Microbes* **2015**, *6*, 321–325. [CrossRef] [PubMed]
35. Bäckhed, F.; Roswall, J.; Peng, Y.; Feng, Q.; Jia, H.; Kovatcheva-Datchary, P.; Li, Y.; Xia, Y.; Xie, H.; Zhong, H.; et al. Dynamics and Stabilization of the Human Gut Microbiome during the First Year of Life. *Cell Host Microbe* **2015**, *17*, 852. [CrossRef]
36. Latorre, R.; Sternini, C.; De Giorgio, R.; Greenwood-Van Meerveld, B. Enteroendocrine cells: A review of their role in brain-gut communication. *Neurogastroenterol. Motil.* **2016**, *28*, 620–630. [CrossRef]
37. Mayer, E.A.; Knight, R.; Mazmanian, S.K.; Cryan, J.F.; Tillisch, K. Gut microbes and the brain: Paradigm shift in neuroscience. *J. Neurosci.* **2014**, *34*, 15490–15496. [CrossRef]
38. Cryan, J.F.; Dinan, T.G. Mind-altering microorganisms: The impact of the gut microbiota on brain and behaviour. *Nat. Rev. Neurosci.* **2012**, *13*, 701–712. [CrossRef]
39. Shaw, P.; Stringaris, A.; Nigg, J.; Leibenluft, E. Emotion dysregulation in attention deficit hyperactivity disorder. *Am. J. Psychiatry* **2014**, *171*, 276–293. [CrossRef]
40. Cortese, S.; Brown, T.E.; Corkum, P.; Gruber, R.; O'Brien, L.M.; Stein, M.; Weiss, M.; Owens, J. Assessment and Management of Sleep Problems in Youths With Attention-Deficit/Hyperactivity Disorder. *J. Am. Acad. Child. Adolesc. Psychiatry* **2013**, *52*, 784–796. [CrossRef]
41. Baird, A.L.; Coogan, A.N.; Siddiqui, A.; Donev, R.M.; Thome, J. Adult attention-deficit hyperactivity disorder is associated with alterations in circadian rhythms at the behavioural, endocrine and molecular levels. *Mol. Psychiatry* **2012**, *17*, 988–995. [CrossRef]
42. Van Lenten, S.A.; Doane, L.D. Examining multiple sleep behaviors and diurnal salivary cortisol and alpha-amylase: Within- and between-person associations. *Psychoneuroendocrinology* **2016**, *68*, 100–110. [CrossRef] [PubMed]
43. Tsigos, C.; Chrousos, G.P. Hypothalamic–pituitary–adrenal axis, neuroendocrine factors and stress. *J. Psychosom. Res.* **2002**, *53*, 865–871. [CrossRef]
44. Freitag, C.M.; Hänig, S.; Palmason, H.; Meyer, J.; Wüst, S.; Seitz, C. Cortisol awakening response in healthy children and children with ADHD: Impact of comorbid disorders and psychosocial risk factors. *Psychoneuroendocrinology* **2009**, *34*, 1019–1028. [CrossRef] [PubMed]
45. Blomqvist, M.; Holmberg, K.; Lindblad, F.; Fernell, E.; Ek, U.; Dahllöf, G. Salivary cortisol levels and dental anxiety in children with attention deficit hyperactivity disorder. *Eur. J. Oral Sci.* **2007**, *115*, 1–6. [CrossRef]
46. Corominas-Roso, M.; Palomar, G.; Ferrer, R.; Real, A.; Nogueira, M.; Corrales, M.; Casas, M.; Ramos-Quiroga, J.A. Cortisol Response to Stress in Adults with Attention Deficit Hyperactivity Disorder. *Int. J. Neuropsychopharmacol.* **2015**, *18*, 18. [CrossRef]
47. Lackschewitz, H.; Hüther, G.; Kröner-Herwig, B. Physiological and psychological stress responses in adults with attention-deficit/hyperactivity disorder (ADHD). *Psychoneuroendocrinology* **2008**, *33*, 612–624. [CrossRef]
48. Principi, N.; Esposito, S. Gut microbiota and central nervous system development. *J. Infect.* **2016**, *73*, 536–546. [CrossRef]
49. Sato, K. Effects of Microglia on Neurogenesis. *Glia* **2015**, *63*, 1394–1405. [CrossRef]
50. Erny, D.; De Angelis, A.L.H.; Jaitin, D.; Wieghofer, P.; Staszewski, O.; David, E.; Keren-Shaul, H.; Mahlakoiv, T.; Jakobshagen, K.; Buch, T.; et al. Host microbiota constantly control maturation and function of microglia in the CNS. *Nat. Neurosci.* **2015**, *18*, 965–977. [CrossRef]
51. Critchley, H.D.; Eccles, J.; Garfinkel, S.N. Interaction between cognition, emotion, and the autonomic nervous system. *Stroke* **2013**, *117*, 59–77.
52. Koopman, F.A.; Stoof, S.P.; Straub, R.H.; Van Maanen, M.A.; Vervoordeldonk, M.J.; Tak, P.P. Restoring the Balance of the Autonomic Nervous System as an Innovative Approach to the Treatment of Rheumatoid Arthritis. *Mol. Med.* **2011**, *17*, 937–948. [CrossRef] [PubMed]
53. Lyte, M. Microbial Endocrinology and the Microbiota-Gut-Brain Axis. *Adv. Exp. Med. Biol.* **2014**, *817*, 3–24. [PubMed]

54. Negrao, B.L.; Bipath, P.; Van Der Westhuizen, D.; Viljoen, M. Autonomic Correlates at Rest and during Evoked Attention in Children with Attention-Deficit/Hyperactivity Disorder and Effects of Methylphenidate. *Neuropsychobiology* **2011**, *63*, 82–91. [CrossRef] [PubMed]
55. Musser, E.D.; Backs, R.W.; Schmitt, C.F.; Ablow, J.C.; Measelle, J.R.; Nigg, J.T. Emotion regulation via the autonomic nervous system in children with attention-deficit/hyperactivity disorder (ADHD). *J. Abnorm. Child. Psychol.* **2011**, *39*, 841–852. [CrossRef] [PubMed]
56. Tandon, M.; Pergjika, A. Attention Deficit Hyperactivity Disorder in Preschool-Age Children. *Child Adolesc. Psychiatr Clin. N. Am.* **2017**, *26*, 523–538. [CrossRef] [PubMed]
57. Willcutt, E.G.; Nigg, J.T.; Pennington, B.F.; Solanto, M.V.; Rohde, L.A.; Tannock, R.; Loo, S.K.; Carlson, C.L.; McBurnett, K.; Lahey, B.B. Validity of DSM-IV attention deficit/hyperactivity disorder symptom dimensions and subtypes. *J. Abnorm. Psychol.* **2012**, *121*, 991–1010. [CrossRef]
58. Thapar, A.; Cooper, M.; Eyre, O.; Langley, K. What have we learnt about the causes of ADHD? *J. Child. Psychol. Psychiatry* **2013**, *54*, 3–16. [CrossRef]
59. Starobrat-Hermelin, B. The effect of deficiency of selected bioelements on hyperactivity in children with certain specified mental disorders. *Ann. Acad. Med. Stetin.* **1998**, *44*, 297–314.
60. Sciberras, E.; Mulraney, M.; Silva, D.; Coghill, D. Prenatal Risk Factors and the Etiology of ADHD—Review of Existing Evidence. *Curr. Psychiatry Rep.* **2017**, *19*, 1. [CrossRef]
61. Dias, T.G.C.; Kieling, C.; Graeff-Martins, A.S.; Moriyama, T.S.; Rohde, L.A.; Polanczyk, G.V. Developments and challenges in the diagnosis and treatment of ADHD. *Braz. J. Psychiatry* **2013**, *35*, S40–S50. [CrossRef]
62. Sharma, A.; Couture, J. A review of the pathophysiology, etiology, and treatment of attention-deficit hyperactivity disorder (ADHD). *Ann. Pharmacother.* **2014**, *48*, 209–225. [CrossRef] [PubMed]
63. Daubner, S.C.; Le, T.; Wang, S. Tyrosine hydroxylase and regulation of dopamine synthesis. *Arch. Biochem. Biophys.* **2011**, *508*, 1–12. [CrossRef] [PubMed]
64. Arias-Carrión, O.; Stamelou, M.; Murillo-Rodriguez, E.; Menéndez-González, M.; Pöppel, E. Dopaminergic reward system: A short integrative review. *Int. Arch. Med.* **2010**, *3*, 24. [CrossRef] [PubMed]
65. Dougherty, D.D.; Bonab, A.A.; Spencer, T.J.; Rauch, S.L.; Madras, B.K.; Fischman, A.J. Dopamine transporter density in patients with attention deficit hyperactivity disorder. *Lancet* **1999**, *354*, 2132–2133. [CrossRef]
66. Tong, J.; Meyer, J.H.; Furukawa, Y.; Boileau, I.; Chang, L.-J.; Wilson, A.A.; Houle, S.; Kish, S.J. Distribution of monoamine oxidase proteins in human brain: Implications for brain imaging studies. *Br. J. Pharmacol.* **2013**, *33*, 863–871. [CrossRef]
67. Seiden, L.S.; Sabol, K.E.; Ricaurte, G.A. Amphetamine: Effects on catecholamine systems and behavior. *Annu. Rev. Pharmacol. Toxicol.* **1993**, *33*, 639–677. [CrossRef]
68. Strandwitz, P. Neurotransmitter modulation by the gut microbiota. *Brain Res.* **2018**, *1693*, 128–133. [CrossRef]
69. Aarts, E.; Ederveen, T.H.A.; Naaijen, J.; Zwiers, M.P.; Boekhorst, J.; Timmerman, H.M.; Smeekens, S.P.; Netea, M.G.; Buitelaar, J.K.; Franke, B.; et al. Gut microbiome in ADHD and its relation to neural reward anticipation. *PLoS ONE* **2017**, *12*, e0183509. [CrossRef]
70. Lou, H. Dopamine precursors and brain function in phenylalanine hydroxylase deficiency. *Acta Paediatr.* **1994**, *83*, 86–88. [CrossRef]
71. Scheres, A.; Milham, M.P.; Knutson, B.; Castellanos, F.X. Ventral Striatal Hyporesponsiveness During Reward Anticipation in Attention-Deficit/Hyperactivity Disorder. *Boil. Psychiatry* **2007**, *61*, 720–724. [CrossRef]
72. Ming, X.; Chen, N.; Ray, C.; Brewer, G.; Kornitzer, J.; Steer, R.A. A Gut Feeling: A Hypothesis of the Role of the Microbiome in Attention-Deficit/Hyperactivity Disorders. *Child Neurol. Open* **2018**, *5*, 2329048X18786799. [CrossRef] [PubMed]
73. Antshel, K.M.; Waisbren, S.E. Developmental timing of exposure to elevated levels of phenylalanine is associated with ADHD symptom expression. *J. Abnorm. Child Psychol.* **2003**, *31*, 565–574. [CrossRef] [PubMed]
74. Baker, G.; Bornstein, R.; Rouget, A.; Ashton, S.; Van Muyden, J.; Coutts, R. Phenylethylaminergic mechanisms in attention-deficit disorder. *Boil. Psychiatry* **1991**, *29*, 15–22. [CrossRef]
75. Bornstein, R.; Baker, G.B.; Carroll, A.; King, G.; Wong, J.T.; Douglass, A.B. Plasma amino acids in attention deficit disorder. *Psychiatry Res.* **1990**, *33*, 301–306. [CrossRef]
76. Bergwerff, C.E.; Luman, M.; Blom, H.J.; Oosterlaan, J. No Tryptophan, Tyrosine and Phenylalanine Abnormalities in Children with Attention-Deficit/Hyperactivity Disorder. *PLoS ONE* **2016**, *11*, e0151100. [CrossRef]

77. O'Mahony, S.; Clarke, G.; Borre, Y.; Dinan, T.; Cryan, J.; Dinan, T. Serotonin, tryptophan metabolism and the brain-gut-microbiome axis. *Behav. Brain Res.* **2015**, *277*, 32–48. [CrossRef]
78. Dinan, T.G.; Stanton, C.; Cryan, J.F. Psychobiotics: A Novel Class of Psychotropic. *Boil. Psychiatry* **2013**, *74*, 720–726. [CrossRef]
79. Mawe, G.M.; Hoffman, J.M. Serotonin signalling in the gut—Functions, dysfunctions and therapeutic targets. *Nat. Rev. Gastroenterol. Hepatol.* **2013**, *10*, 473–486. [CrossRef]
80. Mechan, A.O.; Fowler, A.; Seifert, N.; Rieger, H.; Wöhrle, T.; Etheve, S.; Wyss, A.; Schüler, G.; Colletto, B.; Kilpert, C.; et al. Monoamine reuptake inhibition and mood-enhancing potential of a specified oregano extract. *Br. J. Nutr.* **2011**, *105*, 1150–1163. [CrossRef]
81. Banerjee, E.; Nandagopal, K. Does serotonin deficit mediate susceptibility to ADHD? *Neurochem. Int.* **2015**, *82*, 52–68. [CrossRef]
82. Johansson, J.; Landgren, M.; Fernell, E.; Vumma, R.; Åhlin, A.; Bjerkenstedt, L.; Venizelos, N. Altered tryptophan and alanine transport in fibroblasts from boys with attention-deficit/hyperactivity disorder (ADHD): An in vitro study. *Behav. Brain Funct.* **2011**, *7*, 40. [CrossRef] [PubMed]
83. Clarke, G.; Grenham, S.; Scully, P.; Fitzgerald, P.; Moloney, R.D.; Shanahan, F.; Dinan, T.G.; Cryan, J.F. The microbiome-gut-brain axis during early life regulates the hippocampal serotonergic system in a sex-dependent manner. *Mol. Psychiatry* **2013**, *18*, 666–673. [CrossRef] [PubMed]
84. Badawy, A.A. Tryptophan metabolism, disposition and utilization in pregnancy. *Biosci. Rep.* **2015**, *35*, e00261. [CrossRef] [PubMed]
85. Wu, H.Q.; Okuyama, M.; Kajii, Y.; Pocivavsek, A.; Bruno, J.P.; Schwarcz, R. Targeting kynurenine aminotransferase II in psychiatric diseases: Promising effects of an orally active enzyme inhibitor. *Schizophr. Bull.* **2014**, *40*, S152–S158. [CrossRef] [PubMed]
86. Aarsland, T.I.M.; Landaas, E.T.; Hegvik, T.-A.; Ulvik, A.; Halmøy, A.; Ueland, P.M.; Haavik, J. Serum concentrations of kynurenines in adult patients with attention-deficit hyperactivity disorder (ADHD): A case-control study. *Behav. Brain Funct.* **2015**, *11*, 36. [CrossRef] [PubMed]
87. Maes, M.; Mihaylova, I.; De Ruyter, M.; Kubera, M.; Bosmans, E. The immune effects of TRYCATs (tryptophan catabolites along the IDO pathway): Relevance for depression- and other conditions characterized by tryptophan depletion induced by inflammation. *Neuro Endocrinol. Lett.* **2007**, *28*, 826–831. [PubMed]
88. Moroni, F.; Cozzi, A.; Sili, M.; Mannaioni, G. Kynurenic acid: A metabolite with multiple actions and multiple targets in brain and periphery. *J. Neural Transm.* **2012**, *119*, 133–139. [CrossRef]
89. Neale, S.A.; Copeland, C.S.; Uebele, V.N.; Thomson, F.J.; Salt, T.E. Modulation of Hippocampal Synaptic Transmission by the Kynurenine Pathway Member Xanthurenic Acid and Other VGLUT Inhibitors. *Neuropsychopharmacology* **2013**, *38*, 1060–1067. [CrossRef]
90. Cenit, M.C.; Nuevo, I.C.; Codoñer-Franch, P.; Sanz, Y.; Dinan, T.G. Gut microbiota and attention deficit hyperactivity disorder: New perspectives for a challenging condition. *Eur. Child. Adolesc. Psychiatry* **2017**, *8*, 429–1092. [CrossRef]
91. Kozak, R.; Campbell, B.M.; Strick, C.A.; Horner, W.; Hoffmann, W.E.; Kiss, T.; Chapin, D.S.; McGinnis, D.; Abbott, A.L.; Roberts, B.M.; et al. Reduction of Brain Kynurenic Acid Improves Cognitive Function. *J. Neurosci.* **2014**, *34*, 10592–10602. [CrossRef]
92. Vécsei, L.; Szalárdy, L.; Fülöp, F.; Toldi, J. Kynurenines in the CNS: Recent advances and new questions. *Nat. Rev. Drug Discov.* **2013**, *12*, 64–82. [CrossRef] [PubMed]
93. Evangelisti, M.; De Rossi, P.; Rabasco, J.; Donfrancesco, R.; Lionetto, L.; Capi, M.; Sani, G.; Simmaco, M.; Nicoletti, F.; Villa, M.P. Changes in serum levels of kynurenine metabolites in paediatric patients affected by ADHD. *Eur. Child. Adolesc. Psychiatry* **2017**, *26*, 1433–1441. [CrossRef] [PubMed]
94. Landaas, E.T.; Aarsland, T.I.; Ulvik, A.; Halmøy, A.; Ueland, P.M.; Haavik, J. Vitamin levels in adults with ADHD. *BJPsych Open* **2016**, *2*, 377–384. [CrossRef] [PubMed]
95. Dolina, S.; Margalit, D.; Malitsky, S.; Rabinkov, A. Attention-deficit hyperactivity disorder (ADHD) as a pyridoxine-dependent condition: Urinary diagnostic biomarkers. *Med. Hypotheses* **2014**, *82*, 111–116. [CrossRef]
96. Said, Z.M.; Subramanian, V.S.; Vaziri, N.D.; Said, H.M. T1881 Pyridoxine Uptake By Colonocytes: A Specific and Regulated Carrier-Mediated Process. *Am. J. Physiol. Cell Physiol.* **2008**, *294*, C1192–C1197. [CrossRef]

97. Gagliardi, A.; Totino, V.; Cacciotti, F.; Iebba, V.; Neroni, B.; Bonfiglio, G.; Trancassini, M.; Passariello, C.; Pantanella, F.; Schippa, S. Rebuilding the Gut Microbiota Ecosystem. *Int. J. Environ. Res. Public Health* **2018**, *15*, 1679. [CrossRef]
98. Fond, G.; Boukouaci, W.; Chevalier, G.; Regnault, A.; Eberl, G.; Hamdani, N.; Dickerson, F.; MacGregor, A.; Boyer, L.; Dargel, A.; et al. The "psychomicrobiotic": Targeting microbiota in major psychiatric disorders: A systematic review. *Pathol. Boil.* **2015**, *63*, 35–42. [CrossRef]
99. Saltzman, E.T.; Palacios, T.; Thomsen, M.; Vitetta, L. Intestinal Microbiome Shifts, Dysbiosis, Inflammation, and Non-alcoholic Fatty Liver Disease. *Front. Microbiol.* **2018**, *9*, 61. [CrossRef]
100. Varatharaj, A.; Galea, I. The blood-brain barrier in systemic inflammation. *Brain Behav. Immun.* **2017**, *60*, 1–12. [CrossRef]
101. Verlaet, A.A.J.; Noriega, D.B.; Hermans, N.; Savelkoul, H.F.J. Nutrition, immunological mechanisms and dietary immunomodulation in ADHD. *Eur. Child. Adolesc. Psychiatry* **2014**, *23*, 519–529. [CrossRef]
102. Mitchell, R.H.; Goldstein, B.I. Inflammation in children and adolescents with neuropsychiatric disorders: A systematic review. *J. Am. Acad. Child Adolesc. Psychiatry* **2014**, *53*, 274–296. [CrossRef] [PubMed]
103. Di Cesare, A.; Di Meglio, P.; Nestle, F.O. A role for Th17 cells in the immunopathogenesis of atopic dermatitis? *J. Investig. Dermatol.* **2008**, *128*, 2569–2571. [CrossRef] [PubMed]
104. Chen, M.H.; Su, T.P.; Chen, Y.S.; Hsu, J.W.; Huang, K.L.; Chang, W.H.; Bai, Y.M. Attention deficit hyperactivity disorder, tic disorder, and allergy: Is there a link? A nationwide population-based study. *J. Child. Psychol. Psychiatry* **2013**, *54*, 545–551. [CrossRef] [PubMed]
105. Tsai, M.C.; Lin, H.K.; Lin, C.H.; Fu, L.S. Prevalence of attention deficit/hyperactivity disorder in pediatric allergic rhinitis: A nationwide population-based study. *Allergy Asthma Proc.* **2011**, *32*, 41–46. [CrossRef] [PubMed]
106. Genuneit, J.; Braig, S.; Brandt, S.; Wabitsch, M.; Florath, I.; Brenner, H.; Rothenbacher, D. Infant atopic eczema and subsequent attention-deficit/hyperactivity disorder–a prospective birth cohort study. *Pediatr. Allergy Immunol.* **2014**, *25*, 51–56. [CrossRef] [PubMed]
107. Lynch, S.V. Gut Microbiota and Allergic Disease. New Insights. *Ann. Am. Thorac. Soc.* **2016**, *13*, S51–S54.
108. Martínez, I.; Lattimer, J.M.; Hubach, K.L.; Case, J.A.; Yang, J.; Weber, C.G.; Louk, J.A.; Rose, D.J.; Kyureghian, G.; Peterson, D.A.; et al. Gut microbiome composition is linked to whole grain-induced immunological improvements. *ISME J.* **2013**, *7*, 269–280. [CrossRef]
109. Christian, L.M.; Galley, J.D.; Hade, E.M.; Schoppe-Sullivan, S.; Kamp Dush, C.; Bailey, M.T. Gut microbiome composition is associated with temperament during early childhood. *Brain Behav. Immun.* **2015**, *45*, 118–127. [CrossRef]
110. Buske-Kirschbaum, A.; Schmitt, J.; Plessow, F.; Romanos, M.; Weidinger, S.; Roessner, V. Psychoendocrine and psychoneuroimmunological mechanisms in the comorbidity of atopic eczema and attention deficit/hyperactivity disorder. *Psychoneuroendocrinology* **2013**, *38*, 12–23. [CrossRef]
111. Jiang, H.-Y.; Zhou, Y.-Y.; Zhou, G.-L.; Li, Y.-C.; Yuan, J.; Li, X.-H.; Ruan, B. Gut microbiota profiles in treatment-naïve children with attention deficit hyperactivity disorder. *Behav. Brain Res.* **2018**, *347*, 408–413. [CrossRef]
112. Marshall, P. Attention deficit disorder and allergy: A neurochemical model of the relation between the illnesses. *Psychol. Bull.* **1989**, *106*, 434–446. [CrossRef]
113. Van Der Schans, J.; De Vries, T.W.; Hak, E.; Hoekstra, P.J.; Çiçek, R. Association of atopic diseases and attention-deficit/hyperactivity disorder: A systematic review and meta-analyses. *Neurosci. Biobehav. Rev.* **2017**, *74*, 139–148. [CrossRef] [PubMed]
114. Schmitt, J.; Romanos, M.; Meurer, M.; Kirch, W. Atopic Eczema and Attention-Deficit/Hyperactivity Disorder in a Population-Based Sample of Children and Adolescents. *JAMA* **2009**, *301*, 724. [CrossRef] [PubMed]
115. Strachan, D.; Sibbald, B.; Weiland, S.; Aït-Khaled, N.; Anabwani, G.; Anderson, H.R.; Asher, M.I.; Beasley, R.; Björkstén, B.; Burr, M.; et al. Worldwide variations in prevalence of symptoms of allergic rhinoconjunctivitis in children: The International Study of Asthma and Allergies in Childhood (ISAAC). *Pediatr. Allergy Immunol.* **1997**, *8*, 161–176. [CrossRef] [PubMed]
116. Leung, D.Y.; Bieber, T. Atopic dermatitis. *Lancet* **2003**, *361*, 151–160. [CrossRef]
117. Novak, N. Immune mechanisms leading to atopic dermatitis. *J. Allergy Clin. Immunol.* **2003**, *112*, S128–S139. [CrossRef]

118. Penders, J.; Thijs, C.; van den Brandt, P.A.; Kummeling, I.; Snijders, B.; Stelma, F.; Adams, H.; van Ree, R.; Stobberingh, E.E. Gut microbiota composition and development of atopic manifestations in infancy: The KOALA Birth Cohort Study. *Gut* **2007**, *56*, 661–667. [CrossRef]
119. Qiu, X.; Zhang, M.; Yang, X.; Hong, N.; Yu, C. Faecalibacterium prausnitzii upregulates regulatory T cells and anti-inflammatory cytokines in treating TNBS-induced colitis. *J. Crohns Colitis* **2013**, *7*, e558–e568. [CrossRef]
120. Quévrain, E.; Maubert, M.A.; Michon, C.; Chain, F.; Marquant, R.; Tailhades, J.; Miquel, S.; Carlier, L.; Bermúdez-Humarán, L.G.; Pigneur, B.; et al. Identification of an anti-inflammatory protein from Faecalibacterium prausnitzii, a commensal bacterium deficient in Crohn's disease. *Gut* **2016**, *65*, 415–425.
121. Dominguez-Bello, M.G.; Costello, E.K.; Contreras, M.; Magris, M.; Hidalgo, G.; Fierer, N.; Knight, R. Delivery mode shapes the acquisition and structure of the initial microbiota across multiple body habitats in newborns. *Proc. Natl. Acad. Sci. USA* **2010**, *107*, 11971–11975. [CrossRef]
122. Penders, J.; Thijs, C.; Vink, C.; Stelma, F.F.; Snijders, B.; Kummeling, I.; Brandt, P.A.V.D.; Stobberingh, E.E. Factors Influencing the Composition of the Intestinal Microbiota in Early Infancy. *Pediatrics* **2006**, *118*, 511–521. [CrossRef] [PubMed]
123. Jakobsson, H.E.; Abrahamsson, T.R.; Jenmalm, M.C.; Harris, K.; Quince, C.; Jernberg, C.; Björkstén, B.; Engstrand, L.; Andersson, A.F. Decreased gut microbiota diversity, delayed Bacteroidetes colonisation and reduced Th1 responses in infants delivered by caesarean section. *Gut* **2014**, *63*, 559–566. [CrossRef] [PubMed]
124. Boksa, P.; El-Khodor, B.F. Birth insult interacts with stress at adulthood to alter dopaminergic function in animal models: Possible implications for schizophrenia and other disorders. *Neurosci. Biobehav. Rev.* **2003**, *27*, 91–101. [CrossRef]
125. Salas, M.; Hotman, A.; Stricker, B.H. Confounding by Indication: An Example of Variation in the Use of Epidemiologic Terminology. *Am. J. Epidemiol.* **1999**, *149*, 981–983. [CrossRef] [PubMed]
126. Ketzer, C.R.; Gallois, C.; Martinez, A.L.; Rohde, L.A.; Schmitz, M. Is there an association between perinatal complications and attention-deficit/hyperactivity disorder-inattentive type in children and adolescents? *Braz. J. Psychiatry* **2012**, *34*, 321–328. [CrossRef] [PubMed]
127. Silva, D.; Colvin, L.; Hagemann, E.; Bower, C. Environmental risk factors by gender associated with attention-deficit/hyperactivity disorder. *Pediatrics* **2014**, *133*, e14–e22. [CrossRef] [PubMed]
128. Curran, E.A.; O'Neill, S.M.; Cryan, J.F.; Kenny, L.C.; Dinan, T.G.; Khashan, A.S.; Kearney, P.M. Research review: Birth by caesarean section and development of autism spectrum disorder and attention-deficit/hyperactivity disorder: A systematic review and meta-analysis. *J. Child Psychol. Psychiatry* **2015**, *56*, 500–508. [CrossRef]
129. Curran, E.A.; Khashan, A.S.; Dalman, C.; Kenny, L.C.; Cryan, J.F.; Dinan, T.G.; Kearney, P.M. Obstetric mode of delivery and attention-deficit/hyperactivity disorder: A sibling-matched study. *Int. J. Epidemiol.* **2016**, *45*, 532–542. [CrossRef]
130. Axelsson, P.B.; Clausen, T.D.; Petersen, A.H.; Hageman, I.; Pinborg, A.; Kessing, L.V.; Bergholt, T.; Rasmussen, S.C.; Keiding, N.; Løkkegaard, E.C.L. Investigating the effects of cesarean delivery and antibiotic use in early childhood on risk of later attention deficit hyperactivity disorder. *J. Child Psychol. Psychiatry* **2019**, *60*, 151–159. [CrossRef]
131. Curran, E.A.; Cryan, J.F.; Kenny, L.C.; Dinan, T.G.; Kearney, P.M.; Khashan, A.S. Obstetrical Mode of Delivery and Childhood Behavior and Psychological Development in a British Cohort. *J. Autism Dev. Disord.* **2016**, *46*, 603–614. [CrossRef]
132. Li, J.; Olsen, J.; Vestergaard, M.; Obel, C. Attention-deficit/hyperactivity disorder in the offspring following prenatal maternal bereavement: A nationwide follow-up study in Denmark. *Eur. Child. Adolesc. Psychiatry* **2010**, *19*, 747–753. [CrossRef] [PubMed]
133. Van den Bergh, B.R.; Marcoen, A. High antenatal maternal anxiety is related to ADHD symptoms, externalizing problems, and anxiety in 8- and 9-year-olds. *Child Dev.* **2004**, *75*, 1085–1097. [CrossRef] [PubMed]
134. Grizenko, N.; Shayan, Y.R.; Polotskaia, A.; Ter-Stepanian, M.; Joober, R. Relation of maternal stress during pregnancy to symptom severity and response to treatment in children with ADHD. *J. Psychiatry Neurosci.* **2008**, *33*, 10–16. [PubMed]
135. Jašarević, E.; Howerton, C.L.; Howard, C.D.; Bale, T.L. Alterations in the Vaginal Microbiome by Maternal Stress Are Associated With Metabolic Reprogramming of the Offspring Gut and Brain. *Endocrinology* **2015**, *156*, 3265–3276. [CrossRef] [PubMed]
136. Galley, J.D.; Bailey, M.T. Impact of stressor exposure on the interplay between commensal microbiota and host inflammation. *Gut Microbes* **2014**, *5*, 390–396. [CrossRef] [PubMed]

137. Barrett, E.; Ross, R.P.; O'Toole, P.W.; Fitzgerald, G.F.; Stanton, C. γ-Aminobutyric acid production by culturable bacteria from the human intestine. *J. Appl. Microbiol.* **2012**, *113*, 411–417. [CrossRef]
138. Edden, R.A.E.; Crocetti, D.; Zhu, H.; Gilbert, D.L.; Mostofsky, S.H. Reduced GABA concentration in attention-deficit/hyperactivity disorder. *Arch. Gen. Psychiatry* **2012**, *69*, 750–753. [CrossRef]
139. Bollmann, S.; Ghisleni, C.; Poil, S.-S.; Martin, E.; Ball, J.; Eich-Höchli, D.; Edden, R.A.E.; Klaver, P.; Michels, L.; Brandeis, D.; et al. Developmental changes in gamma-aminobutyric acid levels in attention-deficit/hyperactivity disorder. *Transl. Psychiatry* **2015**, *5*, e589. [CrossRef]
140. Sumner, P.; Edden, R.A.E.; Bompas, A.; Evans, C.J.; Singh, K.D. More GABA, less distraction: A neurochemical predictor of motor decision speed. *Nat. Neurosci.* **2010**, *13*, 825–827. [CrossRef]
141. Wiebking, C.; Duncan, N.W.; Tiret, B.; Hayes, D.J.; Marjańska, M.; Doyon, J.; Bajbouj, M.; Northoff, G. GABA in the insula—A predictor of the neural response to interoceptive awareness. *Neuroimage* **2014**, *86*, 10–18. [CrossRef]
142. Pärtty, A.; Kalliomäki, M.; Wacklin, P.; Salminen, S.; Isolauri, E. A possible link between early probiotic intervention and the risk of neuropsychiatric disorders later in childhood: A randomized trial. *Pediatr. Res.* **2015**, *77*, 823–828. [CrossRef]
143. Kalliomäki, M.; Salminen, S.; Arvilommi, H.; Kero, P.; Koskinen, P.; Isolauri, E. Probiotics in primary prevention of atopic disease: A randomised placebo-controlled trial. *Lancet* **2001**, *357*, 1076–1079. [CrossRef]
144. Barrett, E.; Kerr, C.; Murphy, K.; O'Sullivan, O.; Ryan, C.A.; Dempsey, E.M.; Murphy, B.P.; O'Toole, P.W.; Cotter, P.D.; Fitzgerald, G.F.; et al. The individual-specific and diverse nature of the preterm infant microbiota. *Arch. Dis. Child Fetal Neonatal Ed.* **2013**, *98*, F334–F340. [CrossRef] [PubMed]
145. Bhutta, A.T.; Cleves, M.A.; Casey, P.H.; Cradock, M.M.; Anand, K.J.S. Cognitive and behavioral outcomes of school-aged children who were born preterm: A meta-analysis. *JAMA* **2002**, *288*, 728–737. [CrossRef] [PubMed]
146. Johnson, S.; Hollis, C.; Kochhar, P.; Hennessy, E.; Wolke, D.; Marlow, N. Psychiatric disorders in extremely preterm children: Longitudinal finding at age 11 years in the EPICure study. *J. Am. Acad. Child Adolesc. Psychiatry* **2010**, *49*, 453–463.e1. [CrossRef]
147. Ask, H.; Gustavson, K.; Ystrom, E.; Havdahl, K.A.; Tesli, M.; Askeland, R.B.; Reichborn-Kjennerud, T. Association of Gestational Age at Birth With Symptoms of Attention-Deficit/Hyperactivity Disorder in Children. *JAMA Pediatr.* **2018**, *172*, 749–756. [CrossRef]
148. Chou, I.-C.; Kuo, H.-T.; Chang, J.-S.; Wu, S.-F.; Chiu, H.-Y.; Su, B.-H.; Lin, H.-C. Lack of Effects of Oral Probiotics on Growth and Neurodevelopmental Outcomes in Preterm Very Low Birth Weight Infants. *J. Pediatr.* **2010**, *156*, 393–396. [CrossRef]
149. Melville, J.M.; Moss, T.J. The immune consequences of preterm birth. *Front. Neurosci.* **2013**, *7*, 79. [CrossRef]
150. Quinn, J.-A.; Munoz, F.M.; Gonik, B.; Frau, L.; Cutland, C.; Mallett-Moore, T.; Kissou, A.; Wittke, F.; Das, M.; Nunes, T.; et al. Preterm birth: Case definition & guidelines for data collection, analysis, and presentation of immunisation safety data. *Vaccine* **2016**, *34*, 6047–6056.
151. Lindström, K.; Lindblad, F.; Hjern, A. Preterm birth and attention-deficit/hyperactivity disorder in schoolchildren. *Pediatrics* **2011**, *127*, 858–865. [CrossRef]
152. D'Onofrio, B.M.; Class, Q.A.; Rickert, M.E.; Larsson, H.; Langström, N.; Lichtenstein, P. Preterm birth and mortality and morbidity: A population-based quasi-experimental study. *JAMA Psychiatry* **2013**, *70*, 1231–1240. [CrossRef] [PubMed]
153. Farooqi, A.; Hägglöf, B.; Sedin, G.; Gothefors, L.; Serenius, F. Mental Health and Social Competencies of 10- to 12-Year-Old Children Born at 23 to 25 Weeks of Gestation in the 1990s: A Swedish National Prospective Follow-up Study. *Pediatrics* **2007**, *120*, 118–133. [CrossRef] [PubMed]
154. Sternbach, H.; State, R. Antibiotics: Neuropsychiatric effects and psychotropic interactions. *Harv. Rev. Psychiatry* **1997**, *5*, 214–226. [CrossRef] [PubMed]
155. Becattini, S.; Taur, Y.; Pamer, E.G. Antibiotic-Induced Changes in the Intestinal Microbiota and Disease. *Trends Mol. Med.* **2016**, *22*, 458–478. [CrossRef] [PubMed]
156. Park, S.; Kim, B.N.; Kim, J.W.; Shin, M.S.; Yoo, H.J.; Cho, S.C. Protective effect of breastfeeding with regard to children's behavioral and cognitive problems. *Nutr. J.* **2014**, *13*, 111. [CrossRef] [PubMed]
157. Mimouni-Bloch, A.; Kachevanskaya, A.; Mimouni, F.B.; Shuper, A.; Raveh, E.; Linder, N. Breastfeeding may protect from developing attention-deficit/hyperactivity disorder. *Breastfeed Med.* **2013**, *8*, 363–367. [CrossRef] [PubMed]

158. Stadler, D.D.; Musser, E.D.; Holton, K.F.; Shannon, J.; Nigg, J.T. Recalled Initiation and Duration of Maternal Breastfeeding Among Children with and Without ADHD in a Well Characterized Case-Control Sample. *J. Abnorm. Child. Psychol.* **2016**, *44*, 347–355. [CrossRef]
159. Golmirzaei, J.; Namazi, S.; Amiri, S.; Zare, S.; Rastikerdar, N.; Hesam, A.A.; Rahami, Z.; Ghasemian, F.; Namazi, S.S.; Paknahad, A.; et al. Evaluation of Attention-Deficit Hyperactivity Disorder Risk Factors. *Int. J. Pediatr.* **2013**, *2013*, 1–6. [CrossRef]
160. Newburg, D.S.; Walker, W.A. Protection of the neonate by the innate immune system of developing gut and of human milk. *Pediatr. Res.* **2007**, *61*, 2–8. [CrossRef]
161. Cacho, N.T.; Lawrence, R.M. Innate Immunity and Breast Milk. *Front. Immunol.* **2017**, *8*, 584. [CrossRef]
162. Richardson, A.; Puri, B. The potential role of fatty acids in attention-deficit/hyperactivity disorder. *Prostaglandins Leukot. Essent. Fat. Acids* **2000**, *63*, 79–87. [CrossRef] [PubMed]
163. Richardson, A.J. Omega-3 fatty acids in ADHD and related neurodevelopmental disorders. *Int. Rev. Psychiatry* **2006**, *18*, 155–172. [CrossRef] [PubMed]
164. Bezirtzoglou, E.; Tsiotsias, A.; Welling, G.W. Microbiota profile in feces of breast- and formula-fed newborns by using fluorescence in situ hybridization (FISH). *Anaerobe* **2011**, *17*, 478–482. [CrossRef] [PubMed]
165. Fallani, M.; Young, D.; Scott, J.; Norin, E.; Amarri, S.; Adam, R.; Aguilera, M.; Khanna, S.; Gil, A.; Edwards, C.A.; et al. Intestinal Microbiota of 6-week-old Infants Across Europe: Geographic Influence Beyond Delivery Mode, Breast-feeding, and Antibiotics. *J. Pediatr. Gastroenterol. Nutr.* **2010**, *51*, 77–84. [CrossRef]
166. Guaraldi, F.; Salvatori, G. Effect of Breast and Formula Feeding on Gut Microbiota Shaping in Newborns. *Front. Microbiol.* **2012**, *2*, 94. [CrossRef]
167. Underwood, M.A.; Kalanetra, K.M.; Bokulich, N.A.; Lewis, Z.T.; Mirmiran, M.; Tancredi, D.J.; Mills, D.A. A comparison of two probiotic strains of bifidobacteria in premature infants. *J. Pediatr.* **2013**, *163*, 1585–1591.e9. [CrossRef]
168. Underwood, M.A.; German, J.B.; Lebrilla, C.B.; Mills, D.A. Bifidobacterium longum subspecies infantis: Champion colonizer of the infant gut. *Pediatr. Res.* **2015**, *77*, 229–235. [CrossRef]
169. Adesman, A.; Soled, D.; Rosen, L. Formula Feeding as a Risk Factor for Attention-Deficit/Hyperactivity Disorder: Is Bisphenol A Exposure a Smoking Gun? *J. Dev. Behav. Pediatr.* **2017**, *38*, 545–551.e9. [CrossRef]
170. Mariadason, J.M.; Corner, G.A.; Augenlicht, L.H. Genetic reprogramming in pathways of colonic cell maturation induced by short chain fatty acids: Comparison with trichostatin A, sulindac, and curcumin and implications for chemoprevention of colon cancer. *Cancer Res.* **2000**, *60*, 4561–4572.
171. Canani, R.B.; Di Costanzo, M.; Leone, L.; Pedata, M.; Meli, R.; Calignano, A. Potential beneficial effects of butyrate in intestinal and extraintestinal diseases. *World J. Gastroenterol.* **2011**, *17*, 1519–1528. [CrossRef]
172. Macfabe, D.F. Enteric short-chain fatty acids: Microbial messengers of metabolism, mitochondria, and mind: Implications in autism spectrum disorders. *Microb. Ecol. Heal. Dis.* **2015**, *26*, 28177. [CrossRef] [PubMed]
173. Bercik, P.; Denou, E.; Collins, J.; Jackson, W.; Lu, J.; Jury, J.; Deng, Y.; Blennerhassett, P.; Macri, J.; McCoy, K.D.; et al. The Intestinal Microbiota Affect Central Levels of Brain-Derived Neurotropic Factor and Behavior in Mice. *Gastroenterology* **2011**, *141*, 599–609.e3. [CrossRef] [PubMed]
174. Corominas-Roso, M.; Ramos-Quiroga, J.A.; Ribases, M.; Sanchez-Mora, C.; Palomar, G.; Valero, S.; Bosch, R.; Casas, M. Decreased serum levels of brain-derived neurotrophic factor in adults with attention-deficit hyperactivity disorder. *Int. J. Neuropsychopharmacol.* **2013**, *16*, 1267–1275. [CrossRef] [PubMed]
175. Akay, A.P.; Resmi, H.; Güney, S.A.; Erkuran, H.; Özyurt, G.; Sargin, E.; Topuzoglu, A.; Tufan, A.E. Serum brain-derived neurotrophic factor levels in treatment-naïve boys with attention-deficit/hyperactivity disorder treated with methylphenidate: An 8-week, observational pretest-posttest study. *Eur. Child Adolesc. Psychiatry* **2018**, *27*, 127–135. [CrossRef]
176. Amiri, A.; Torabi Parizi, G.; Kousha, M.; Saadat, F.; Modabbernia, M.J.; Najafi, K.; Atrkar Roushan, Z. Changes in plasma Brain-derived neurotrophic factor (BDNF) levels induced by methylphenidate in children with Attention deficit-hyperactivity disorder (ADHD). *Prog. Neuropsychopharmacol. Biol. Psychiatry* **2013**, *47*, 20–24. [CrossRef]
177. Shim, S.H.; Hwangbo, Y.; Kwon, Y.J.; Jeong, H.Y.; Lee, B.H.; Lee, H.J.; Kim, Y.K. Increased levels of plasma brain-derived neurotrophic factor (BDNF) in children with attention deficit-hyperactivity disorder (ADHD). *Prog. Neuropsychopharmacol. Biol. Psychiatry* **2008**, *32*, 1824–1828. [CrossRef]

178. Fujimura, H.; Chen, R.; Nakamura, T.; Nakahashi, T.; Kambayashi, J.-I.; Sun, B.; Altar, C.A.; Tandon, N.N. Brain-derived neurotrophic factor is stored in human platelets and released by agonist stimulation. *Thromb. Haemost.* **2002**, *87*, 728–734. [CrossRef]
179. Amjad Khan, W.; Chun-Mei, H.; Khan, N.; Iqbal, A.; Lyu, S.W.; Shah, F. Bioengineered Plants Can Be a Useful Source of Omega-3 Fatty Acids. *Biomed. Res. Int.* **2017**, *2017*, 7348919. [CrossRef]
180. Cryan, J.F.; O'Mahony, S.M. The microbiome-gut-brain axis: From bowel to behavior. *Neurogastroenterol. Motil.* **2011**, *23*, 187–192. [CrossRef]
181. Weiser, M.J.; Butt, C.M.; Mohajeri, M.H. Docosahexaenoic Acid and Cognition throughout the Lifespan. *Nutrients* **2016**, *8*, 99. [CrossRef]
182. Robertson, R.C.; Oriach, C.S.; Murphy, K.; Moloney, G.M.; Cryan, J.F.; Dinan, T.G.; Ross, R.P.; Stanton, C. Omega-3 polyunsaturated fatty acids critically regulate behaviour and gut microbiota development in adolescence and adulthood. *Brain Behav. Immun.* **2017**, *59*, 21–37. [CrossRef] [PubMed]
183. Choi-Lundberg, D.L.; Lin, Q.; Chang, Y.-N.; Chiang, Y.L.; Hay, C.M.; Mohajeri, H.; Davidson, B.L.; Bohn, M.C. Dopaminergic Neurons Protected from Degeneration by GDNF Gene Therapy. *Science* **1997**, *275*, 838–841. [CrossRef] [PubMed]
184. Bohn, M.C.; Connor, B.; Kozlowski, D.A.; Mohajeri, M.H. Gene transfer for neuroprotection in animal models of Parkinson's disease and amyotrophic lateral sclerosis. *Novartis Found Symp.* **2000**, *231*, 70–93. [PubMed]
185. Rao, J.S.; Ertley, R.N.; Lee, H.J.; DeMar, J.C.; Arnold, J.T.; Rapoport, S.I.; Bazinet, R.P. N-3 polyunsaturated fatty acid deprivation in rats decreases frontal cortex BDNF via a p38 MAPK-dependent mechanism. *Mol. Psychiatry* **2007**, *12*, 36–46. [CrossRef]
186. Soares, J.C.; Kochunov, P.; Monkul, E.S.; Nicoletti, M.A.; Brambilla, P.; Sassi, R.B.; Mallinger, A.G.; Frank, E.; Kupfer, D.J.; Lancaster, J.; et al. Structural brain changes in bipolar disorder using deformation field morphometry. *NeuroReport* **2005**, *16*, 541–544. [CrossRef]
187. Costantini, L.; Molinari, R.; Farinon, B.; Merendino, N. Impact of Omega-3 Fatty Acids on the Gut Microbiota. *Int. J. Mol. Sci.* **2017**, *18*, 2645. [CrossRef]
188. Yan, Y.; Jiang, W.; Spinetti, T.; Tardivel, A.; Castillo, R.; Bourquin, C.; Guarda, G.; Tian, Z.; Tschopp, J.; Zhou, R. Omega-3 Fatty Acids Prevent Inflammation and Metabolic Disorder through Inhibition of NLRP3 Inflammasome Activation. *Immunity* **2013**, *38*, 1154–1163. [CrossRef]
189. Kaliannan, K.; Li, X.-Y.; Wang, B.; Pan, Q.; Chen, C.-Y.; Hao, L.; Xie, S.; Kang, J.X. Multi-omic analysis in transgenic mice implicates omega-6/omega-3 fatty acid imbalance as a risk factor for chronic disease. *Commun. Boil.* **2019**, *2*, 276. [CrossRef]
190. Kaliannan, K.; Wang, B.; Li, X.Y.; Kim, K.J.; Kang, J.X. A host-microbiome interaction mediates the opposing effects of omega-6 and omega-3 fatty acids on metabolic endotoxemia. *Sci. Rep.* **2015**, *5*, 11276. [CrossRef]
191. Crippa, A.; Agostoni, C.; Mauri, M.; Molteni, M.; Nobile, M. Polyunsaturated Fatty Acids Are Associated With Behavior But Not With Cognition in Children With and Without ADHD: An Italian study. *J. Atten. Disord.* **2018**, *22*, 971–983. [CrossRef]
192. Chang, J.P.; Su, K.P.; Mondelli, V.; Pariante, C.M. Omega-3 Polyunsaturated Fatty Acids in Youths with Attention Deficit Hyperactivity Disorder: A Systematic Review and Meta-Analysis of Clinical Trials and Biological Studies. *Neuropsychopharmacology* **2018**, *43*, 534–545. [CrossRef] [PubMed]
193. Anand, P.; Sachdeva, A. Effect of Poly Unsaturated Fatty Acids Administration on Children with Attention Deficit Hyperactivity Disorder: A Randomized Controlled Trial. *J. Clin. Diagn. Res.* **2016**, *10*, OC01–OC05. [CrossRef] [PubMed]
194. Gillies, D.; Sinn, J.K.; Lad, S.S.; Leach, M.J.; Ross, M.J. Polyunsaturated fatty acids (PUFA) for attention deficit hyperactivity disorder (ADHD) in children and adolescents. *Cochrane Database Syst. Rev.* **2012**, *7*, CD007986. [CrossRef] [PubMed]
195. Watson, H.; Mitra, S.; Croden, F.C.; Taylor, M.; Wood, H.M.; Perry, S.L.; Spencer, J.A.; Quirke, P.; Toogood, G.J.; Lawton, C.L.; et al. A randomised trial of the effect of omega-3 polyunsaturated fatty acid supplements on the human intestinal microbiota. *Gut* **2018**, *67*, 1974–1983. [CrossRef] [PubMed]
196. Ilag, L.L. Are Long-Chain Polyunsaturated Fatty Acids the Link between the Immune System and the Microbiome towards Modulating Cancer? *Medicines* **2018**, *5*, 102. [CrossRef] [PubMed]
197. Bennet, R.; Eriksson, M.; Nord, C.E. The fecal microflora of 1-3-month-old infants during treatment with eight oral antibiotics. *Infection* **2002**, *30*, 158–160. [CrossRef] [PubMed]

198. Hussey, S.; Wall, R.; Gruffman, E.; O'Sullivan, L.; Ryan, C.A.; Murphy, B.; Fitzgerald, G.; Stanton, C.; Ross, R.P. Parenteral antibiotics reduce bifidobacteria colonization and diversity in neonates. *Int. J. Microbiol.* **2011**, *2011*, 130574. [CrossRef] [PubMed]
199. Slykerman, R.F.; Thompson, J.; Waldie, K.E.; Murphy, R.; Wall, C.; Mitchell, E.A. Antibiotics in the first year of life and subsequent neurocognitive outcomes. *Acta Paediatr.* **2017**, *106*, 87–94. [CrossRef]
200. Reid, G.; Hammond, J.A. Probiotics. Some evidence of their effectiveness. *Can. Fam. Physician* **2005**, *51*, 1487–1493.
201. Hill, C.; Guarner, F.; Reid, G.; Gibson, G.R.; Merenstein, D.J.; Pot, B.; Morelli, L.; Canani, R.B.; Flint, H.J.; Salminen, S.; et al. Expert consensus document. The International Scientific Association for Probiotics and Prebiotics consensus statement on the scope and appropriate use of the term probiotic. *Nat. Rev. Gastroenterol. Hepatol.* **2014**, *11*, 506–514. [CrossRef]
202. Kumar, M.; Nagpal, R.; Verma, V.; Kumar, A.; Kaur, N.; Hemalatha, R.; Gautam, S.K.; Singh, B. Probiotic metabolites as epigenetic targets in the prevention of colon cancer. *Nutr. Rev.* **2013**, *71*, 23–34. [CrossRef] [PubMed]
203. Reid, G.; Younes, J.A.; Van der Mei, H.C.; Gloor, G.B.; Knight, R.; Busscher, H.J. Microbiota restoration: Natural and supplemented recovery of human microbial communities. *Nat. Rev. Microbiol.* **2011**, *9*, 27–38. [CrossRef] [PubMed]
204. Rezac, S.; Kok, C.R.; Heermann, M.; Hutkins, R. Fermented Foods as a Dietary Source of Live Organisms. *Front. Microbiol.* **2018**, *9*, 1785. [CrossRef]
205. Savignac, H.M.; Kiely, B.; Dinan, T.G.; Cryan, J.F. Bifidobacteria exert strain-specific effects on stress-related behavior and physiology in BALB/c mice. *Neurogastroenterol. Motil.* **2014**, *26*, 1615–1627. [CrossRef] [PubMed]
206. Felice, V.D.; O'Mahony, S.M. The microbiome and disorders of the central nervous system. *Pharmacol. Biochem. Behav.* **2017**, *160*, 1–13. [CrossRef] [PubMed]
207. Tsai, S.J. Attention-deficit hyperactivity disorder may be associated with decreased central brain-derived neurotrophic factor activity: Clinical and therapeutic implications. *Med. Hypotheses* **2007**, *68*, 896–899. [CrossRef] [PubMed]
208. Pelsser, L.M.; Frankena, K.; Toorman, J.; Rodrigues Pereira, R. Diet and ADHD, Reviewing the Evidence: A Systematic Review of Meta-Analyses of Double-Blind Placebo-Controlled Trials Evaluating the Efficacy of Diet Interventions on the Behavior of Children with ADHD. *PLoS ONE* **2017**, *12*, e0169277. [CrossRef] [PubMed]

6

Chronic Monosodium Glutamate Administration Induced Hyperalgesia in Mice

Anca Zanfirescu, Aurelia Nicoleta Cristea †, George Mihai Nitulescu *, Bruno Stefan Velescu and Daniela Gradinaru

Faculty of Pharmacy, "Carol Davila" University of Medicine and Pharmacy, TraianVuia 6, 020956 Bucharest, Romania; zanfirescuanca@yahoo.com (A.Z.); anicoletacristea@yahoo.com (A.N.C); bruno_velescu@yahoo.co.uk (B.S.V.); danielagrdnr@yahoo.com (D.G.)

* Correspondence: nitulescu_mihai@yahoo.com

† In Memoriam: The authors would like to respectfully dedicate this article to Prof. Aurelia Nicoleta Cristea who passed away on 24 November 2017.

Abstract: Monosodium glutamate (MSG) is a widely used food additive. Although it is generally considered safe, some questions regarding the impact of its use on general health have arisen. Several reports correlate MSG consumption with a series of unwanted reactions, including headaches and mechanical sensitivity in pericranial muscles. Endogenous glutamate plays a significant role in nociceptive processing, this neurotransmitter being associated with hyperalgesia and central sensitization. One of the mechanisms underlying these phenomena is the stimulation of Ca^{2+}/calmodulin sensitive nitric oxide synthase, and a subsequent increase in nitric oxide production. This molecule is a key player in nociceptive processing, with implications in acute and chronic pain states. Our purpose was to investigate the effect of this food additive on the nociceptive threshold when given orally to mice. Hot-plate and formalin tests were used to assess nociceptive behaviour. We also tried to determine if a correlation between chronic administration of MSG and variations in central nitric oxide (NO) concentration could be established. We found that a dose of 300 mg/kg MSG given for 21 days reduces the pain threshold and is associated with a significant increase in brain NO level. The implications of these findings on food additive-drug interaction, and on pain perception in healthy humans, as well as in those suffering from affections involving chronic pain, are still to be investigated.

Keywords: monosodium glutamate; hyperalgesia; hot-plate test; formalin test; nitric oxide synthase

---

1. Introduction

Monosodium glutamate (MSG), the salt of glutamic acid, is widely used as a food additive (E621). Two enantiomers are known, but only the naturally occurring isomer *L* is used as a flavor enhancer. Kwok, in 1968 [1], reported transient subjective symptoms (flushing, headache, numbness, general weakness, palpitation) following consumption of Chinese dishes known to contain high concentrations of E621. Several human studies were conducted afterwards to determine if a causal relationship existed between MSG and this symptom complex, but the results were inconsistent. The Joint FAO/WHO Expert Committee on Food Additives in 1971 [2], 1974 [3], and 1987 allocated it an "acceptable daily intake (ADI) not specified", considering MSG consumption to be safe [4]. The total intake of glutamate from food in European countries was assessed to range between 5 and 12 g/day, taking into account both natural and added glutamate [5].

Although MSG consumption is believed to be safe, several reports correlate MSG consumption with a series of unwanted reactions, including headache and mechanical sensitivity in pericranial muscles [5,6]. Clinical reports state that MSG consumption increases the frequency of fibromyalgia symptoms [7].

L-glutamate is a fast excitatory neurotransmitter with a significant role in nociceptive processing [8]. Two types of glutamate receptors are currently known: ligand-gated ion channels (NMDA, AMPA, kainate), and G protein-coupled receptors (metabotropic receptors) [9]. These receptors are well expressed in the central and peripheral nervous system, and have a high distribution in pain pathways [10–12]. Intraperitoneal or intrathecal administration of glutamate or agonists selective for one type of glutamate receptor induces nociceptive behaviors. Treatments with NMDA and AMPA antagonists or with inhibitors of glutamate release significantly reduce the hyperalgesia induced in experimental rodent models of acute inflammatory and neuropathic pain [13,14].

One of the mechanisms linked with NMDA-mediated hyperalgesia is stimulation of Ca^{2+}/calmodulin sensitive nitric oxide synthase, and a subsequent increase in nitric oxide (NO) production [15]. This molecule is a key player in nociceptive processing, with implications in acute [16] and chronic pain states [13]. The peripheral and central (mostly spinal) role of NO in nociceptive response was investigated in different animal models. Rat response to mechanical stimuli in a paradoxical sleep deprivation hyperalgesia model has been associated to nitric oxide synthase (NOS) activity enhancement in dorsolateral grey matter, leading to changes in the descendent modulating pain pathways [17]. Knock-out mice, lacking NOS encoding genes, showed a decrease of the tactile allodyniain mechanical stimulus test [18]. Nx-nitro-L-arginine methyl ester (L-NAME), a non-selective NOS inhibitor reduced the behavioral signs of neuropathic pain induced in rats by constricting the spinal [19] and sciatic [20] nerves. Intrathecal administration of L-NAME or of methylene blue, a soluble guanylatecyclase inhibitor, suppresses the thermal hyperalgesia induced in the sciatic nerve constriction model. Pretreatment with NOS inhibitors significantly attenuated the thermal hyperalgesia induced by the intraplantar injection of complete Freund's adjuvant in mice [21].

Taking into account the involvement of endogenous glutamate in pain processing and the different existing reports on MSG, we hypothesized that oral administration of this flavor enhancer would modify the nociceptive threshold when orally administered in mice. We also tried to determine some of the molecular changes underlying this effect.

2. Materials and Methods

2.1. Chemicals

Drugs and reagents employed were as follows: L-glutamic acid monosodium salt monohydrate, L-arginine, formaldehyde solution for molecular biology (36.5–38% in water), phosphate-buffered saline (PBS), Folin & Ciocalteu's phenol reagent, *N*-(1-naphthyl)-ethylenediaminedihydrochloride, cadmium chloride. All reagents were purchased from Sigma-Aldrich (St. Louis, MO, USA).

2.2. Animals

All experiments were performed in 5 weeks male NMRI mice ($n = 60$; 30 ± 3.6 g), purchased from UMF Biobase (Bucharest, Romania). They were housed 10 animals per cage (35.5 cm × 22.9 cm × 15.2 cm), in a ventilated cage system, with a bedding of wood sawdust, under controlled light/dark cycle conditions (12 h light/12 h dark; lights on at 6:00 a.m.), with free access to water and food pellets. The temperature ranged between 20 and 22 °C, and the relative humidity was maintained at 35–45%. All reagents were purchased from Sigma-Aldrich (St. Louis, MO, USA). All procedures were carried out according to EU Directive 2010/63/UE, and with the approval of the Institutional Animal Care and Use Committee. The study was approved by the Bioethics Commission of the University of Medicine and Pharmacy Bucharest with the ethical approval code 589/04.09.2016. For each experiment we used 30 mice, divided in three equal groups. The animals received the test solutions for 21 days by means of a straight animal ball-tipped feeding needle. The body weight evolution was constant during the experiment for all three groups, exhibiting no significant differences. After 21 days the mice body weight was 41 ± 4 g.

2.3. Formalin-Induced Nociception

Group I represented the control, and was given distilled water 1 mL/100 g, group II received 150 mg/kg MSG (1.5% MSG solution), and group III 300 mg/kg MSG (3.0% MSG solution). All solutions were prepared in distilled water. The doses of MSG used were selected following multiple tests, as reported previously [22]. Mice were injected with 20 μL of formalin reagent containing formaldehyde 1.2% in PBS into the plantar surface of the left hind-paw with a 30-gauge needle. They were then placed in a Plexiglas box (30 cm × 30 cm × 30 cm) with a mirror below the floor at a 45 degree angle to allow an unobstructed view of the paws. The total time spent by animal either licking or biting the injected paw (reaction time) was recorded for the following 50 min. We took into account the biphasic behavior induced by formalin: an initial acute phase (with a duration of 0–5 min, neurogenic pain), followed by a prolonged tonic response (between 25 and 50 min, inflammatory pain). Between phases 1 and 2, there was an intermittent period where little nociceptive behavior was observed. The total time spent by animal licking or biting the paw injected with formalin was considered an index of nociception in the formalin test.

2.4. Hot-Plate Latency Assay

Groups of ten mice received doses of 150 and 300 mg/kg MSG orally for 21 days, while the control group was administered with the vehicle. On day 21, animals were treated and brought into the testing room one hour before testing. Animals were placed in the testing chamber and allowed to acclimate for 1 h. For testing, mice were put into a fiberglass cylinder (15 cm diameter, 30 cm high) on a metal base, maintained at a temperature of 53 ± 1 °C. Paw withdrawal latency to thermal noxious stimuli and latency of jumping response were used to assess the effects of substances on the thermal nociceptive threshold (Hot Plate, UgoBasile, Italy). In the absence of a response, the cut-off time was set to 45 s to prevent extensive damage of tissue. Hind-paw lifting was defined as lifting a hind-paw completely off the hot-plate. After 2 h, animals were sacrificed by decapitation, and the brain was harvested on ice. The biological material was used for the biochemical assays.

2.5. Assay of NO-Synthase (NOS) Activity

Total NOS activity was determined in crude tissue homogenates using the Griess method for human plasma adapted for brain tissue [23]. Using this method, we determined the concentration of NO metabolites: nitrites and nitrates (NOx). Freshly harvested brains were homogenized with PBS 1:5, centrifuged 10× *g* min/2000 rpm and the supernatant further used. The brains were homogenized, centrifuged and then kept on ice until all culls were complete. Cofactors and substrate were added according to Table 1.

Table 1. Working method for NO metabolites (NOx) determination.

Reagents (μL)	Test	Control
Supernatant	360	360
PBS	310	540
L-Arginine [1]	60	-
FAD [2]	60	-
NADPH [3]	10	-
37 °C, 60 min		
Cadmium chloride	0.5 g/mL	0.5 g/mL
25 °C, 30 min		
Griess reagent	1000	1000

[1] 1.3 mg L-arginine/10 mL solution; [2] 0.6 mg FAD/10 mL solution; [3] 12.5 mg NADPH/1 mL solution. PBS, phosphate-buffered saline.

The reagents were stored on ice. Between each addition of cofactor/substrate, the aliquots were vortexed. The cofactors/substrates were prepared in PBS. When left for 60 or 30 min, the aliquots were left on a rocker. The nitrates were reduced to nitrites in the presence of cadmium, and treated with a diazotizing reagent, sulfanilamide, in acidic media to form a transient diazonium salt. This intermediate reacts with the coupling reagent, *N*-(1-naphthyl)-ethylenediaminedihydrochloride, to form a stable azo compound. The intense purple color of the product allows nitrite assay with high sensitivity, which was used to measure nitrite concentration spectrophotometrically at 660 nm (Chemwell2010, Awareness Technology, Inc., Palm City, FL, USA).

2.6. Total Protein Assay

The total protein concentration for the same samples of brain tissue was determined using the Lowry protein assay [24]. Diluted protein solutions treated with copper salts in basic pH and Folin & Ciocalteu's phenol reagent (hexavalent phosphomolybdic/phosphotungstic acid complexes) lead to the formation of blue compounds, whose concentration is linearly proportional to the protein concentration in the sample. NOx concentration was expressed for 1mg of protein.

2.7. Statistical Analysis

Statistical analysis was performed using GraphPad Prism version 5.00 for Windows, (GraphPad Software, San Diego, CA, USA). The type of distribution of the animal response was established with D'Agostino & Pearson test. Data are reported as means ± standard error of the mean (SEM), and were analyzed statistically using parametrical Student's *t*-Test, a confidence interval (CI) of 90%, and with *p* values of 0.05 or less being considered to be significant.

3. Results

3.1. Formalin-Induced Nociception

The control group exhibited a typical biphasic nociceptive response: increased time of reaction in the first 5 min, a reduction in response for approximately 10 min, and a subsequent increased level of nociceptive response, which began 15 min after formalin injection, and lasted until the end of the experiment. The results (Figure 1) showed that, in the first phase of the formalin test, there were no significant differences between the tested groups, although a slight increase in reaction time (7.05%) was noticed for group III-MSG 300 mg/kg vs. control.

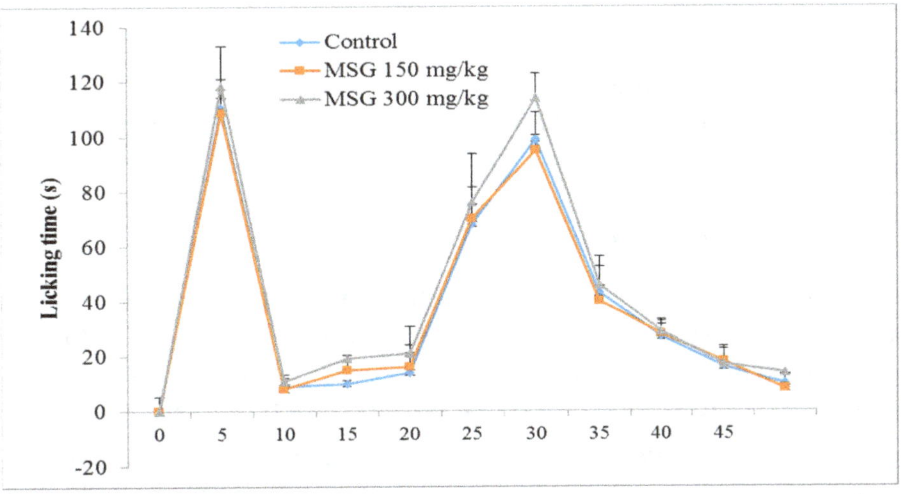

Figure 1. Time course of the formalin test in control (—◆—) and in Monosodium glutamate (MSG) treated mice (—■— MSG 150mg/kg; —▲— MSG 300 mg/kg). Values represent means ± standard error of the mean (SEM) of 10 animals.

For phase 2, characterized by inflammatory pain, MSG administered in a dose of 300 mg/kg determined a significant increase in the mean reaction time vs. the control group (11.31%, $p < 0.05$). In addition, the frequency of nociceptive responses during the normally quiet intermediate phase was similar to that of the late phase of the formalin test.

3.2. Hot-Plate Latency Assay

We tested the effects of oral dosing of MSG on baseline heat pain thresholds in mice. Previous studies showed no significant changes vs. the control group in hot-plate assay after seven days of MSG oral administration, for either 150 mg/kg or 300 mg/kg dosage. Only a slight, non-significant, reduction of the pain threshold was seen, after 14 days of MSG 300 mg/kg administration (data not published). Oral administration of MSG in doses of 150 mg/kg and 300 mg/kg significantly reduced the average latency of hind-paw lifting vs. baseline (−29.69% and −40.43%, respectively, all $p < 0.05$), following 21 days of administration. However, only the dose of 300 mg/kg MSG significantly reduced (−30.03%, $p < 0.05$) the average latency of hind-paw lifting vs. control (Figure 2). For the latency of jumping time, a significantly larger number of animals jumped when compared to the control group (data not shown).

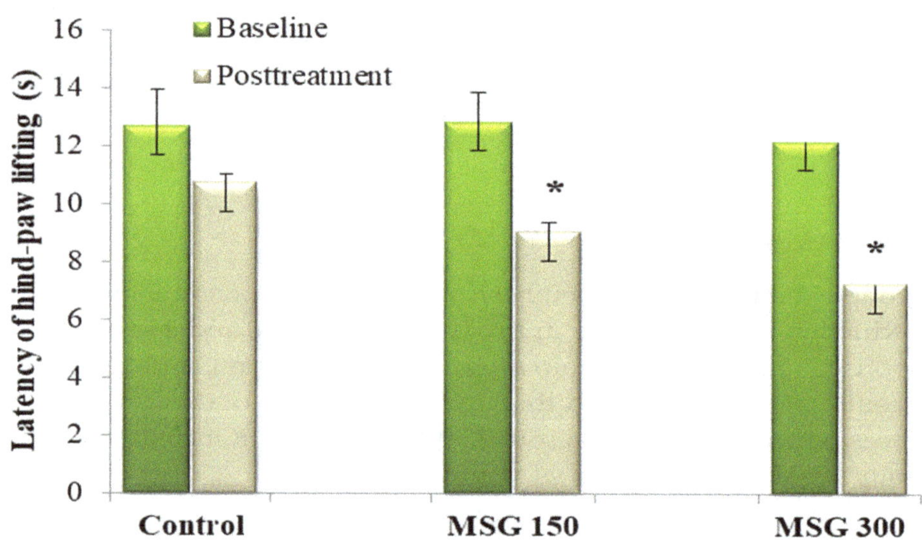

Figure 2. Medium latency of hind-paw lifting ± SEM before and after 21 days of MSG exposure. * Statistical significance vs. baseline (Student's *t*-Test, 90% CI, $p < 0.05$) and control group (Student's *t*-Test, 90% CI, $p < 0.05$).

3.3. Assay of NO-Synthase (NOS) Activity

NOS activity was assessed indirectly, by determining the concentration of NO metabolites (NOx). Administration of 300 mg/kg MSG for 21 days determined an increase of NOx concentration in the brain, and therefore an intensification of NOS activity in brain tissue (Figure 3). There were no changes in the total concentration of brain proteins when compared with the control.

We established a direct correlation between the increase in NOx concentration and the hyperalgic response to repeated administration of MSG (Spearman correlation, $p < 0.05$). Further studies will establish the effect of MSG administration on NOx in nociceptive behavior-naïve mice.

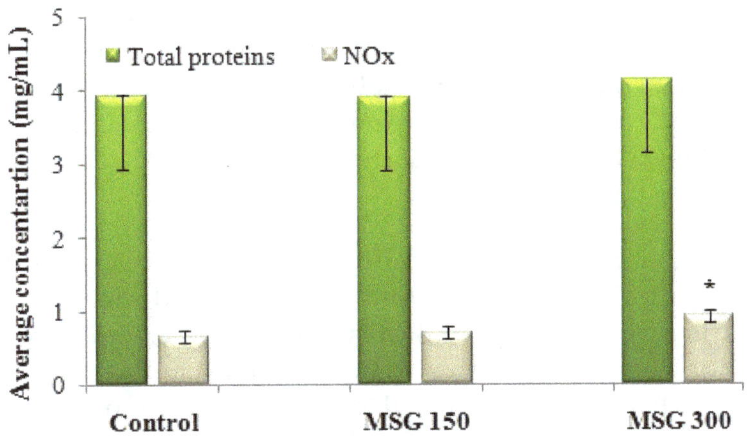

Figure 3. Average concentration of NO metabolites (NOx) in brain tissue after 21 days of exposure to distilled water (control) or MSG (150 mg/kg or 300 mg/kg). NOx concentration, as determined with the Griess method (x), is reported against the total protein concentration assessed in the same sample of brain tissue (y). The NOx concentration per 1 mg of protein = x/y. * Statistical significance vs. control (Student's *t*-Test, 90% CI, $p < 0.05$).

4. Discussion

Administration of MSG in a dosage of 300 mg/kg reduces the thermal nociceptive threshold and increases nociceptive behavior. The effect of MSG on the thermal threshold was correlated with an increase in NOx concentration, which suggests that the hyperalgic effect of MSG could be mediated via this messenger.

There is no literature data on the effect of MSG oral administration on the thermal threshold, as far as we know. Hot-plate is an objective, quantifiable, specific central antinociceptive test used to study the response to a noxious thermal stimulus [25,26]. The involvement of nitric oxide in nociceptive processing is generally recognized, with this molecule playing a pivotal role in hyperalgesia and central sensitization [27].

The formalin test assesses nociception as well as inflammation. Injection of formalin induces a biphasic response; the early first phase is neurogenic, and results from direct stimulation of nociceptors. This leads to the activation of sensory C-fibers through the transient receptor potential A1 receptors [28] in the paw, and the consequent release of substance P and bradykinin [29]. The late phase is inflammatory, and is due to the release of histamine, serotonin, bradykinin, prostaglandins, sympathomimetic amines, tumor necrosis factor-alpha and interleukins [30,31]. Central sensitization is partly responsible for the prolonged second phase of this test [32].

MSG administered in a dose of 300 mg/kg determined a significant increase in the mean reaction time vs. the control group for phase 2 of the formalin test. More importantly, a similar pattern of nociceptive response was seen during the normally quiet intermediate phase, as in the late phase of the formalin test. This may suggest MSG treatment shifts the tonic phase of formalin nociception to an earlier time point, possibly by enhancing the processes involved in mediating the sensitization in the spinal cord. Data from the literature support our findings regarding the correlation between the administration of MSG and the results of the formalin test. The enhancement of hyperalgesia in rats treated with L-glutamate was reversed by pretreatment with L-NAME. L-glutamate enhances hyperalgesia and persistent nociception following formalin-induced tissue injury, which seems to be mediated by intracellular messengers, including nitric oxide. Intrathecal pretreatment with inhibitors of nitric oxide synthase reduced formalin injury-induced nociceptive behaviors. L-NAME affected the tonic, but not the acute, phase of the formalin response. Conversely, formalin-induced nociceptive responses were enhanced by stimulators of nitric oxide such as sodium nitroprusside [33].

The increase in response during the inflammatory phase could be explained by a NO-induced rise in peripheral concentrations of prostaglandin E2 and prostacyclin, a phenomenon reported by several authors [13,16]. This increase was completely impeded by the NOS inhibitors. In vitro assays support the hypothesis that NO activates cyclooxygenases [34]. These results indicate that NO can also induce peripheral hyperalgesia by regulation of the expression and/or activity of cyclooxygenases, resulting in an increase of prostaglandins release.

The implications of MSG consumption could go further than hyperalgesia, since glutamate induces astrocyte mitochondrial apoptosis. Glutamate increased the expression of representative apoptotic markers, including cleaved caspase-8, cleaved caspase-9, and cleaved caspase-3, as well as level key markers in endoplasmic reticulum stress, in primary cultured spinal cord astrocytes [35]. This opens the way for further investigations: Does administration of MSG impacts spinal cord astrocytes? And what would the consequence be, taking into account the multiple roles of these cells in central nervous system CNS, and given that their apoptosis subsequently leads to CNS injury?

Our findings raise some questions regarding the safety of long-term MSG consumption, and represent a good starting point for any clinical tests focused on examining the impact of MSG nutritional intake on hyperalgesia.

One of these questions concerns the possible interactions between MSG and some analgesics; opioids, non-steroidal anti-inflammatory drugs, and natural products have peripheral and central antinociceptive effect mediated via L-arginine/NO-cGMP pathway [36,37]. Ventura-Martinez et al. showed that acute or chronic administration of L-arginine to mice decreases morphine analgesia. The inhibitory effect of L-arginine on morphine-analgesia and entry into the CNS is blocked by the NOS inhibitor L-NNA [38].

Another issue regards the effect of MSG consumption on pain perception in healthy humans, as well as in those suffering from maladies involving chronic pain. Already, this food additive is classified as a causative substance of headache in the International Classification of Headache Disorders, 3rd edition (ICHD-III beta), and has been found to increase the frequency of fibromyalgia symptoms [7]. Further studies need to be made in order to evaluate the impact of MSG consumption on pain associated with injuries, nerve lesions and degenerative diseases such as osteoarthritis.

Acknowledgments: The authors acknowledge the financial support offered by Romanian National Authority for Scientific Research UEFISCDI through grant PN-II-RU-TE-2014-4-1670, No. 342/2015. The costs to publish in open access were supported by the aforementioned grant.

Author Contributions: A.Z. literature research, performed the pharmacological assays, article preparation; A.N.C. experimental design of pharmacological tests; G.M.N. statistical analysis, literature research, article preparation; B.S.V. performed the biological assays; D.G. development of biochemical assays.

References

1. Kwok, R.H.M. Chinese-Restaurant Syndrome. *N. Engl. J. Med.* **1968**, *278*, 796. [PubMed]
2. Evaluation of Food Additives. Specifications for the identity and purity of food additives and their toxocological evaluation: Some extraction solvents and certain other substances; and a review of the technological efficacy of some antimicrobial agents. *World Health Organ. Tech. Rep. Ser.* **1971**, *462*, 1–36.
3. Joint FAO/WHO Expert Committee on Food Additives; World Health Organization; Food and Agriculture Organization of the United Nations. Toxicological evaluation of certain food additives with a review of general principles and of specifications. Seventeenth report of the joint FAO-WHO Expert Committee on Food Additives. *World Health Organ. Tech. Rep. Ser.* **1974**, *539*, 1–40.
4. Walker, R.; Lupien, J.R. The safety evaluation of monosodium glutamate. *J. Nutr.* **2000**, *130*, 1049S–1052S. [PubMed]

5. Beyreuther, K.; Biesalski, H.K.; Fernstrom, J.D.; Grimm, P.; Hammes, W.P.; Heinemann, U.; Kempski, O.; Stehle, P.; Steinhart, H.; Walker, R. Consensus meeting: Monosodium glutamate—An update. *Eur. J. Clin. Nutr.* **2006**, *61*, 304–313. [CrossRef] [PubMed]
6. Shimada, A.; Baad-Hansen, L.; Castrillon, E.; Ghafouri, B.; Stensson, N.; Gerdle, B.; Ernberg, M.; Cairns, B.; Svensson, P.; Svensson Odont, P. Differential effects of repetitive oral administration of monosodium glutamate on interstitial glutamate concentration and muscle pain sensitivity. *Nutrition* **2015**, *31*, 315–323. [CrossRef] [PubMed]
7. Holton, K.F.; Taren, D.L.; Thomson, C.A.; Bennett, R.M.; Jones, K.D. The effect of dietary glutamate on fibromyalgia and irritable bowel symptoms. *Clin. Exp. Rheumatol.* **2012**, *30*, 10–17. [PubMed]
8. Hoffman, E.M.; Zhang, Z.; Schechter, R.; Miller, K.E. Glutaminase increases in rat dorsal root ganglion neurons after unilateral adjuvant-induced hind paw inflammation. *Biomolecules* **2016**, *6*, 10. [CrossRef] [PubMed]
9. Szekely, J.I.; Torok, K.; Mate, G. The Role of Ionotropic Glutamate Receptors in Nociception with Special Regard to the AMPA Binding Sites. *Curr. Pharm. Des.* **2002**, *8*, 887–912. [CrossRef] [PubMed]
10. Larsson, M. Ionotropic Glutamate Receptors in Spinal Nociceptive Processing. *Mol. Neurobiol.* **2009**, *40*, 260–288. [CrossRef] [PubMed]
11. Neugebauer, V. Metabotropic glutamate receptors–important modulators of nociception and pain behavior. *Pain* **2002**, *98*, 1–8. [CrossRef]
12. Chiechio, S. Chapter Three-Modulation of Chronic Pain by Metabotropic Glutamate Receptors. *Adv. Pharm.* **2016**, *75*, 63–89.
13. Chen, Z.; Muscoli, C.; Doyle, T.; Bryant, L.; Cuzzocrea, S.; Mollace, V.; Mastroianni, R.; Masini, E.; Salvemini, D. NMDA receptor activation and nitroxidative regulation of the glutamatergic pathway during nociceptive processing. *Pain* **2010**, *149*, 100–106. [CrossRef] [PubMed]
14. Gangadharan, V.; Wang, R.; Ulzhöfer, B.; Luo, C.; Bardoni, R.; Bali, K.K.; Agarwal, N.; Tegeder, I.; Hildebrandt, U.; Nagy, G.G.; et al. Peripheral calcium-permeable AMPA receptors regulate chronic inflammatory pain in mice. *J. Clin. Investig.* **2011**, *121*, 1608–1623. [CrossRef] [PubMed]
15. Luo, Z.D.; Cizkova, D. The role of nitric oxide in nociception. *Curr. Rev. Pain* **2000**, *4*, 459–466. [CrossRef] [PubMed]
16. Toriyabe, M.; Omote, K.; Kawamata, T.; Namiki, A. Contribution of Interaction between Nitric Oxide and Cyclooxygenases to the Production of Prostaglandins in Carrageenan-induced Inflammation. *Anesthesiology* **2004**, *101*, 983–990. [CrossRef] [PubMed]
17. Damasceno, F.; Skinner, G.O.; Araújo, P.C.; Ferraz, M.M.D.; Tenório, F.; de Almeida, O.M.M.S. Nitric oxide modulates the hyperalgesic response to mechanical noxious stimuli in sleep-deprived rats. *BMC Neurosci.* **2013**, *14*, 92. [CrossRef] [PubMed]
18. Kuboyama, K.; Tsuda, M.; Tsutsui, M.; Toyohara, Y.; Tozaki-Saitoh, H.; Shimokawa, H.; Yanagihara, N.; Inoue, K. Reduced spinal microglial activation and neuropathic pain after nerve injury in mice lacking all three nitric oxide synthases. *Mol. Pain* **2011**, *7*, 50. [CrossRef] [PubMed]
19. Yoon, Y.W.; Sung, B.; Chung, J.M. Nitric oxide mediates behavioral signs of neuropathic pain in an experimental rat model. *Neuroreport* **1998**, *9*, 367–372. [CrossRef] [PubMed]
20. Chacur, M.; Matos, R.J.B.; Alves, A.S.; Rodrigues, A.C.; Gutierrez, V.; Cury, Y.; Britto, L.R.G. Participation of neuronal nitric oxide synthase in experimental neuropathic pain induced by sciatic nerve transection. *Brazilian J. Med. Biol. Res.* **2010**, *43*, 367–376. [CrossRef] [PubMed]
21. Chen, Y.; Boettger, M.K.; Reif, A.; Schmitt, A.; Üçeyler, N.; Sommer, C. Nitric oxide synthase modulates CFA-induced thermal hyperalgesia through cytokine regulation in mice. *Mol. Pain* **2010**, *6*, 13. [CrossRef] [PubMed]
22. Buzescu, A.; Negres, S.; Călin, O.; Chiriță, C. Experimental demonstration of hyperalgesia induced by repeated ingestion of dietary monosodium glutamate. *Farmacia* **2013**, *61*, 1009–1017.
23. Tsikas, D. Analysis of nitrite and nitrate in biological fluids by assays based on the Griess reaction: Appraisal of the Griess reaction in the L-arginine/nitric oxide area of research. *J. Chromatogr. B* **2007**, *851*, 51–70. [CrossRef] [PubMed]
24. Krohn, R.I. The Colorimetric Detection and Quantitation of Total Protein. In *Current Protocols in Cell Biology*; John Wiley & Sons, Inc.: Hoboken, NJ, USA, 2001.

25. Gunn, A.; Bobeck, E.N.; Weber, C.; Morgan, M.M. The influence of non-nociceptive factors on hot-plate latency in rats. *J. Pain* **2011**, *12*, 222–227. [CrossRef] [PubMed]
26. De Sousa, D.P. Analgesic-like activity of essential oils constituents. *Molecules* **2011**, *16*, 2233–2252. [CrossRef] [PubMed]
27. Cury, Y.; Picolo, G.; Gutierrez, V.P.; Ferreira, S.H. Pain and analgesia: The dual effect of nitric oxide in the nociceptive system. *Nitric Oxide* **2011**, *25*, 243–254. [CrossRef] [PubMed]
28. McNamara, C.R.; Mandel-Brehm, J.; Bautista, D.M.; Siemens, J.; Deranian, K.L.; Zhao, M.; Hayward, N.J.; Chong, J.A.; Julius, D.; Moran, M.M.; et al. TRPA1 mediates formalin-induced pain. *Proc. Natl. Acad. Sci. USA* **2007**, *104*, 13525–13530. [CrossRef] [PubMed]
29. Parada, C.A.; Tambeli, C.H.; Cunha, F.Q.; Ferreira, S.H. The major role of peripheral release of histamine and 5-hydroxytryptamine in formalin-induced nociception. *Neuroscience* **2001**, *102*, 937–944. [CrossRef]
30. Milano, J.; Oliveira, S.M.; Rossato, M.F.; Sauzem, P.D.; Machado, P.; Beck, P.; Zanatta, N.; Martins, M.A.P.; Mello, C.F.; Rubin, M.A.; et al. Antinociceptive effect of novel trihalomethyl-substituted pyrazoline methyl esters in formalin and hot-plate tests in mice. *Eur. J. Pharmacol.* **2008**, *581*, 86–96. [CrossRef] [PubMed]
31. Zeashan, H.; Amresh, G.; Rao, C.V.; Singh, S. Antinociceptive activity of Amaranthus spinosus in experimental animals. *J. Ethnopharmacol.* **2009**, *122*, 492–496. [CrossRef] [PubMed]
32. Coderre, T.J.; Melzack, R. The contribution of excitatory amino acids to central sensitization and persistent nociception after formalin-induced tissue injury. *J. Neurosci.* **1992**, *12*, 3665–3670. [PubMed]
33. Coderre, T.J.; Yashpal, K. Intracellular Messengers Contributing to Persistent Nociception and Hyperalgesia Induced by L-Glutamate and Substance P in the Rat Formalin Pain Model. *Eur. J. Neurosci.* **1994**, *6*, 1328–1334. [CrossRef] [PubMed]
34. Little, J.W.; Doyle, T.; Salvemini, D. Reactive nitroxidative species and nociceptive processing: Determining the roles for nitric oxide, superoxide, and peroxynitrite in pain. *Amino Acids* **2012**, *42*, 75–94. [CrossRef] [PubMed]
35. Zhang, C.; Wang, C.; Ren, J.; Guo, X.; Yun, K. Morphine Protects Spinal Cord Astrocytes from Glutamate-Induced Apoptosis via Reducing Endoplasmic Reticulum Stress. *Int. J. Mol. Sci.* **2016**, *17*, 1523. [CrossRef] [PubMed]
36. Ventura-Martínez, R.; Déciga-Campos, M.; Díaz-Reval, M.I.; González-Trujano, M.E.; López-Muñoz, F.J. Peripheral involvement of the nitric oxide-cGMP pathway in the indomethacin-induced antinociception in rat. *Eur. J. Pharmacol.* **2004**, *503*, 43–48. [CrossRef] [PubMed]
37. Déciga-Campos, M.; López-Muñoz, F.J. Participation of the L-arginine-nitric oxide-cyclic GMP-ATP-sensitive K^+ channel cascade in the antinociceptive effect of rofecoxib. *Eur. J. Pharmacol.* **2004**, *484*, 193–199. [CrossRef] [PubMed]
38. Hishikawa, K.; Nakaki, T.; Tsuda, M.; Esumi, H.; Ohshima, H.; Suzuki, H.; Saruta, T.; Kato, R. Effect of systemic L-arginine administration on hemodynamics and nitric oxide release in man. *Jpn. Heart J.* **1992**, *33*, 41–48. [CrossRef] [PubMed]

7

Natural Dietary Supplementation of Curcumin Protects Mice Brains against Ethanol-Induced Oxidative Stress-Mediated Neurodegeneration and Memory Impairment via Nrf2/TLR4/RAGE Signaling

Muhammad Ikram †, Kamran Saeed †, Amjad Khan, Tahir Muhammad, Muhammad Sohail Khan, Min Gi Jo, Shafiq Ur Rehman and Myeong Ok Kim *

Division of Applied Life Science (BK 21), College of Natural Sciences, Gyeongsang National University, Jinju 52828, Korea; qazafi417@gnu.ac.kr (M.I.); kamran.biochem@gnu.ac.kr (K.S.); amjadkhan@gnu.ac.kr (A.K.); mtahir.khan@gnu.ac.kr (T.M.); sohail.bannu@gnu.ac.kr (M.S.K.); mingi.cho@gnu.ac.kr (M.G.J.); shafiq12@gnu.ac.kr (S.U.R.)

* Correspondence: mokim@gnu.ac.kr

† These authors contributed equally to this paper.

Abstract: The aim of the current study was to explore the underlying neuroprotective mechanisms of curcumin (50 mg/kg, for six weeks) against ethanol (5 mg/kg i.p., for six weeks) induced oxidative stress and inflammation-mediated cognitive dysfunction in mice. According to our findings, ethanol triggered reactive oxygen species (ROS), apoptosis, neuroinflammation, and memory impairment, which were significantly inhibited with the administration of curcumin, as assessed by ROS, lipid peroxidation (LPO), and Nrf2/HO-1 (nuclear factor erythroid 2-related factor 2/Heme-oxygenase-1) expression in the experimental mice brains. Moreover, curcumin regulated the expression of the glial cell markers in ethanol-treated mice brains, as analyzed by the relative expression TLR4 (Toll like Receptor 4), RAGE (Receptor for Advanced Glycations End products), GFAP (Glial fibrillary acidic protein), and Iba-1 (Ionized calcium binding adaptor molecule 1), through Western blot and confocal microscopic analysis. Moreover, our results showed that curcumin downregulated the expression of p-JNK (Phospo c-Jun N-Terminal Kinase), p-NF-kB (nuclear factor kappa-light-chain-enhancer of activated B cells), and its downstream targets, as assessed by Western blot and confocal microscopic analysis. Finally, the expression of synaptic proteins and the behavioral results also supported the hypothesis that curcumin may inhibit memory dysfunction and behavioral alterations associated with ethanol intoxication. Altogether, to the best of our knowledge, we believe that curcumin may serve as a potential, promising, and cheaply available neuroprotective compound against ethanol-associated neurodegenerative diseases.

Keywords: neurodegenerative diseases; oxidative stress; neuroinflammation; apoptosis; synaptic dysfunction

---

1. Introduction

Alcohol is a sedative agent and is pharmacologically similar to other hypnotic drugs, which makes it a potential candidate for abuse worldwide. In Western, European, and North American populations, the percentage of alcoholics among the adult population varies from 2% to 12% [1]. Alcohol and its derivatives promote physiological, behavioral, and cognitive dysfunctions in consumers [2], so worldwide alcohol dependence is considered to be a serious health issue in the modern world [3]. Ethanol has shown strong neurodegenerative consequences in experimental animal brains [4,5]. The neurodegenerative effects are associated with neuroinflammation, apoptotic cell death [6], and synaptic dysfunction [7,8]. Moreover, it has been shown that the consumption of alcohol leads to the generation of free radicals and to the chain reaction of lipid peroxidation that causes damage to the brain and other vital organs [9,10]. To combat the challenges of free radical generation, a potent antioxidant defense mechanism is of crucial importance. In the journey to find a novel, potent, and effective antioxidant system, naturally occurring compounds have always drawn more attention because of their ease of availability, safety, and efficacy. Many natural compounds and their derivatives have shown efficacy in the management of different neurological disorders [11–13], and are under consideration and evaluation for these disorders. Curcumin, a compound known to inhibit neuroinflammation, reduces plaque deposition in AD (Alzheimer's Disease) models and improves vascular dysfunction [14]. It has been shown to antagonize many steps in the inflammatory cascade [15], including the suppression of nuclear factor-B, iNOS (Inducible nitric oxide synthase), and JNK (c-Jun N-terminal kinases) [13,16]. Moreover, it has shown the best antioxidant effects in mice [17]. It has shown effectiveness against the MPTP (1-methyl-4-phenyl-1,2,3,6-tetrahydropyridine) model of Parkinson's disease [18] and the MCAO (middle cerebral artery occlusion) animal model of the ischemic brain [19]. Based on the promising therapeutic potentials of naturally occurring curcumin, we hypothesized that chronic curcumin administration may inhibit ethanol-induced neurodegeneration and memory impairment in mice, by regulating reactive oxygen species (ROS), toll-like receptor-4 (TLR4), and Receptor for advanced glycation end products (RAGE)-mediated neuroinflammation, while p-JNK and p-NF-kB triggered the release of cytokines and synaptic dysfunction. The main target of the current study is oxidative stress, regulated by nuclear factor erythroid-2 (Nrf2; an endogenous antioxidant enzyme), and neuroinflammation, initiated by the activation of the innate immune response, mostly tailored by the activation of TLR4 and RAGE, playing a role in recognizing the microbial-associated molecular patterns initiating and modulating the immune response. The activation of the TLR4 signaling promotes the phosphorylation of NF-kB, thereby promoting the inflammatory effects [20]. The signals generated by both the RAGE and TLR4 receptors funnel to the same pathway of neuroinflammation [21]. Compounds counteracting the abnormal ROS generation, inhibition of TLR4/RAGE, and inhibition of the phosphorylation of JNK/NF-kB signaling may render protection to the brain against the mediators of neurodegeneration. Here, we have made an attempt to explore the underlying neuroprotective mechanisms of chronic curcumin administration against ethanol-induced neurodegeneration and memory impairment, by targeting the oxidative stress, neuroinflammation, and apoptotic cell death.

2. Materials and Methods

2.1. Chemicals and Antibodies

The antibodies used in the Western blot and immunofluorescence studies were anti-Nrf2 (sc-722), anti-HO1 (sc-136,961), anti-synaptosomal-associated protein 23 (SNAP-23) (sc-374,215), anti-PSD-95 (sc-71,933), anti-Syntaxin (sc-12,736), anti-tumor necrosis factor-α (TNF-α) (sc-52,746), anti-PARP-1 (sc-8007), TLR4 (sc-16240), Synaptophysin (sc-17750), anti-interleukin (IL)-1β (sc-32,294), anti-Bax (sc-7480), anti-Bcl2 (sc-7382), anti-p-NF-κB (sc-136,548), anti-Iba-1 (sc-32,725), anti-Glial fibrillary acidic protein (GFAP; sc-33,673), and anti-β- actin (sc-47,778) (Santa Cruz Biotechnology, Dallas, TX, USA). In addition, the anti-Cleaved Caspase-3 (#9664) antibodies were obtained from Cell Signaling Technology (Danvers, MA, USA). For Syntaxin and β-actin, the antibodies were diluted in TBST (1:10000) (Santa Cruz Biotechnology, Dallas, TX, USA). Other primary antibodies were diluted in 1x TBST (1:1000), and Secondary anti-mouse HRP (Horseradish peroxidase) conjugated (Promega Ref# W402) and anti-rabbit HRP conjugated (Promega Ref# W401) were diluted 1:10,000 in 1× TBST and were purchased from Promega, (Fitchburg, WI, USA). TAK242, Resatorvid (CAS 243984-11-4), the specific inhibitor of TLR4. For the confocal microscopic studies, the secondary fluorescent antibodies used were goat anti-mouse (Ref# A11029) and goat anti-rabbit (Ref# 32732) diluted in 1× PBS.

2.2. *Animals Grouping and Drugs Administration*

Male mice (C57BL/6N, $n = 60$, mice 25 ± 3 g, eight old weeks) were acclimatized to the animal house environment for one week, at 12/12 h light/dark cycles at room temperature. The study was approved and conducted in accordance with the guidelines of the Institutional Animal Care and Use Committee (IACUC) of the Division of Applied Life Science, Gyeongsang National University, South Korea (approval ID: 125). Efforts were made to minimize the number of animals used, as well as their suffering. The mice were randomly divided into three groups. (1) The control group mice were treated with an equal volume of vehicle intraperitoneally (physiological saline 0.1 mL/100 g/day) for six weeks, and the mice were freely allowed water and food ad-libitum. (2) The ethanol group mice were treated with an intraperitoneal injection of ethanol for six weeks (5 g/kg i.p., for six weeks, daily). (3) The ethanol and curcumin group mice were treated with curcumin 50 mg/kg for six weeks, daily. The doses of ethanol and curcumin were purely selected on the bases of previously published papers [22]. After the completion of the treatment and behavioral analysis, the mice were sacrificed.

2.3. *Tissues Collections for Molecular and Morphological Analysis*

For biochemical studies, the mice (8–10/group) were anesthetized, sacrificed, and the brain sections were separated. Next, the brain tissue was homogenized in a protein extraction solution (PRO-PREP^{TM}), according to the instructions (iNtRON Biotechnology, Inc., Sungnam, South Korea). After homogenization, the samples were centrifuged at 13,000 r.p.m. at 4 °C for 25 min. The supernatants were collected and stored at −80 °C.

For the morphological studies, the mice (seven to eight per group) were anesthetized and perfused transcardially with saline at a flow rate of 10 mL/min for 3 min, followed by perfusion with a 4% paraformaldehyde solution for 8 min using a peristaltic pump, as provided [23]. The brains were removed and fixed in 4% cold neutral buffer paraformaldehyde for 48 h, and cryoprotected by immersing into a 30% sucrose phosphate buffer for 48 h at 4 °C [23]. After that, the whole brain was frozen in an OCT (optimal cutting temperature compound) compound (Sakura, Torrance, CA, USA), and 14 µm sections were made in the coronal planes using a microtome (Leica cryostat CM 3050S, Nussloch, Germany). The sections were mounted on the probe-on plus charged slides (Fisher, Pittsburgh, PA, USA), and were stored at −70 °C for further analyses.

2.4. *In Vitro Cell Culturing, Drug Treatment, Nuclear Factor-2 Erythroid-2 (Nrf2) Gene Silencing by Small Interfering RNA (siRNA) and Western Blot Analysis*

The mouse hippocampal HT22 and murine BV2 microglial cells were cultured in Dulbecco's modified Eagle's medium (DMEM) supplemented with FBS (Fetal bovine serum) (10%) and penicillin/streptomycin (1%) in a 5% CO2 incubator at 37 °C. After attaining a confluency of 70%, the cells were pretreated for 1 h with ethanol (100 µM), followed by curcumin (2 µM) or Nrf2 siRNA for 24 h, or TAK242 (TLR4 specific inhibitor). The Nrf2 gene was knocked down with Nrf2 siRNA at a concentration of 10 µM per transfection for 36 h, as directed (SC: 37049, Santa Cruz Biotechnology, Inc., Dallas, TX, USA). The transfection was conducted with lipofectamine™2000 reagent (Invitrogen, Waltham, MA, USA) when the cells culture reached to 75–80%. The control group cells were treated with 0.01% Dimethyl sulfoxide (DMSO).

2.5. *Western Blot Analysis*

Western blot was performed as described previously, with some modifications [24,25]. The proteins were loaded and separated by SDS–PAGE (sodium dodecyl sulfate-polyacrylamide gel electrophoresis), and transferred to a polyvinylidene difluoride (PVDF) membrane (Immobilon-P^{SQ}, Transfer membrane, Merck Millipore, Burlington, MA, USA). The immunoreaction was carried out for 16 h at 4 °C using an appropriate ratio of the primary antibodies. After that, the membranes were washed with 1× TBST three times for 10 min, and reacted with a horseradish peroxidase-conjugated secondary antibody for

2 h, as appropriate. The expression of the respective proteins was detected using an ECL (Enhanced chemiluminescence) -detection reagent, according to the manufacturer's instructions. The expressions of the different proteins were obtained on X-ray films and were scanned, and the optical densities of the bands were analyzed by densitometry, using the computer-based ImageJ software (version 1.50, NIH, https://imagej.nih.gov/ij/, Bethesda, MD, USA).

2.6. *Immunofluorescence Staining*

The fluorescence assay was performed as mentioned previously [26,27]. The slides were dried overnight at room temperature, washed with PBS (0.01 mM) for 8–10 min (two times), treated with proteinase K for 5 min, rinsed with PBS, and blocked with normal serum (2% goat/rabbit, as appropriate) in PBS, added with 0.1% Triton X-100. After that, the slides were incubated with primary antibodies overnight at 4 °C. The slides were then incubated with tetramethylrhodamine isothiocyanate–fluorescein isothiocyanate (FITC)-labeled secondary antibodies (antirabbit and antimouse, as appropriate), at room temperature for 95 min. The slides were covered using the fluorescent mounting medium. Images were taken using a confocal laser-microscope (FluoView FV 1000 MPE, Olympus, Tokyo, Japan). Integrated density was used for the quantification of the staining intensity and for the amount in the immunofluorescent microscopic image. ImageJ software (wsr@nih.gov., https://imagej.nih.gov/ij/) was used to quantify the integrated density, which represents the sum of the pixel values in an image.

2.7. *ROS Assay*

To analyze the effects of curcumin against ethanol-induced oxidative stress, we conducted a ROS assay, as described previously [28,29]. The assay is based on the oxidation of 2′,7′-dichlorodihydrofluorescein diacetate (CAS 4091-99-0, Santa Cruz Biotechnology, Dallas, TX, USA) to 2′ 7′ dichlorofluorescein (DCF). The brain homogenates were diluted with cold Lock's buffer at 1:20, to yield the final concentration of 2.5 mg tissue/500 μL. The reaction mixture of Lock's buffer (1 mL; pH ± 7.4), 0.2 mL of homogenate, and 10 mL of DCFH-DA (dichlorodihydrofluorescein diacetate) (5 mM) was incubated at room temperature for 15 min, to convert the DCFH-DA to the fluorescent product DCF. The conversion of DCFH-DA to the DCF was analyzed using a spectrofluorimeter (Promega, Fitchburg, WI, USA), with excitation at 484 nm and emission at 530 nm. For the background fluorescence (conversion of DCFH-DA in the absence of homogenate), parallel blanks were measured. The quantitative expression of ROS has been shown with a histogram.

2.8. *Determination of Lipid Peroxidation*

Lipid peroxidation (LPO) is used to assess oxidative stress. Free malondialdehyde (MDA), which is an indicator of LPO, was analyzed in the tissue homogenates, by using a lipid peroxidation (MDA) colorimetric/fluorometric assay kit (BioVision, San Francesco, CA, USA, Cat#739-100), according to the manufacturer's instructions.

2.9. *Morris Water Maze Test*

The behavioral analysis was done by the MWM (Morris Water Maze) and Y-maze test (n = 12 mice/group), as performed previously [30,31]. The apparatus used for the analysis was made of a circular tank (100 cm in diameter, 40 cm in height), containing water (23 ± 1 °C) to a depth of 15.5 cm. The water was made opaque by adding a non-toxic white color. A platform made of white plastic was kept 1 cm below the water surface, at one quadrant. For five consecutive days, the mice were trained consecutively. The latency to escape from the water (searching the hidden platform) was calculated for each trial. On the sixth day, the probe test was conducted for the evaluation of the memory effects. The probe test was conducted by removing the platform and allowing the mice to explore the tank freely for one hour. The time spent by the mice in the target quadrant and the number of crossings over the position of the platform were recorded. The time spent in the target quadrant was taken to show the degree of memory changes. The data were recorded using video-tracking software (SMART Panlab, Harvard Apparatus, Holliston, MA, USA).

2.10. Y-Maze Test

The apparatus used for the evaluation of the Y-maze was made of black-painted wood, and the dimensions of the arms were 50 cm long and 20 cm height and 10 cm width, as already used by our group [32] and others [33]. The mice were allowed to move freely in the Y-maze, and for that, the mice were kept in the center of the apparatus for 8 min, three times. The arm entries were visualized and observed carefully. The successive entry of the mice into the arms was defined as spontaneous alternations. The alternation behaviors were considered as (successive triplet sets (entries into three different arms consecutively)/total number of arm entries (2)) × 100. A higher percentage (%) of spontaneous alternations was considered to be an indicator of the improved cognitive performance of the experimental mice, and vice versa.

2.11. Fluoro-Jade B Staining

The Fluoro-Jade B staining was done as described previously [28], and according to the instructions provided (Burlington, MA, USA, Cat #AG310, Lot #2159662). The slides were dried at room temperature for 24 h. Furthermore, the slides were dipped in a solution of 1% sodium hydroxide and 80% ethanol, for five min. After that, the slides were kept in 70% ethanol for 2 min and in D-water for 2 min, transferred into a potassium permanganate solution (0.06%) for 10 min, rinsed with D-water, and kept in 0.1% acetic acid solution and 0.01% Fluoro-Jade B solution for 20 min, washed with D-water, and dried for 10 min. The sections were covered using a DPX mounting medium, and the images were taken using a confocal laser microscope (FV 1000, Olympus, Tokyo, Japan). Integrated density was used for the quantification of the staining intensity and for the amount in the immunofluorescent microscopic image. ImageJ software (wsr@nih.gov, https://imagej.nih.gov/ij/) was used to quantify the integrated density, which represents the sum of the pixel values in an image.

2.12. Nissl Staining

Nissl staining was performed according to the previously used methods [34], so as to visualize the histological changes in the brain. The slides were washed with 0.01 M BPS, twice for 15 min, and stained with 0.5% cresyl violet solution (containing a few drops of glacial acetic acid) for 12 to 15 min. Then, the sections were washed with D-water and dehydrated in ethanols (70%, 95%, and 100%), and xylene was dropped on the slides and covered by using the non-fluorescent mounting medium. The neurodegeneration was visualized by light microscope, and the densities of the cells were counted by using ImageJ software.

2.13. Data Analysis and Statistics

The densities of the bands were analyzed by densitometry using the ImageJ software. We performed one-way ANOVA (Analysis of variance) with Tukey's post-hoc test for comparisons among the different experimental groups. The data are presented as the "mean (SD)" of 7–10 mice per group, and are representative of three independent experiments. The calculations and graphs were generated by using Prism 6 software (GraphPad Software, San Diego, CA, USA). Ω is significantly different from the vehicle-treated, Φ is significantly different from the ethanol-treated group. Significance = Ω, $p < 0.05$, Φ, $p < 0.05$, and Ψ, $p < 0.05$.

3. Results

3.1. Chronic Administration of Curcumin Inhibits Ethanol-Induced Oxidative Stress in Mice Brains and In-Vitro HT22 Cells

Oxidative stress has been a significant player in ethanol [35] and other neurotoxins-induced neurodegenerative disorders [36,37]. To find the potential effects of curcumin against ethanol-induced oxidative stress, we performed ROS and LPO assays. According to our findings, curcumin inhibits the elevated level of LPO and ROS (Figure 1A,B). Similarly, the other main antioxidant genes, Nrf2/HO-1, were also analyzed in the experimental groups. According to our Western blot and confocal findings, the chronic co-administration of curcumin with ethanol inhibited the suppression of Nrf2/HO-1 in the mice brains, thereby preserving the endogenous antioxidant mechanism of the brains (Figure 2C,D). Furthermore, we observed a reduced expression of Nrf2 and its target genes HO-1, in the ethanol (100 μM) exposed HT22 cells, which was markedly reversed by curcumin (2 μM), thereby upregulating the expression of Nrf2 and HO-1 in the cells. Interestingly, curcumin could not upregulate the expression of Nrf2/HO-1 in the ethanol-treated cell lines, where the Nrf2 genes were knocked down by Nrf2 siRNA (Figure 1E), indicating that curcumin abrogated the elevated ROS, by upregulating the Nrf2 genes, and the downstream targets of Nrf2.

3.2. Chronic Administration of Curcumin Attenuates Ethanol-Induced Astrocytes and Microglia Activation in Ethanol-Treated Mouse Brains and In-Vitro Microglial Cells

Previous literature has shown that there is activated microglia and astrocytes with ethanol intoxication [4], which may promote neurological disorders such as AD and dementia [38]. TLR4, a receptor for innate immune response, has been shown to be upregulated with ethanol; another receptor is RAGE, which has been shown to be playing a similar role in the inflammatory signaling. Our findings demonstrate that there was a significant reduction in the activation of both of the receptors in the curcumin-treated group. The Glial fibrillary acidic protein (GFAP) and ionized calcium-binding adaptor 1 (Iba-1) are assigned markers for the activities of astrocytes and microglia, respectively [28]. According to our Western blot and confocal microscopic results, there was an increased expression of GFAP and Iba-1 in the ethanol-treated mice brains, which was significantly rescued with the administration of curcumin (Figure 2). Furthermore, the in vitro findings also showed an enhanced expression of TLR4 and Iba-1 in the ethanol treated BV-2 microglial cells, which were significantly reduced in the curcumin and TAK242 (a specific inhibitor of TLR4) treated cells.

3.3. Chronic Administration of Curcumin Regulated Ethanol-Induced Inflammatory Markers in Mouse Brains

Previous studies have shown that ethanol intoxication is responsible for the activation of stress-markers and inducing inflammatory cytokines [39]. To explore whether these markers may be inhibited with the administration of curcumin, we analyzed the expression of stress and inflammatory markers, such as p-JNK, p-NF-κB, cyclooxygenase-2 (COX-2), interleukin-1β (IL-1β), and tissue necrosis factor-α (TNF-α), in the mice brains. As shown here, treatment with ethanol elevated the expression of p-JNK, p-Nf-κB, IL-1β, COX-2, and TNF-α. However, the mice that were co-administered the curcumin and ethanol had a lower expression of these markers compared with the ethanol-treated group, supporting the hypothesis that curcumin inhibits the expression of inflammatory cytokines, thereby rendering protection to mice brains against ethanol-induced neurodegeneration. The Western blot results were further supported by the confocal microscopic analysis, which showed that curcumin inhibits the effects of ethanol against the activation of p-JNK in mice brains (Figure 3).

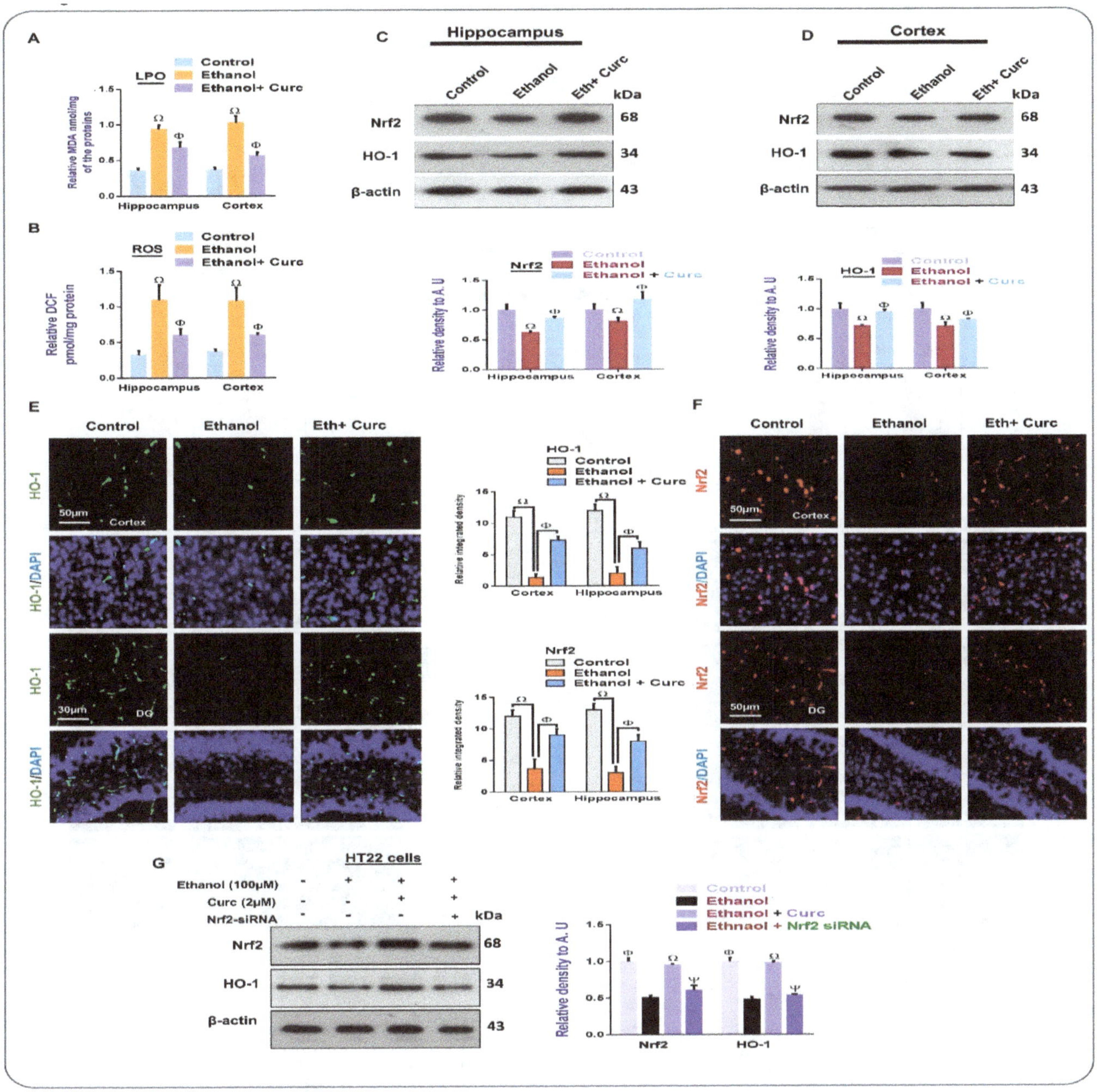

Figure 1. Chronic administration of curcumin inhibits ethanol-induced oxidative stress in mice brain: (**A** & **B**) Results of lipid peroxidation (LPO) and reactive oxygen species (ROS) assays, respectively; (**C** & **D**) Western blot results of nuclear factor erythroid 2-related factor 2 (Nrf2) & heme-oxygenase 1 (HO-1), in the mice brain; (**E** & **F**) Confocal microscopic results of HO-1, and Nrf2 in the experimental groups, with bar graphs, magnification 30×, scale bar 50 μm; (**G**) In vitro HT22 cells treated with ethanol. Curcumin or ethanol + curcumin, and Ω, significantly different from the vehicle-treated, Φ, significantly different from the ethanol-treated group, and Ψ, significantly different from the ethanol + Curc treated group. DG means dentate gyrus, Significance = Φ $p < 0.05$; Ω, $p < 0.05$; Ψ, $p < 0.05$. MDA: malondialdehyde, DCF: 2′ 7′ dichlorofluorescein, eth: ethanol, curc: curcumin.

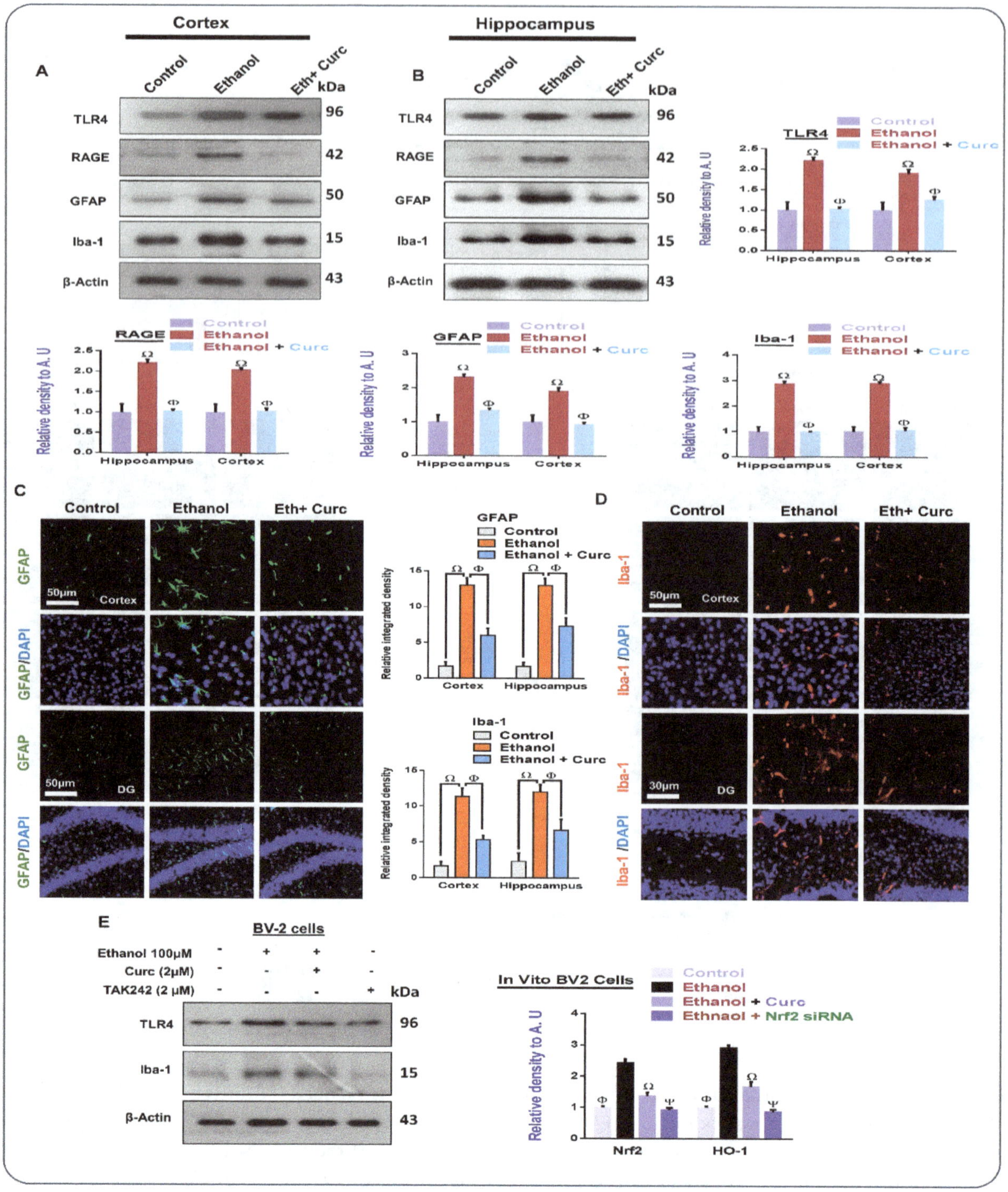

Figure 2. Curcumin Rescued activated Microglia and Astrocytes in the ethanol-treated Mouse Brains: (**A & B**) The Western blot results of toll-like receptor 4 (TLR4), Receptor for Advanced Glycations End Product (RAGE), glial fibrillary acidic protein (GFAP), and ionized calcium binding adaptor molecule 1 (Iba-1) in the brains of the experimental groups; (**C**) Immunofluorescence images of the expression of GFAP in the experimental groups; (**D**) Immunofluorescence images of Iba-1 in the experimental groups ($n = 12$ mice per group); (**E**) Immunoblot results of TLR4 and Iba-1 in BV-2 Cells, in different experimental groups. Magnification 30× objective field, scale bar = 50 μm & 30 μm. Ω, significantly different from the vehicle-treated, Φ, significantly different from the ethanol-treated group and Ψ, significantly different from the ethanol + Curc treated group. DG means dentate gyrus, Significance = Φ $p < 0.05$; Ω, $p < 0.05$; Ψ, $p < 0.05$. eth: ethanol, curc: curcumin, DAPI: 4′,6-diamidino-2-phenylindole dihydrochloride.

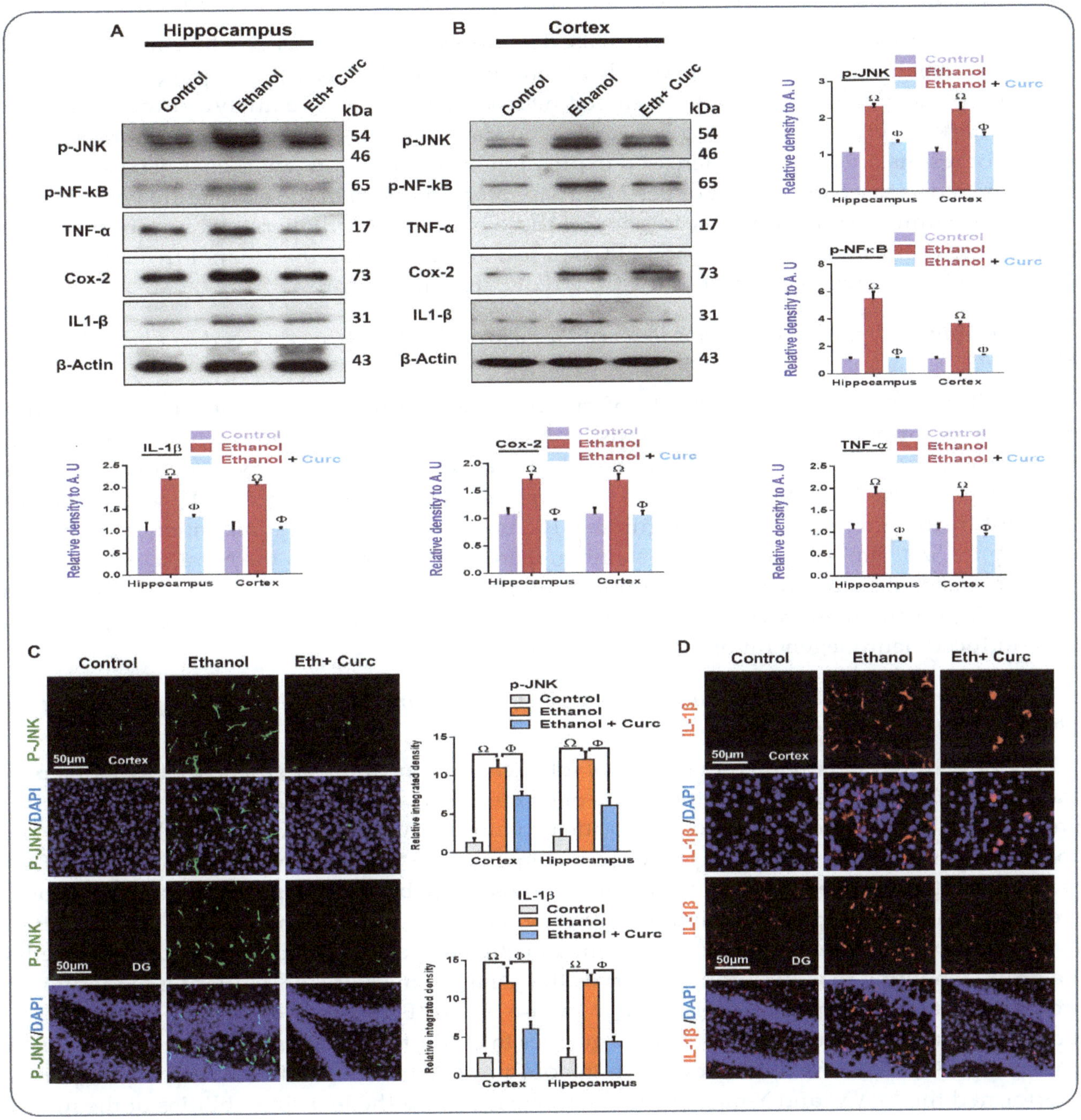

Figure 3. Curcumin Abrogates the Phosphorylation of c-Jun N-Terminal Kinase (JNK) and its Downstream Targets in Ethanol-Treated Mouse Brain: (**A** & **B**) Immunoblot results, showing the expression of active phospho c-Jun N-terminal kinase (p-JNK), nuclear factor kappa-light-chain enhancer of activated B cells (p-NF-kB), tumor necrosis factor alpha (TNF-α), cyclooxygenase-2 (COX-2), and IL- 1β and in mice that received saline, ethanol, and ethanol plus Curcumin for 6 weeks (n = 12 mice per group), normalized with its β-actin, as a loading control, with its Histograms; (**C** & **D**). Confocal images, showing active JNK and interleukin-1β (IL-1β) in the mouse brain. Magnification 30× objective field, scale bar = 50 μm, Ω, significantly different from the vehicle-treated, Φ, significantly different from the ethanol-treated group. DG means dentate gyrus, Significance = Φ $p < 0.05$, Ω, $p < 0.05$. eth: ethanol, curc: curcumin.

3.4. Chronic Administration of Curcumin Rescued Apoptotic Cell Death and Neurodegeneration

Studies have shown that there is an increased expression of apoptotic markers in ethanol-treated mice brains, which leads to apoptotic cell death and neuronal loss [4,40]. Keeping in mind the role of these apoptotic markers in ethanol-induced neurodegeneration, we analyzed the expression of apoptotic markers, including Bax and Bcl-2, Cleaved Caspase-3, and PARP-1 in mice brains. Per our Western blot results, there was an increased expression of pro-apoptotic markers Caspase-3, Bax, and PARP-1, and a decreased expression of Bcl-2 (anti-apoptotic marker) in the ethanol-treated mice brains. However, curcumin regulated the expression of these markers. Moreover, the immunofluorescence results indicated the increased expression of Caspase-3 and PARP-1 in the ethanol-treated mice brains, which were inhibited with chronic administration of curcumin (Figure 4).

3.5. Chronic Administration of Curcumin Rescued the Neuronal Cell Loss, as Assessed by Fluoro-Jade B and Nissl staining

Overall, the neuroprotective effects of curcumin were further confirmed by visualizing the morphology of hippocampal neurons, by using Nissl and FJB staining on the mice brains, as these staining protocols have extensively been used to visualize the morphology of neurons in different experimental settings [41,42]. According to FJB staining, there were increased FJB stained neurons in the ethanol-treated group, which was significantly inhibited with the administration of curcumin, as shown (Figure 5A). Similarly, in the Nissl staining, there was a decrease in the Nissl stained neurons in the ethanol injected group, which was significantly preserved with the administration of curcumin, as shown (Figure 5B), thereby confirming the hypothesis that curcumin plays a rescuing role against ethanol-induced neurodegeneration and memory impairment.

3.6. Chronic Administration of Curcumin Reversed Synaptic Dysfunction and Memory Impairment in the Ethanol-Treated Mouse Brain

Previous studies have shown that ethanol intoxication contributes to the loss of synaptic protein in animal models [39,43]. To explore the effects of curcumin on synaptic marker ethanol-treated mouse brains, we evaluated the expression of synaptic proteins via Western blot and confocal microscopy. According to our findings, the synaptic proteins, including PSD-95, synaptophysin, and SNAP-25, were significantly downregulated in the ethanol-treated mice brains compared with the control mice. Interestingly, curcumin significantly inhibited these effects. The confocal microscopic results of PSD-95 showed significant fluorescence in the curcumin- and ethanol-treated group compared with the ethanol alone group, showing that curcumin preserves the synaptic markers by regulating oxidative stress, neuroinflammation, and apoptotic cell death in mouse brains (Figure 6). Previously, it has been shown that chronic ethanol intoxication causes abnormalities in motor functions and impaired spatial learning and memory [39]. To show whether curcumin could rescue ethanol-induced memory impairment, we performed the MWM and Y-maze tests. First, we recorded the learning abilities of the mice (n = 12 mice/group) with the MWM test. We found that ethanol-treated mice had an enhanced latency to reach to the platform, and the mice that had received curcumin (50 mg/kg, i.p., six weeks) showed a decreased escape latency (Figure 6). Twenty-four hours after the fifth day of training, the platform was removed and the mice were allowed to swim freely. We found that the ethanol-treated mice spent less time in the target quadrant and showed less platform crossings, highlighting that ethanol induces memory impairments. Interestingly, curcumin improved the ethanol-induced memory impairments by increasing the total time spent in the target quadrant, and the number of crossings of the platform (Figure 6F,G). After that, we checked the spontaneous alternation behaviors (showing the spatial working memory or short-term memory) of mice (n = 12 mice/group) in the Y-maze test. In the ethanol-treated mice, there was a reduction in the spontaneous alternation behaviors compared with the saline-treated mice, showing a cognition decline in the ethanol treated mice. Interestingly, curcumin significantly increased the spontaneous alternation behaviors in the ethanol-treated mice compared with the ethanol-treated group (Figure 6H). Collectively, our findings showed that the co-administration of curcumin with ethanol significantly prevents cognitive dysfunctions in mice.

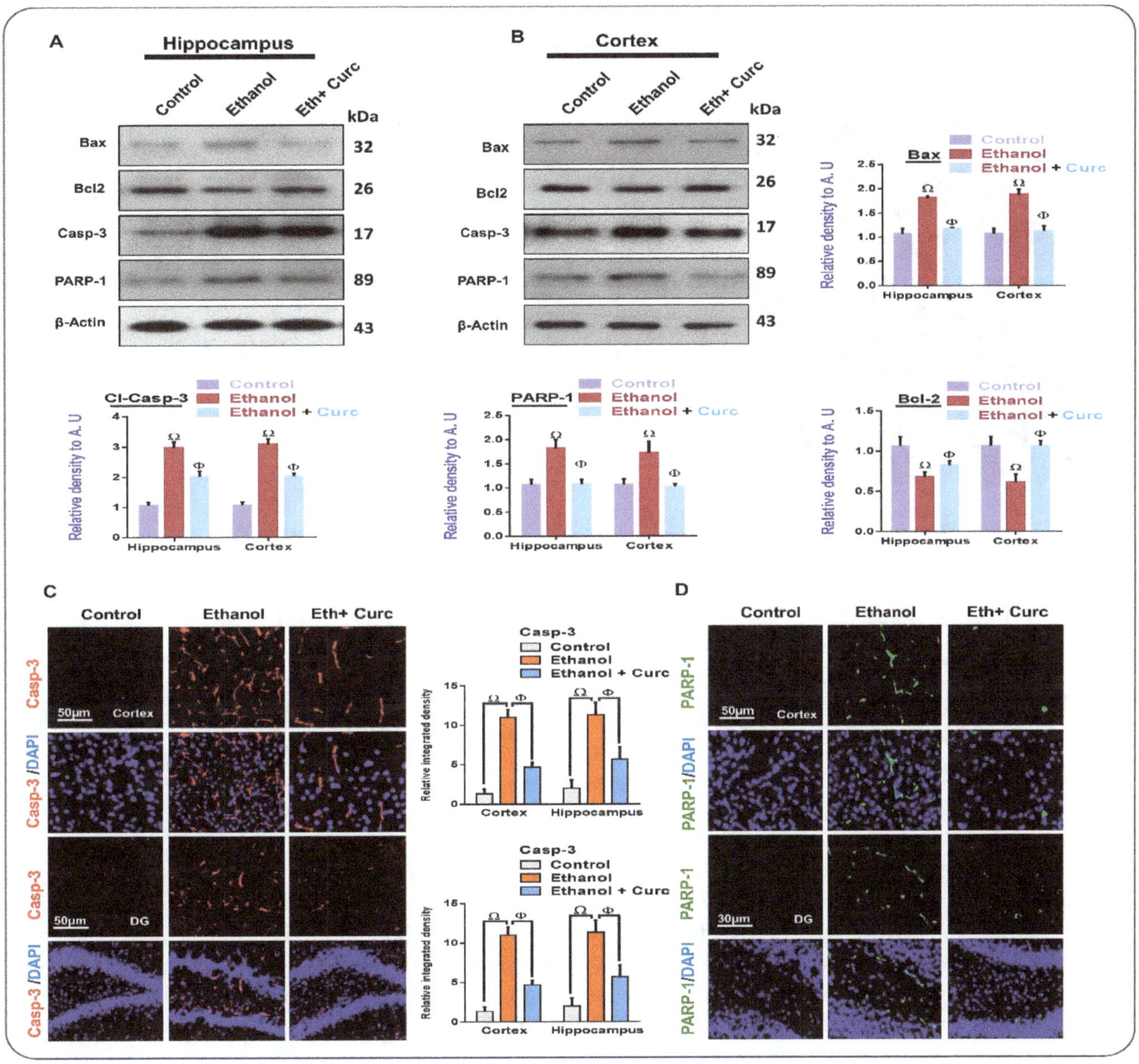

Figure 4. Curcumin Abrogated Ethanol-Induced Apoptotic Cell Death in Mouse Brain: (**A & B**) Immunoblot results of B-cell lymphoma 2-associated X (Bax); , B-cell lymphoma 2 (Bcl-2), Caspase-3, and PARP-1 in the brains of the experimental groups, with their relative bra graphs; (**C & D**) Immunofluorescence results of activated Caspase-3 and poly (ADP-ribose)polymerase 1 (PARP-1) in the brains of the experimental mice, with their histograms ($n = 12$ mice/group), Magnification, 40×, scale bar 50 µm & 30 µm. Ω, significantly different from the vehicle-treated, Φ, significantly different from the ethanol-treated group. DG means dentate gyrus, Significance = Φ $p < 0.05$, Ω, $p < 0.05$. eth: ethanol, curc: curcumin.

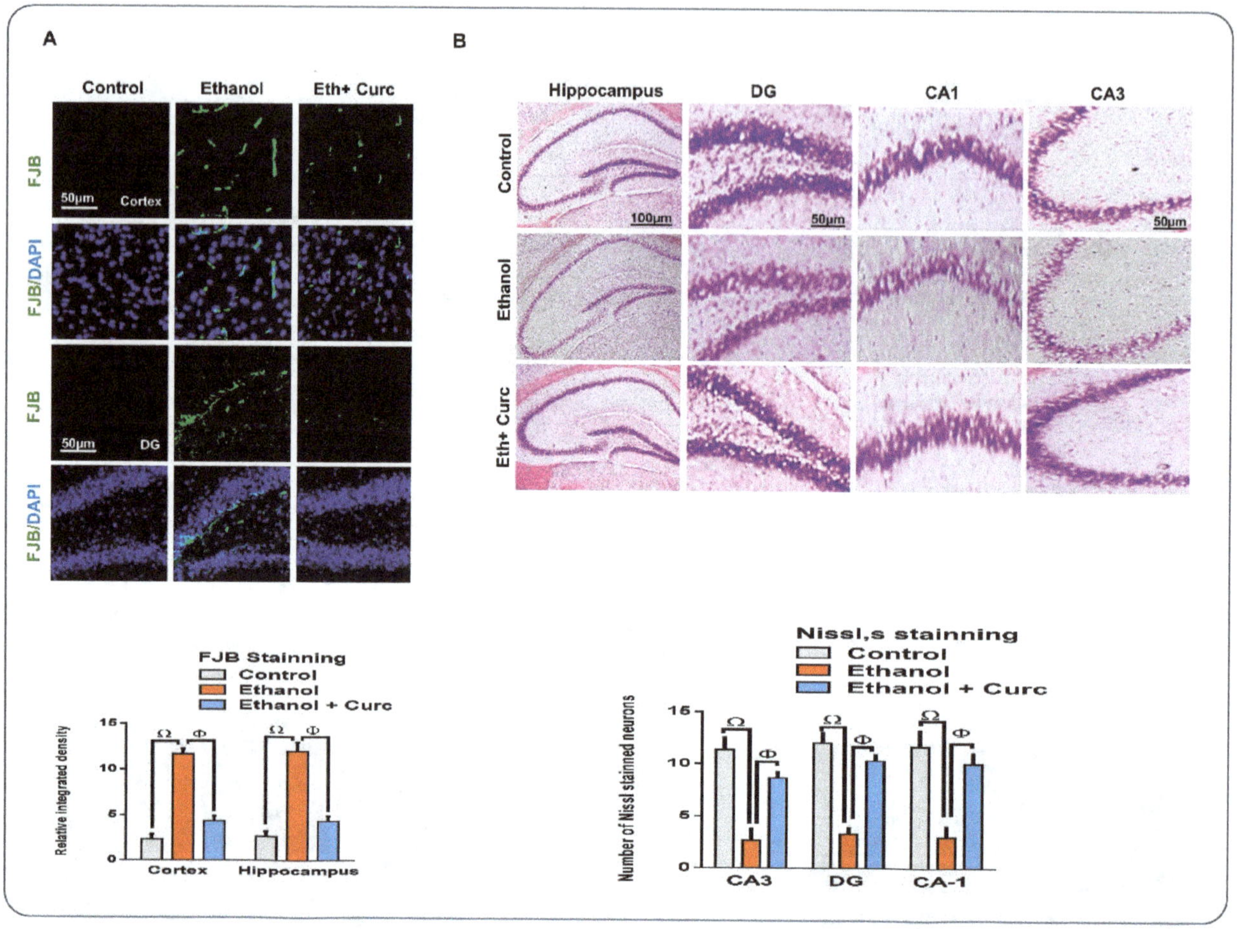

Figure 5. Curcumin Ameliorates Neurodegeneration in Mouse Brains, as visualized by Nissl and FJB staining: (**A**) FJB stained sections from mice hippocampus, co-stained with DAPI and its histogram, the differences have been shown in the histogram; (**B**) Images of the Nissl stained sections (CA1, CA3 and DG) from different experimental groups with histograms, $n = 12$ mice/group, scale bar 50 μm & 100 μm, Ω, significantly different from the vehicle-treated, Φ, significantly different from the ethanol-treated group. DG means dentate gyrus, Significance = Φ, $p < 0.05$, Ω, $p < 0.05$. eth: ethanol, curc: curcumin.

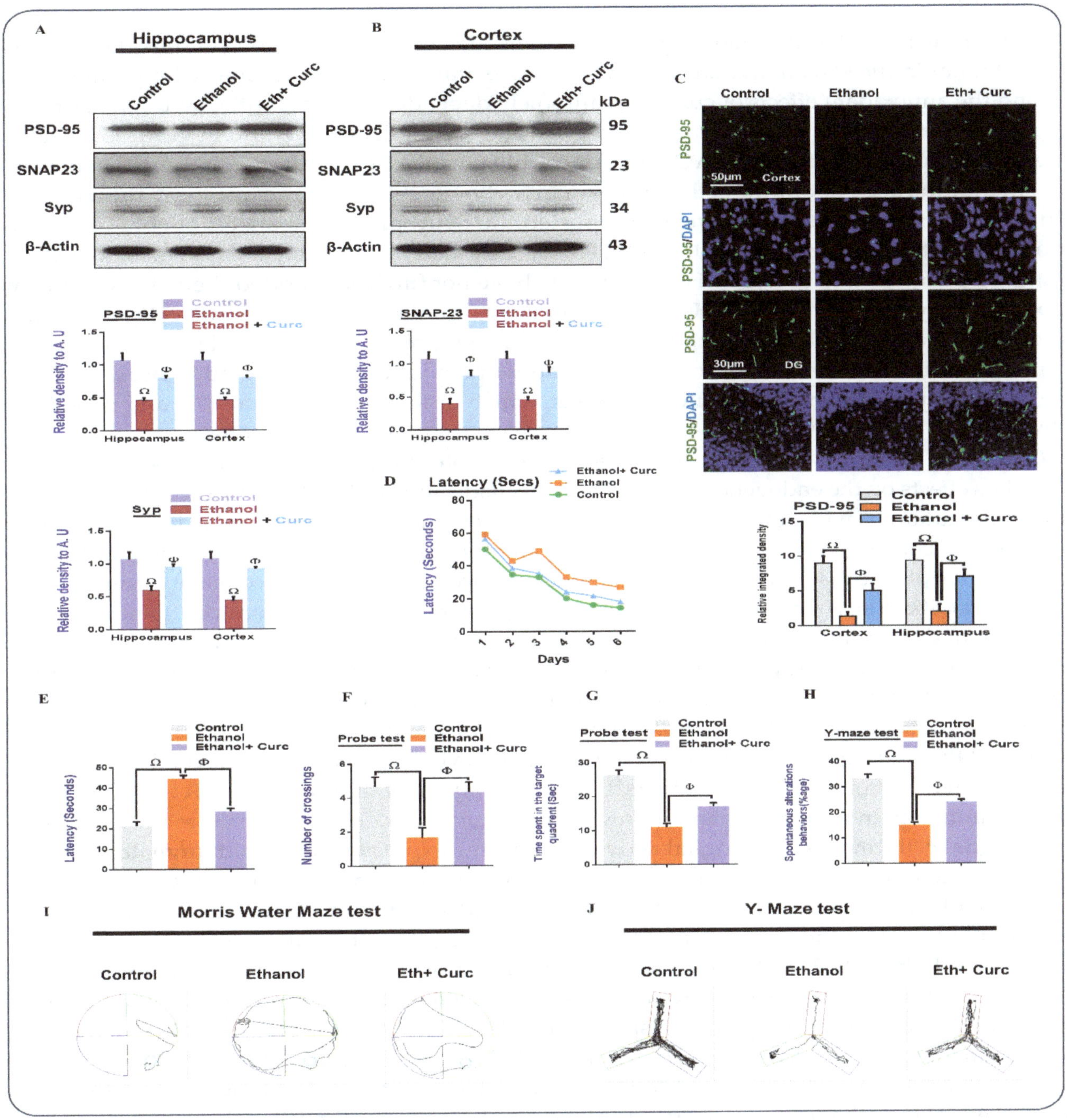

Figure 6. Curcumin Rescued Ethanol-Induced Synaptic Dysfunction and Memory Impairment in Mouse: (**A** & **B**) Immunoblot results of PSD95, SNAP23 and synaptophysin in mice brain ($n = 10$), with histograms; (**C**) Confocal images of PSD-95 in mouse brains, with its bar graph. Magnification, 40×, scale bar up to 50 μm; (**D**). Mean escape latency (shown in seconds) to the platform during a training session, $n = 12$ mice/group; (**E**). Latency on the final day of the probe test; (**F**). Histograms showing the number of platform crossings during the probe test; (**G**) Time spent in the target quadrant during the probe trial; (**H**) Spontaneous alternations (in percent) in the Y-maze test; (**I** & **J**). Trajectories of the MWM tests & Y-maze tests, respectively ($n = 12$ mice/group). Ω, significantly different from the vehicle-treated, Φ, significantly different from the ethanol-treated group. Significance = Φ $p < 0.05$, Ω, $p < 0.05$. eth: ethanol, curc: curcumin.

4. Discussion

The current study has the following main findings. (i) Curcumin has strong anti-oxidant potentials against ethanol-induced oxidative stress, in vivo mouse brains, and in vitro mouse hippocampal HT22 cells, and the antioxidant effects of curcumin are solely dependent on Nrf2. (ii) Curcumin has rescuing effects against ethanol induced activated astrocytes and microglia, in vivo and in vitro, as revealed by the reduced expression of TLR4/RAGE, GFAP, and Iba-1. (iii) Curcumin may rescue the mice brain from ethanol-induced apoptotic cell death, synaptic dysfunction, and memory impairment in mice brains. Several lines of studies have also reported the neuroprotective effects of curcumin against neuroinflammation and apoptotic cell death [44–46]. One study completely focused on oxidative stress mediated neuroinflammation [47]. However, they have not further extended their study to the main antioxidant enzymes, such as Nrf2/HO-1. Curcumin was administered intraperitoneally, and although it is considered a parenteral route of administration, the pharmacokinetics of substances administered intraperitoneally are more similar to those seen after oral administration. In both cases, the primary route of absorption is into the mesenteric vessels, which drain into the portal vein and pass through the liver [48].

Curcumin has long since been reported to be a potent antioxidant, but no studies have yet reported its effects on the endogenous antioxidant mechanisms (Nrf2/HO-1) and TLR4/RAGE mediated neurodegeneration. A wide range of effects are associated with ethanol intoxication, including oxidative stress, apoptotic neurodegeneration, excitotoxicity, and the disruption of cell to cell interactions [40,49]. The production of ROS may cause other serious consequences, such as an altered metabolism, deleterious structural modifications of proteins, DNA mishandlings, and altered mitochondrial homeostasis. Here, we report that ethanol-induced oxidative stress mediated neuroinflammation via Nrf-2/TLR4 signaling. The induction of oxidative stress with the administration of ethanol is in accordance with previous studies [50]. Interestingly, the in vitro findings also support the results, showing antioxidant effects against ethanol induced oxidative stress. For more confirmatory purposes, we used specific Nrf2 siRNA, and the findings showed that curcumin may relieve the elevated ROS level through Nrf2.

The other outcome of our study is that curcumin may inhibit the TLR4/RAGE triggered neuroinflammation in mice brains and in in vitro microglial cells. TLR4, which is mainly expressed in the microglial cells, induces microglial activation and the expression of proinflammatory cytokines, such as TNF-α and p-NF-kB, in response to a variety of stimuli [51]. Besides TLR4, other receptors are also involved in neurodegenerative conditions, such as RAGE. Here, we also evaluated the expression of RAGE in the experimental groups. According to our findings, there was an enhanced expression of TLR4/RAGE and its downstream inflammatory mediators in the ethanol-treated mice brain. Interestingly, these markers were significantly reduced with the administration of curcumin. For more confirmatory purposes, we used a specific TLR4 inhibitor (TAK242). Interestingly, the rescuing effects of curcumin against TLR4/iba-1 in the microglial cells were comparable to TAK 242. GFAP and Iba-1, which are the assigned markers for the activated astrocytes and microglia, were significantly upregulated in the ethanol-treated group, however, there was a significantly lower expression in the curcumin-treated group. The upregulation of GFAP and Iba1 in the ethanol-treated group is in accordance with the previous reports [4]. The inhibition of TLR4 further inhibited the expression of its downstream effectors (Iba-1) in the microglial cells. The upregulation of TLR4, RAGE, and the iba-1 in the ethanol-treated mice brains is in accordance with the previous reported effects of ethanol [52].

The other inducer of the neurodegenerative conditions are as follows: the phosphorylation of MAP kinases, which phosphorylates and translocates the NF-kB to the nucleus, playing a pivotal role in the release of inflammatory mediators [53]. According to our findings, there were enhanced expressions of p-JNK and p-NF-kB, as well as other inflammatory mediators (TNF-α, Cox-2, and IL-1β) in the ethanol treated mice, which is in accordance with previous studies [39]. Another main contributor to the neurodegeneration is apoptotic cell death in neurodegenerative conditions [54], as apoptotic cell death has closely been linked to the oxidative damage [55]. For the evaluation of the effects of curcumin against apoptotic cell death, the expression of proapoptotic (Bax, Caspase-3, and PARP-1) and antiapoptotic (Bcl-2) markers were evaluated; according to our findings, ethanol promoted proapoptotic cell death, which was significantly inhibited with the administration of curcumin. For more confirmatory purposes, we performed Nissl and FJB staining, which showed that curcumin significantly inhibited the neurotoxic effects of ethanol on mice brains. The ultimate consequence of neurodegeneration is synaptic dysfunction and loss of memory, which have been extensively reported with ethanol intoxication [56].

For the evaluation of synaptic dysfunction and memory impairment, we performed behavioral studies in Morris water maze and Y-maze tests, as well as the protein markers related to synaptotoxicity. According to our results, curcumin significantly improved the behavioral alterations and synaptic markers (postsynaptic density protein-95, SNAP-23, and synaptophysin) in the mice brain. The protective effects of curcumin on the behavioral changes and synaptic dysfunction are in accordance with previous studies [43,57].

5. Conclusions

Altogether, our findings support the hypothesis that the chronic administration of curcumin may protect mice brains against the detrimental effects of ethanol, by serving as a strong antioxidant, anti-inflammatory, and antiapoptotic agent in vivo mice brains and in vitro cells.

Author Contributions: M.I designed and conducted the experiments, and wrote manuscript; K.S., and M.S.K. conducted the experiments; A.K., T.M., M.G.J., and S.U.R. conducted the statistical analysis, reviewed and edited the manuscripts; M.O.K. supervised and organized the final version of the manuscript. All of the authors reviewed and approved the paper.

References

1. Kohnke, M.D. Approach to the genetics of alcoholism: A review based on pathophysiology. *Biochem. Pharmacol.* **2008**, *75*, 160–177. [CrossRef] [PubMed]
2. Lee, J.W.; Lee, Y.K.; Lee, B.J.; Nam, S.Y.; Lee, S.I.; Kim, Y.H.; Kim, K.H.; Oh, K.W.; Hong, J.T. Inhibitory effect of ethanol extract of Magnolia officinalis and 4-O-methylhonokiol on memory impairment and neuronal toxicity induced by β-amyloid. *Pharmacol. Biochem. Behav.* **2010**, *95*, 31–40. [CrossRef] [PubMed]
3. Badshah, H.; Kim, T.H.; Kim, M.J.; Ahmad, A.; Ali, T.; Yoon, G.H.; Naseer, M.I.; Kim, M.O. Apomorphine attenuates ethanol-induced neurodegeneration in the adult rat cortex. *Neurochem. Int.* **2014**, *74*, 8–15. [CrossRef] [PubMed]
4. Saito, M.; Chakraborty, G.; Hui, M.; Masiello, K.; Saito, M. Ethanol-induced neurodegeneration and glial activation in the developing brain. *Brain Sci.* **2016**, *6*. [CrossRef]
5. Naseer, M.I.; Ullah, I.; Narasimhan, M.L.; Lee, H.Y.; Bressan, R.A.; Yoon, G.H.; Yun, D.J.; Kim, M.O. Neuroprotective effect of osmotin against ethanol-induced apoptotic neurodegeneration in the developing rat brain. *Cell Death Dis.* **2014**, *5*, e1150. [CrossRef] [PubMed]
6. von Haefen, C.; Sifringer, M.; Menk, M.; Spies, C.D. Ethanol enhances susceptibility to apoptotic cell death via down-regulation of autophagy-related proteins. *Alcohol. Clin. Exp. Res.* **2011**, *35*, 1381–1391. [CrossRef]
7. Menetski, J.; Mistry, S.; Lu, M.; Mudgett, J.S.; Ransohoff, R.M.; Demartino, J.A.; Macintyre, D.E.; Abbadie, C. Mice overexpressing chemokine ligand 2 (CCL2) in astrocytes display enhanced nociceptive responses. *Neuroscience* **2007**, *149*, 706–714. [CrossRef] [PubMed]
8. Lucas, S.M.; Rothwell, N.J.; Gibson, R.M. The role of inflammation in CNS injury and disease. *Br. J. Pharmacol.* **2006**, *147* (Suppl. 1), S232–S240. [CrossRef]
9. Manoharan, J.P.S.; Subramaniyan, A.V.D. Neuroprotective Effects of pterois volitans venom against alcohol induced oxidative dysfunction in Rats. *J. Environ. Anal. Toxicol.* **2015**, *5*. [CrossRef]
10. Ojala, J.; Sutinen, E. The role of interleukin-18, oxidative stress and metabolic syndrome in Alzheimer's disease. *J. Clin. Med.* **2017**, *6*, 55. [CrossRef] [PubMed]

11. Bent, S. Herbal medicine in the United States: Review of efficacy, safety, and regulation: Grand rounds at University of California, San Francisco Medical Center. *J. Gen. Intern. Med.* **2008**, *23*, 854–859. [CrossRef]
12. Jun, Y.L.; Bae, C.H.; Kim, D.; Koo, S.; Kim, S. Korean Red Ginseng protects dopaminergic neurons by suppressing the cleavage of p35 to p25 in a Parkinson's disease mouse model. *J. Ginseng Res.* **2015**, *39*, 148–154. [CrossRef] [PubMed]
13. Begum, A.N.; Jones, M.R.; Lim, G.P.; Morihara, T.; Kim, P.; Heath, D.D.; Rock, C.L.; Pruitt, M.A.; Yang, F.; Hudspeth, B.; et al. Curcumin structure-function, bioavailability, and efficacy in models of neuroinflammation and Alzheimer's disease. *J. Pharmacol. Exp. Ther.* **2008**, *326*, 196–208. [CrossRef]
14. Sompamit, K.; Kukongviriyapan, U.; Nakmareong, S.; Pannangpetch, P.; Kukongviriyapan, V. Curcumin improves vascular function and alleviates oxidative stress in non-lethal lipopolysaccharide-induced endotoxaemia in mice. *Eur. J. Pharmacol.* **2009**, *616*, 192–199. [CrossRef] [PubMed]
15. Ng, Q.; Soh, A.; Loke, W.; Venkatanarayanan, N.; Lim, D.; Yeo, W.-S. A meta-analysis of the clinical use of curcumin for irritable bowel syndrome (IBS). *J. Clin. Med.* **2018**, *7*, 298. [CrossRef] [PubMed]
16. Weber, W.M.; Hunsaker, L.A.; Gonzales, A.M.; Heynekamp, J.J.; Orlando, R.A.; Deck, L.M.; Vander Jagt, D.L. TPA-induced up-regulation of activator protein-1 can be inhibited or enhanced by analogs of the natural product curcumin. *Biochem. Pharmacol.* **2006**, *72*, 928–940. [CrossRef]
17. Ataie, A.; Sabetkasaei, M.; Haghparast, A.; Moghaddam, A.H.; Kazeminejad, B. Neuroprotective effects of the polyphenolic antioxidant agent, Curcumin, against homocysteine-induced cognitive impairment and oxidative stress in the rat. *Pharmacol. Biochem. Behav.* **2010**, *96*, 378–385. [CrossRef] [PubMed]
18. Venkatesan, R.; Ji, E.; Kim, S.Y. Phytochemicals that regulate neurodegenerative disease by targeting neurotrophins: A comprehensive review. *BioMed Res. Int.* **2015**, *2015*, 814068. [CrossRef]
19. Thiyagarajan, M.; Sharma, S.S. Neuroprotective effect of curcumin in middle cerebral artery occlusion induced focal cerebral ischemia in rats. *Life Sci.* **2004**, *74*, 969–985. [CrossRef] [PubMed]
20. Nakano, Y.; Shimazawa, M.; Ojino, K.; Izawa, H.; Takeuchi, H.; Inoue, Y.; Tsuruma, K.; Hara, H. Toll-like receptor 4 inhibitor protects against retinal ganglion cell damage induced by optic nerve crush in mice. *J. Pharmacol. Sci.* **2017**, *133*, 176–183. [CrossRef]
21. Frasnelli, S.C.; de Medeiros, M.C.; Bastos Ade, S.; Costa, D.L.; Orrico, S.R.; Rossa Junior, C. Modulation of immune response by RAGE and TLR4 signalling in PBMCs of diabetic and non-diabetic patients. *Scand. J. Immunol.* **2015**, *81*, 66–71. [CrossRef] [PubMed]
22. Sorrenti, V.; Contarini, G.; Sut, S.; Dall'Acqua, S.; Confortin, F.; Pagetta, A.; Giusti, P.; Zusso, M. Curcumin prevents acute neuroinflammation and long-term memory impairment induced by systemic lipopolysaccharide in mice. *Front. Pharmacol.* **2018**, *9*, 183. [CrossRef] [PubMed]
23. Jackson-Lewis, V.; Przedborski, S. Protocol for the MPTP mouse model of Parkinson's disease. *Nat. Protoc.* **2007**, *2*, 141–151. [CrossRef] [PubMed]
24. Badshah, H.; Ullah, I.; Kim, S.E.; Kim, T.H.; Lee, H.Y.; Kim, M.O. Anthocyanins attenuate body weight gain via modulating neuropeptide Y and GABAB1 receptor in rats hypothalamus. *Neuropeptides* **2013**, *47*, 347–353. [CrossRef] [PubMed]
25. Khan, A.; Ali, T.; Rehman, S.U.; Khan, M.S.; Alam, S.I.; Ikram, M.; Muhammad, T.; Saeed, K.; Badshah, H.; Kim, M.O. Neuroprotective effect of quercetin against the detrimental effects of LPS in the adult mouse brain. *Front. Pharmacol.* **2018**, *9*, 1383. [CrossRef]
26. Badshah, H.; Kim, T.H.; Kim, M.O. Protective effects of anthocyanins against amyloid β-induced neurotoxicity in vivo and in vitro. *Neurochem. Int.* **2015**, *80*, 51–59. [CrossRef]
27. Lee, Y.; Chun, H.J.; Lee, K.M.; Jung, Y.S.; Lee, J. Silibinin suppresses astroglial activation in a mouse model of acute Parkinson's disease by modulating the ERK and JNK signaling pathways. *Brain Res.* **2015**, *1627*, 233–242. [CrossRef]
28. Amin, F.U.; Shah, S.A.; Kim, M.O. Vanillic acid attenuates Aβ1-42-induced oxidative stress and cognitive impairment in mice. *Sci. Rep.* **2017**, *7*, 40753. [CrossRef] [PubMed]
29. Ikram, M.; Muhammad, T.; Rehman, S.U.; Khan, A.; Jo, M.G.; Ali, T.; Kim, M.O. Hesperetin confers neuroprotection by regulating Nrf2/TLR4/NF-κB signaling in an Aβ mouse model. In *Molecular Neurobiology*; Springer: Berlin, Germany, 2019.
30. Khan, M.; Shah, S.A.; Kim, M.O. 17β-Estradiol via SIRT1/Acetyl-p53/NF-kB signaling pathway rescued postnatal rat brain against acute ethanol intoxication. *Mol. Neurobiol.* **2017**. [CrossRef] [PubMed]

31. Lin, Y.-T.; Wu, Y.-C.; Sun, G.-C.; Ho, C.-Y.; Wong, T.-Y.; Lin, C.-H.; Chen, H.-H.; Yeh, T.-C.; Li, C.-J.; Tseng, C.-J. Effect of resveratrol on reactive oxygen species-induced cognitive impairment in rats with angiotensin II-induced early alzheimer's disease. *J. Clin. Med.* **2018**, *7*, 329. [CrossRef] [PubMed]
32. Rehman, S.U.; Ahmad, A.; Yoon, G.-H.; Khan, M.; Abid, M.N.; Kim, M.O. Inhibition of c-Jun N-Terminal kinase protects against brain damage and improves learning and memory after traumatic brain injury in adult mice. *Cereb. Cortex* **2017**. [CrossRef] [PubMed]
33. Ayaz, M.; Junaid, M.; Ullah, F.; Subhan, F.; Sadiq, A.; Ali, G.; Ovais, M.; Shahid, M.; Ahmad, A.; Wadood, A.; et al. Anti-Alzheimer's studies on β-Sitosterol isolated from *Polygonum hydropiper* L. *Front. Pharmacol.* **2017**, *8*, 697. [CrossRef]
34. Muhammad, T.; Ali, T.; Ikram, M.; Khan, A.; Alam, S.I.; Kim, M.O. Melatonin rescue oxidative stress-mediated neuroinflammation/neurodegeneration and memory impairment in scopolamine-induced amnesia mice model. *J. Neuroimmune Pharmacol.* **2018**. [CrossRef] [PubMed]
35. Bauer, A.K.; Fitzgerald, M.; Ladzinski, A.T.; Lenhart Sherman, S.; Maddock, B.H.; Norr, Z.M.; Miller, R.R., Jr. Dual behavior of N-acetylcysteine during ethanol-induced oxidative stress in embryonic chick brains. *Nutr. Neurosci.* **2017**, *20*, 478–488. [CrossRef]
36. Jo, M.G.; Ikram, M.; Jo, M.H.; Yoo, L.; Chung, K.C.; Nah, S.Y.; Hwang, H.; Rhim, H.; Kim, M.O. Gintonin mitigates MPTP-induced loss of nigrostriatal dopaminergic neurons and accumulation of alpha-synuclein via the Nrf2/HO-1 pathway. *Mol. Neurobiol.* **2018**. [CrossRef]
37. Ali, T.; Kim, T.; Rehman, S.U.; Khan, M.S.; Amin, F.U.; Khan, M.; Ikram, M.; Kim, M.O. Natural dietary supplementation of anthocyanins via PI3K/Akt/Nrf2/HO-1 pathways mitigate oxidative stress, neurodegeneration, and memory impairment in a mouse model of alzheimer's disease. *Mol. Neurobiol.* **2018**, *55*, 6076–6093. [CrossRef] [PubMed]
38. Fernandez-Lizarbe, S.; Pascual, M.; Guerri, C. Critical role of TLR4 response in the activation of microglia induced by ethanol. *J. Immunol.* **2009**, *183*, 4733–4744. [CrossRef]
39. Shah, S.A.; Yoon, G.H.; Kim, M.O. Protection of the developing brain with anthocyanins against ethanol-induced oxidative stress and neurodegeneration. *Mol. Neurobiol.* **2015**, *51*, 1278–1291. [CrossRef] [PubMed]
40. Crews, F.T.; Nixon, K. Mechanisms of neurodegeneration and regeneration in alcoholism. *Alcohol. Alcohol.* **2009**, *44*, 115–127. [CrossRef] [PubMed]
41. Damjanac, M.; Rioux Bilan, A.; Barrier, L.; Pontcharraud, R.; Anne, C.; Hugon, J.; Page, G. Fluoro-Jade B staining as useful tool to identify activated microglia and astrocytes in a mouse transgenic model of Alzheimer's disease. *Brain Res.* **2007**, *1128*, 40–49. [CrossRef]
42. Ullah, N.; Naseer, M.I.; Ullah, I.; Kim, T.H.; Lee, H.Y.; Kim, M.O. Neuroprotective profile of pyruvate against ethanol-induced neurodegeneration in developing mice brain. *Neurol. Sci.* **2013**, *34*, 2137–2143. [CrossRef]
43. Muhammad, T.; Ikram, M.; Ullah, R.; Rehman, S.U.; Kim, M.O. Hesperetin, a citrus flavonoid, attenuates lps-induced neuroinflammation, apoptosis and memory impairments by modulating TLR4/NF-κB signaling. *Nutrients* **2019**, *11*. [CrossRef] [PubMed]
44. Fan, C.; Song, Q.; Wang, P.; Li, Y.; Yang, M.; Yu, S.Y. Neuroprotective effects of curcumin on IL-1β-induced neuronal apoptosis and depression-like behaviors caused by chronic stress in rats. *Front. Cell. Neurosci.* **2018**, *12*, 516. [CrossRef]
45. Xu, L.; Ding, L.; Su, Y.; Shao, R.; Liu, J.; Huang, Y. Neuroprotective effects of curcumin against rats with focal cerebral ischemia-reperfusion injury. *Int. J. Mol. Med.* **2019**. [CrossRef]
46. Cole, G.M.; Teter, B.; Frautschy, S.A. Neuroprotective effects of curcumin. In *The Molecular Targets and Therapeutic Uses of Curcumin in Health and Disease*; Springer: Boston, MA, USA, 2007; pp. 197–212.
47. Tiwari, V.; Chopra, K. Protective effect of curcumin against chronic alcohol-induced cognitive deficits and neuroinflammation in the adult rat brain. *Neuroscience* **2013**, *244*, 147–158. [CrossRef]
48. Turner, P.V.; Brabb, T.; Pekow, C.; Vasbinder, M.A. Administration of substances to laboratory animals: Routes of administration and factors to consider. *J. Am. Assoc. Lab. Anim. Sci.* **2011**, *50*, 600–613. [PubMed]
49. Goldowitz, D.; Lussier, A.A.; Boyle, J.K.; Wong, K.; Lattimer, S.L.; Dubose, C.; Lu, L.; Kobor, M.S.; Hamre, K.M. Molecular pathways underpinning ethanol-induced neurodegeneration. *Front. Genet.* **2014**, *5*, 203. [CrossRef]
50. Comporti, M.; Signorini, C.; Leoncini, S.; Gardi, C.; Ciccoli, L.; Giardini, A.; Vecchio, D.; Arezzini, B. Ethanol-induced oxidative stress: Basic knowledge. *Genes Nutr.* **2010**, *5*, 101–109. [CrossRef] [PubMed]

51. McColl, B.W.; Allan, S.M.; Rothwell, N.J. Systemic infection, inflammation and acute ischemic stroke. *Neuroscience* **2009**, *158*, 1049–1061. [CrossRef] [PubMed]
52. Crews, F.T.; Vetreno, R.P. Mechanisms of neuroimmune gene induction in alcoholism. *Psychopharmacology* **2016**, *233*, 1543–1557. [CrossRef]
53. Saha, R.N.; Jana, M.; Pahan, K. MAPK p38 regulates transcriptional activity of NF-κB in primary human astrocytes via acetylation of p65. *J. Immunol.* **2007**, *179*, 7101–7109. [CrossRef] [PubMed]
54. Radi, E.; Formichi, P.; Battisti, C.; Federico, A. Apoptosis and oxidative stress in neurodegenerative diseases. *J. Alzheimers Dis.* **2014**, *42* (Suppl. 3), S125–S152. [CrossRef]
55. Khan, A.; Ikram, M.; Muhammad, T.; Park, J.; Kim, M.O. Caffeine modulates cadmium-induced oxidative stress, neuroinflammation, and cognitive impairments by regulating Nrf-2/HO-1 in vivo and in vitro. *J. Clin. Med.* **2019**, *8*, 680. [CrossRef]
56. Wang, P.; Luo, Q.; Qiao, H.; Ding, H.; Cao, Y.; Yu, J.; Liu, R.; Zhang, Q.; Zhu, H.; Qu, L. The neuroprotective effects of carvacrol on ethanol-induced hippocampal neurons impairment via the antioxidative and antiapoptotic pathways. *Oxid. Med. Cell. Longev.* **2017**, *2017*, 4079425. [CrossRef] [PubMed]
57. Wang, X.S.; Zhang, Z.R.; Zhang, M.M.; Sun, M.X.; Wang, W.W.; Xie, C.L. Neuroprotective properties of curcumin in toxin-base animal models of Parkinson's disease: A systematic experiment literatures review. *BMC Complement. Altern. Med.* **2017**, *17*, 412. [CrossRef] [PubMed]

8

Palatability of Goat's versus Cow's Milk: Insights from the Analysis of Eating Behavior and Gene Expression in the Appetite-Relevant Brain Circuit in Laboratory Animal Models

Anica Klockars [1,†], Erin L. Wood [1,†], Sarah N. Gartner [1], Laura K. McColl [1], Allen S. Levine [2], Elizabeth A. Carpenter [3], Colin G. Prosser [3] and Pawel K. Olszewski [1,2,*]

1 Faculty of Science and Engineering, University of Waikato, Hamilton 3240, New Zealand; anica.klockars@waikato.ac.nz (A.K.); elw14@students.waikato.ac.nz (E.L.W.); snm10@students.waikato.ac.nz (S.N.G.); laura.mccoll@waikato.ac.nz (L.K.M.)
2 Department of Food Science and Nutrition, University of Minnesota, St. Paul, MN 55113, USA; aslevine@umn.edu
3 Dairy Goat Cooperative (NZ) Ltd., Hamilton 3206, New Zealand; Liz.Carpenter@dgc.co.nz (E.A.C.); Colin.Prosser@dgc.co.nz (C.G.P.)
* Correspondence: pawel@waikato.ac.nz
† The authors contributed equally to the finished manuscript.

Abstract: Goat's (GM) and cow's milk (CM) are dietary alternatives with select health benefits shown in human and animal studies. Surprisingly, no systematic analysis of palatability or preference for GM vs. CM has been performed to date. Here, we present a comprehensive investigation of short-term intake and palatability profiles of GM and CM in laboratory mice and rats. We studied consumption in no-choice and choice scenarios, including meal microstructure, and by using isocaloric milks and milk-enriched solid diets. Feeding results are accompanied by qPCR data of relevant genes in the energy balance-related hypothalamus and brain stem, and in the nucleus accumbens, which regulates eating for palatability. We found that GM and CM are palatable to juvenile, adult, and aged rodents. Given a choice, animals prefer GM- to CM-based diets. Analysis of meal microstructure using licking patterns points to enhanced palatability of and, possibly, greater motivation toward GM over CM. Most profound changes in gene expression after GM vs. CM were associated with the brain systems driving consumption for reward. We conclude that, while both GM and CM are palatable, GM is preferred over CM by laboratory animals, and this preference is driven by central mechanisms controlling eating for pleasure.

Keywords: milk; hypothalamus; nucleus accumbens; reward; appetite; palatability

---

1. Introduction

Milk is a widely consumed, affordable, and highly nutritive food, which serves as a key source of, among others, protein, calcium, potassium, magnesium, and vitamins (especially A and D) in industrialized countries [1–6]. In Western societies, cow's milk (CM) products represent the largest share of dairy available on the market, and cow's skim milk varieties have become common. However, recent years have generated interest in milk from other species, such as goat's milk (GM). The use of GM as an alternative to CM has been driven by the findings in humans and laboratory animals showing potential beneficial nutritive consequences of GM intake and differences in physiological responses to GM or CM consumption, (for review, see [7]). For example, Bellioni-Businco et al. reported that individuals with a CM allergy were able to drink five times more GM than CM before the symptoms of an allergic response appeared [8]. In studies utilizing rodent models, Barrionuevo et al. demonstrated that GM increases utilization of copper, zinc, and selenium [9]. Bioavailability of iron and copper was found to be improved in GM-fed rodents suffering from malabsorptive syndrome and in healthy controls [9,10]. Finally, GM improved bone turnover in iron-deficient rats compared to rats fed CM [11,12].

Surprisingly, little is known about GM's acceptance and preference relative to the main dairy product in today's food environment in the Western world. There is no systematic analysis of propensity to ingest GM and CM or relative palatability of GM vs. CM in either humans or in laboratory animal models. Consequently, our understanding of acceptance and palatability of GM compared to CM is still mainly based on anecdotal evidence and on market availability, both heavily influenced by local cultural or environmental aspects (such as in Western vs. Asian countries) and habituation-driven intake of a specific milk type [13]. This is a major gap in knowledge as palatability affects, among others, the amount of food eaten in a single meal, the rate of consumption, food anticipation, and satiety. It has a profound effect on activity of brain circuits responsible for processing energy intake (including the hypothalamus (HYP) and brain stem (BS)) and reward (such as the nucleus accumbens; NAcc) [14–16]. These parameters can, in turn, impact a plethora of mechanisms outside the central nervous system (CNS), via neural and hormonal interactions linking the brain and peripheral tissues [17–19].

Here, we present for the first time a comprehensive investigation of short-term intake and palatability profiles of GM and CM in laboratory rodent models (mice and rats) using skim milks. We report consumption data on the acceptance (no-choice) and preference (choice) scenarios of calorie-matched milks and milk-enriched solid diets. Consumption data are accompanied by the analysis of expression of appetite-related genes in the HYP and BS, two brain regions predominantly involved in energy balance control, and in the NAcc, a key site that regulates eating for palatability [15,16]. We examined mRNA levels of genes involved in promoting consumption, such as those encoding neuropeptide Y (NPY), Agouti-related protein (AgRP), ghrelin receptor, orexin, opioid peptides/receptors, and gap junction protein, connexin 36 (Cx36). The analysis also included transcripts related to decreased appetite and termination of consumption, such as oxytocin, melanocortin receptors 3 (MC3R) and 4 (MC4R), and proopiomelanocortin (POMC). Typically, presentation of tastants that differ in palatability and composition, among other traits, evokes some changes in expression within this subset of genes, reflecting a different propensity of an animal to ingest specific diets [16,20]. A number of physiological functions by the brain vary with age, including appetite. Weight is typically gained throughout early and middle age, followed by gradual, age-associated anorexia. In line with that, a drive to consume food (and responsiveness to palatability) is high during the earlier stages of life, whereas in aged animals, anhedonia and decreased responsiveness to rewarding diets and to drugs that promote eating for pleasure ensue (e.g., see [21–23]). Therefore, in our feeding experiments, we studied rodents that belong to three distinct age groups: adolescents, adults, and aged animals. It should also be noted that rats and most mammals, other than select groups of humans, poorly digest lactose post-weaning. Though lactase activity in adult rats is residual, rats fed as much as 30% lactose in their daily diet from post-weaning to day 98 had normal body growth or body weight course (their body weight was somewhat lower) [24]. Taking it into consideration, however, in this current study we focused on short-term rather than long-term exposure to milk or milk containing chow.

2. Materials and Methods

2.1. Animals

Male Sprague-Dawley rats and C57Bl mice (all weaned on day 21) used in these studies were single-housed in a temperature-controlled (22 °C) animal facility with a 12:12-h LD cycle (lights on at 07:00). Standard chow (Diet 86, Sharpes Stock Feed, Wairarapa, New Zealand) and water were available ad libitum unless indicated otherwise. The University of Waikato animal ethics committee had approved the procedures (ethics approval numbers: 1020, 1043, and 1057), and they are compliant with the NIH Guide for the Care and Use of Laboratory Animals (NIH Publ., no. 80–23, rev. 1996). Feeding experiments were performed in separate cohorts of animals unless specified otherwise. The age of animals included in the adolescent (5–6 weeks), adult (3–5 months), and aged (25–27 months) categories was based on previous publications pertaining to the aging process in rodents [25]. It should be noted that despite poor digestibility of lactose post-weaning, we did not observe any signs of gastrointestinal discomfort or sickness, which is in line with previous studies showing that rats fed as much as 30% lactose in their daily diet (thus, more than given here) for several weeks displayed good tolerance of the carbohydrate [24].

2.2. Episodic Intake of Individually Presented GM and CM in Sated Adult Mice and Rats

We based the protocol on previous studies assessing episodic intake of palatable tastants [26–28]. Individually housed mice and rats were accustomed (in homecages) to receiving one of the four isocaloric (0.6 kcal/g) solutions for 2 h/day on 2 days (10:00–12:00) prior to the experiments using their usual 250 mL sized water bottles (used for all bottle scenarios) to avoid neophobia(mice: n = 8–9/group; rats: 8–10/group): GM, CM, an energy-equivalent 15% sucrose solution (a reference palatable solution), or a 15% cornstarch (CS) suspension (a negative control for palatability; as CS is insoluble in water, 0.3% xanthan gum was added to this liquid in this experiment as described previously in [29]). On the experimental day, bottles with the solutions (at room temperature) were placed in the cages and water and chow were removed for the 2-h experimental session. Spillage (g) from each individual bottle was recorded before placement into cage. Intakes were measured after 2 h using a digital scale and expressed in grams per gram of body weight. This feeding experiment was conducted in a separate cohort of animals. Composition of the milks are shown in Table 1.

Table 1. CM and GM milk powder composition.

Sample	Protein	Fat	Carbohydrate (Lactose)	Ash	Moisture
CM	37.1	1.1	51	6.5	4.3
GM	36.1	0.9	49.9	9.5	3.6

2.3. Energy Deprivation-Induced Intake of Individually Presented GM and CM in Mice and Rats

Mice and rats previously exposed in their homecages to GM, CM, cornstarch, and sucrose were deprived of standard chow overnight (food taken away at 16:00). On the next day (10:00), water bottles were removed and replaced with bottles (at room temperature) containing one of the four treatments (mice: n = 8–10/group; rats: 7–8/group). Spillage (g) from each individual bottle was recorded before placement into cage. Intakes were measured using a digital scale after 2 h and expressed in grams per gram of body weight. This feeding experiment was conducted in a separate cohort of animals.

2.4. Episodic Intake of Individually Presented GM- and CM-Enriched Chow in Sated Adult Mice and Rats

Rats and mice were given episodic access to the chow enriched with GM or CM according to the protocol described above, where, instead of GM or CM, a GM- or CM-enriched chow (see Table 2 for composition of GM and CM chow) was presented for 2 h (10:00). Standard chow pellets were removed during this 2-h meal, but water was left in the cages. Intake of chow pellets (at room temperature) was measured using a digital scale after 2 h and expressed in grams per gram of body weight. In order to assess baseline intake, a control group of animals had a fresh batch of the standard chow placed in the hopper for 2 h (n = 7–8/group for both mice and rats). This feeding experiment was conducted in a separate cohort of animals.

Table 2. Composition of CM- and GM-enriched chow.

Base Skim Milk Powder Composition (1% Milk Fat)	Goat Skim Milk Powder (SMP)		Cow SMP	
	%	g/kg	%	g/kg
Protein	37.8	120	37.1	120
Fat	1.7	5.40	0.86	2.78
Ash	9.4	29.84	7.3	23.61
Moisture	4.1	13.02	4.2	13.58
Lactose	47	149.21	50.54	163.47
Total	100	317.46	100	323.45
	Goat SMP		Cow SMP	
Skim Milk Chow—Ingredient	g/kg		g/kg	
Goat SMP—to supply 12% protein	317.46			
Cow SMP—to supply 12% protein			323.45	
Vitamin mix	50.00		50.00	
Salt mix	50.00		50.00	
Corn oil (added to make 5% fat)	44.60		47.22	
Starch	447.15		452.80	
Lactose (added to make 16.5%)	15.79		1.53	
Cellulose	75.00		75.00	
Moisture				
	1000.00		1000.00	
Target Dietary Content				
Protein	12%		12%	
Fat	5%		5%	
Lactose	16.50%		16.50%	
Fiber	7.50%		7.50%	
Starch	44.7%		45.3%	
Calories				
Protein (4 cal/g)	48		48	
Fat (9 cal/g)	45		45	
Lactose (4 cal/g)	66		66	
Fiber (2 cal/g)	15		15	
Starch (4 cal/g)	179		181	
Calories/100 g	353		355	
% calories				
Protein	14%		14%	
Fat	13%		13%	
Lactose	19%		19%	
Fiber	4%		4%	
Starch	51%		51%	
Skim Milk Powder (1% Milk Fat)	**Goat SMP**		**Cow SMP**	
Ingredients	g/kg		g/kg	
Goat SMP	317.46			
Cow SMP			323.45	
Vitamin mix	50.00		50.00	
Salt mix	50.00		50.00	
Corn oil	44.60		47.22	
Starch	447.15		452.80	
Lactose	15.79		1.53	
Cellulose	75.00		75.00	
Moisture				
	1000.00		1000.00	

Table 2. *Cont.*

Base Skim Milk Powder Composition (1% Milk Fat)	Goat Skim Milk Powder (SMP)	Cow SMP
Target Dietary Content		
Protein	12%	12%
Fat	5%	5%
Lactose	16.50%	16.50%
Fiber	7.50%	7.50%
Starch	44.7%	45.3%
Calories		
Protein (4 cal/g)	48	48
Fat (9 cal/g)	45	45
Lactose (4 cal/g)	66	66
Fiber (2 cal/g)	15	15
Starch (4 cal/g)	179	181
Calories/100 g	353	355
% calories		
Protein	14%	14%
Fat	13%	13%
Lactose	19%	19%
Fiber	4%	4%
Starch	51%	51%

2.5. Energy Deprivation-Induced Intake of Individually Presented GM- and CM-Enriched Chow in Sated Adult Mice and Rats

Rats and mice previously exposed to GM- and CM-enriched chow (pre-exposure to both chow types was simultaneous) were deprived of standard chow overnight (food taken away at 16:00). On the next day (10:00), animals received either standard chow, GM- or CM-enriched pellets (mice: n = 7–8/group; rats: n = 8–9/group) at room temperature. Intakes were measured using a digital scale after 2 h and expressed in grams per gram of body weight. This feeding experiment was conducted in a separate cohort of animals.

2.6. Episodic Intake of Individually Presented GM and CM in Sated Adolescent and Aged Rodents

Mice and rats aged 5–6 weeks (n = 9–11/group for each species) were used in the study on adolescent animals, whereas 25-month old mice and 26-month old rats (n = 8–9/group for each species) were used as the aged cohorts. The feeding experiments utilizing individually presented cornstarch, sucrose, GM, and CM solutions followed the protocol described above for the relevant studies in adult sated rodents that received one of the four solutions for 2 h. This feeding experiment was conducted in a separate cohort of animals.

2.7. Episodic Intake of GM and CM Presented Simultaneously in Sated Adolescent, Adult, and Aged Rodents

Mice (n = 20) and rats (n = 21) aged 5–6 weeks were used in the study on adolescent animals, 16–18-week old mice (n = 10) and rats (n = 12) were included in the study on adults, whereas 25-month old mice (n = 12) and 26-month old rats (n = 11) were used as the aged cohorts. Adult and adolescent rats and mice had been previously exposed to GM and CM (pre-exposure to both milk types was simultaneous). The aged animals came from the cohorts described above (pt. 2.6), however, a week-long 'washout' period was allowed between the previous experiment and this study. First, the animals were accustomed to simultaneously receiving GM and CM as a two-bottle choice (bottles placed next to each other; random order) for circa 1 h per day on two days in their homecage. Then, on the experimental day, chow and water were removed from cages and GM and CM (at room temperature) were given to the animals for 2 h (11:00–13:00). Spillage (g) from each individual bottle was recorded before placement into cage. Intakes were measured using a digital scale after 2 h and expressed in grams per gram of body weight. This feeding experiment was conducted in a separate cohort of adolescent and adult animals.

2.8. *Episodic Intake of GM- and CM-Enriched Chow Presented Simultaneously in Sated Adult and Aged Rodents*

Mice and rats aged 18–20 weeks old mice (n = 8) and rats (n = 8) were included in the study on adults, whereas 25-month old mice (n = 9) and 27-month old rats (n = 10) were used as the aged cohorts. Adult rats and mice had been previously exposed to GM and CM chow (pre-exposure to both chow types was simultaneous). The aged animals came from the same cohort as in the GM/CM chow experiment described above (Section 2.5), however, a two-week-long 'washout' period was allowed between the previous experiment and this study. First, the animals were accustomed to receiving simultaneously CM- and GM-enriched chow in a subdivided hopper in their homecages (placement of GM/CM pellets was random; standard chow was removed) for circa 1 h per day on two days. Then, on the experimental day, after removal of standard chow, CM- and GM-enriched pellets (at room temperature) were given to the animals for 2 h (10:00–12:00). Intakes were measured using a digital scale after 2 h and expressed in grams per gram of body weight. This feeding experiment was conducted in a separate cohort of adult animals.

2.9. *Lickometer-Assessed Preference for Simultaneously Presented GM and CM in Sated Adult Rats*

Six 12-week old male rats were housed individually in cages equipped with bottles attached to lickometers (Lafayette Instruments, Lafayette, IN, USA). The animals were previously given GM and CM to prevent neophobia (the pre-exposure was simultaneous). They were accustomed to receiving a choice between GM and CM on two separate days for 30 min (random order of bottles) in lickometer cages. On the experimental day, standard chow and water were removed from the cages and animals were given simultaneous access to GM and CM (room temperature) for 30 min. The number of licks on each bottle was counted and analyzed (Scurry Activity Monitoring software, Lafayette, IN, USA), both as total number of licks as well as number of licks per 5-minute interval. We also assessed the cluster number (number of bouts of licking—each bout was defined as continuous licking interspaced by no more than 0.5 s between each other) and an average cluster length (bout duration measured in seconds) of GM vs. CM. This feeding experiment was conducted in a separate cohort of animals.

2.10. *72-h Cumulative Intake of Simultaneously Presented CM- and GM-Enriched Chow in Adult Rats*

First, the animals were accustomed to receiving two types of chow pellets (room temperature) simultaneously in a subdivided hopper in their homecage (placement of pellets was random) for circa 2 h per day on two days. On the experimental day 1 (17:00), animals received a choice of either standard/CM chow (n = 9), standard/GM chow (n = 10), or GM/CM chow for 72 h (pellets were exchanged daily; n = 16). Cumulative 72-h intakes were recorded in grams. This feeding experiment was conducted in a separate cohort of animals.

2.11. *Effect of 24-h CM vs. GM Consumption on Feeding-Related Gene Expression in the Brain Circuit*

In order to assess the effect of 24-h intake of GM and CM solutions on the expression of feeding-related genes in the brain, mice were given CM or GM (at room temperature) as the only tastant (starting at 10:00). Animals given water served as baseline controls. At 10:00 on the subsequent day (thus, 24 h after milk presentation), the animals were sacrificed via cervical dislocation. Brains were dissected out and the hypothalamus, nucleus accumbens, and brain stem excised and stored in RNAlater at −80 ° C until further processing. This experiment was conducted in a separate cohort of animals.

Tissues were homogenized in Trizol (Ambien), 1 mL per 0.1 g tissue. 0.2 mL chloroform was added and samples were centrifuged at room temperature for 10 min at 10,000× g. The clear phase containing RNA was isolated and 0.5 mL of isopropanol was added. RNA was precipitated in an ice bath for 10 min then centrifuged at 4 °C for 20 min at 10,000× *g*. Aqueous phase was removed from the pellets, which were then resuspended in 0.3 mL of ethanol and centrifuged at 4 °C for 10 min at 10,000× *g*. Liquid was removed and pellets were air-dried.

Pellets were dissolved in 8 μL DEPC water and 1 μL DNAse buffer (dNature). Samples were then incubated with 1 μL DNAse (dNature) at 37 °C for 30 min. DNAse was inactivated via addition of stop buffer (dNature) and incubation at 67 °C for 10 min. Removal of DNA was confirmed via PCR using HOT FIREPol Blend Master Mix (dNature), followed with agarose gel electrophoresis. Concentrations of RNA were measured with a nanodrop.

cDNA was synthesized from RNA samples with iScript Advanced cDNA synthesis kit (BioRad). Synthesis of cDNA was confirmed with PCR followed by agarose gel electrophoresis.

Quantitative RT-PCR (qPCR) was used to determine relative expression levels of housekeeping genes (ActB, GAPDH, β-tubulin) and of genes of interest. Reactions contained 4 μL of 25 ng/μL sample cDNA, 1 μL of each forward and reverse primers (5 μM), 10 μL iTaq Universal SYBR Green Supermix (BioRad) and 4 μL MilliQ water. qPCR experiments were performed in duplicates alongside negative controls of MilliQ water for each primer pair. Amplification protocol was initiated at 95 °C for 15 min, followed by 45 cycles of 15 s at 95 °C, 15 s at the primer-specific annealing temperature and 30 s at 72 °C. Primers used: GADPH F: 5′-AAGGTCATCCCAGAGC TGAA-3′, R: 5′-CTGCTTCACCACCTTCTTGA-3′; ActB F: 5′-AGTGTGACGTTGACATCCGT-3′, R: 5′-TGCTAGGAGCCAGAGCAGTA-3′; POMC F: 5′-GACACTGGCTGCTCTCCAG-3′, R: 5′-AGCAGCCTCCCGAGACA-3′; Agrp F: 5′-GGATCTGTTGCAGGAGGCTCAG-3′, R: 5′-TGAAGAAGCGGCAGTAGCACGT-3′; NPY F: 5′-GGTCTTCAAGCCGAGTTCTG-3′, R: 5′-AACCTCATCACCAGGCAGAG-3′; MC4R F: 5′-CTTATGATGATCCCAACCCG-3′, R: 5′-GTAGCTCCTTGCTTGCATCC-3′; β-tubulin F: 5′-CGGAAGGAGGCGGAGAGC-3′, R: 5′-AGGGTGCCCATGCCAGAGC-3′; GHSR F: 5′-TCCGATCTGCTCATCTTCCT-3′, R: 5′- GGAAGCAGATGGCGAAGTAG-3′; ORX F: 5′-GCCGTCTCTACGAACTGTTGC-3′, R: 5′-CGCTTTCCCAGAGTCAGGATA-3′; OXT F: 5′-CCTACAGCGGATCTCAGACTG-3′, R: 5′-TCAGAGCCAGTAAGCCAAGCA-3′; OXTR F: 5′-TCTTCTTCGTGCAGATGTGG-3′, R: 5′-CCTTCAGGTACCGAGCAGAG-3′; PENK F: 5′-CGACATCAATTTCCTGGCGT-3′, R: 5′-AGATCCTTGCAGGTCTCCCA-3′; DYN F: 5′-GACAGGAGAGGAAGCAGA-3′, R: 5′-AGCAGCACACAAGTCACC-3′; GHRL F: 5′-CCATCTGCAGTTTGCTGCTA-3′, R: 5′-GCTTGTCCTCTGTCCTCTGG-3′; MOR F: 5′-CCTGCCGCTCTTCTCTGG-3′, R: 5′-CGGACTCGGTAGGCTGTAAC-3′; KOR F: 5′-CACCTTGCTGATCCCAAAC-3′, R: 5′-TTCCCAAGTCACCGTCAG-3′; PNOC F: 5′-AGCACCTGAAGAGAATGCCG-3′, R: 5′-CATCTCGCACTTGCACCAAG-3′; ORLP F: 5′-ATGACTAGGCGTGGACCTGC-3′, R: 5′-GATGGGCTCTGTGGACTGACA-3′; GLP1R F: 5′-ATGGCCAGCACCCCAAGCCTCC-3′, R: 5′-TCAGCTGTAGGAACTCTGG-3′; Cx36 F: 5′-CCAGTAAGGAGACAGAACCAGAT-3′, R: 5′-GATGATGTAGAAGCGGGAGATAC-3′.

2.12. Data Analysis

Analyses of qPCR data utilized BioRad CFX Manager software (BioRad); one-way ANOVA followed by Bonferroni's test with the correction for multiple comparisons was used, with $p < 0.05$ set as criterion of statistical significance. Feeding data from studies comparing two groups were analyzed using a *t*-test, whereas comparisons between three or more groups were done with ANOVA followed by Bonferroni's post-hoc test, with differences considered significant when $p < 0.05$.

3. Results

In the non-choice acceptance tests, sated adult mice and rats showed very low levels of consumption of a 'bland' cornstarch emulsion, whereas intakes of the GM (mice, $F(3,30) = 62.8$, $p < 0.001$; rats, $F(3,32) = 25.5$, $p < 0.001$) and CM (mice, $p < 0.001$; rats, $p < 0.001$), as well as of the sucrose solution (mice, $p < 0.001$; rats, $p < 0.001$), were several times higher than of cornstarch. Energy-deprived animals had a higher baseline intake of cornstarch, but consumed significantly more sucrose (mice, $F(3,32) = 9.77$, $p \leq 0.001$; rats, $F(3,26) = 5.5$, $p = 0.039$), GM (mice, $p < 0.001$; rats, $p = 0.0023$), and CM (mice, $p = 0.034$; rats, $p = 0.0083$; Figure 1A–D). Similarly, both deprived and sated adult individuals ate more GM- and CM-enriched pellets than standard chow (sated mice: $F(2,19) = 5.9$, GM, $p = 0.029$ and CM, $p = 0.011$; sated rats: $F(2,19) = 20.5$, GM, $p < 0.001$ and CM, $p = 0.0011$; deprived mice: $F(2,19) = 6.5$, GM, $p = 0.0058$ and CM, $p = 0.034$; deprived rats: $F(2,22) = 10.8$, GM, $p < 0.001$ and CM, $p = 0.0442$; Figure 1E–H). Adolescent and aged sated mice and rats (Figure 2A,B,E,F) given episodic 2-h access to one of the solutions, consumed more GM (adolescent mice, $F(3,35) = 42.7$, $p < 0.001$; rats, $F(3,36) = 16.9$, $p < 0.001$; aged mice, $F(3,29) = 31.2$, $p < 0.001$; rats, $F(3,29) = 18.9$, $p < 0.001$), CM (adolescent mice, $p < 0.001$; rats, $p < 0.001$; aged mice, $p < 0.001$; rats, $p < 0.001$) and sucrose (adolescent mice, $p < 0.001$; rats, $p < 0.001$; aged mice, $p < 0.001$; rats, $p < 0.001$) than cornstarch.

When given a 2-h episodic choice between GM and CM, all age cohorts of rats (adolescent, $p < 0.001$; adult, $p < 0.001$; aged, $p < 0.001$) and adult and aged mice ($p = 0.012$ and 0.011, respectively) preferred GM (Figure 2C,D,G,H and Figure 3A,B). During a brief, 30-min exposure to both GM and CM in cages equipped with lickometers, adult rats exhibited a more robust response to GM cumulatively over that period ($p = 0.01$) as well as during the first ($p = 0.037$) and second ($p = 0.05$) 5-min time interval of the meal (Figure 3C,D). There was a trend approaching significance ($p = 0.088$) toward an increase in the cluster number (number of licking bouts) of GM over CM, and a significantly greater cluster length of each GM than CM bout ($p = 0.022$; Figure 3E,F). In choice experiments involving GM- and CM-enriched chow, adult and aged rats ($p = 0.009$ and 0.023, respectively) and adult mice ($p = 0.028$) preferred GM chow, whereas in aged mice, a trend toward GM preference was detected ($p = 0.059$) (Figure 4A,B). Adult rats given a 72-h uninterrupted access to a choice between GM and CM chow preferred GM chow ($p < 0.001$), while both GM ($p = 0.015$) and CM pellets ($p < 0.001$) were preferred over standard food during a similar time of exposure (Figure 4C).

Real-time PCR analysis after consumption of the two milk formulations (GM: 19.27 +/− 0.18 g; CM: 18.44 +/− 0.17 g) revealed that GM upregulated in the nucleus accumbens PNOC ($p = 0.0164$), ORL1 ($p = 0.0042$), Cx36 ($p = 0.0017$), GLP1R ($p = 0.0015$), MC4R ($p = 0.002$), OXT ($p < 0.001$), and GHSR ($p < 0.001$) genes, whereas mRNA levels of PENK were lower (though it did not reach significance with a p value of 0.01), compared with CM consumption. In the hypothalamus, MOR ($p = 0.045$) and KOR ($p = 0.017$) transcript levels were higher after GM consumption, and in the brain stem there was a trend toward upregulation of the MC4R ($p = 0.099$) and the MC3R was upregulated ($p = 0.0275$; Figure 5). Compared to water controls, in the nucleus accumbens, GM affected expression of ORL1 ($p = 0.012$), Cx36 ($p = 0.0052$), GLP1R ($p = 0.0042$), MC4R ($p = 0.0053$), OXT ($p = 0.0149$), and GHSR ($p < 0.001$); in the hypothalamus, ORX ($p = 0.0164$), KOR ($p = 0.0399$), and MC4R ($p = 0.0403$). On the other hand, hypothalamic expression of the MC4R gene was elevated by CM intake ($p = 0.041$; Figure 5).

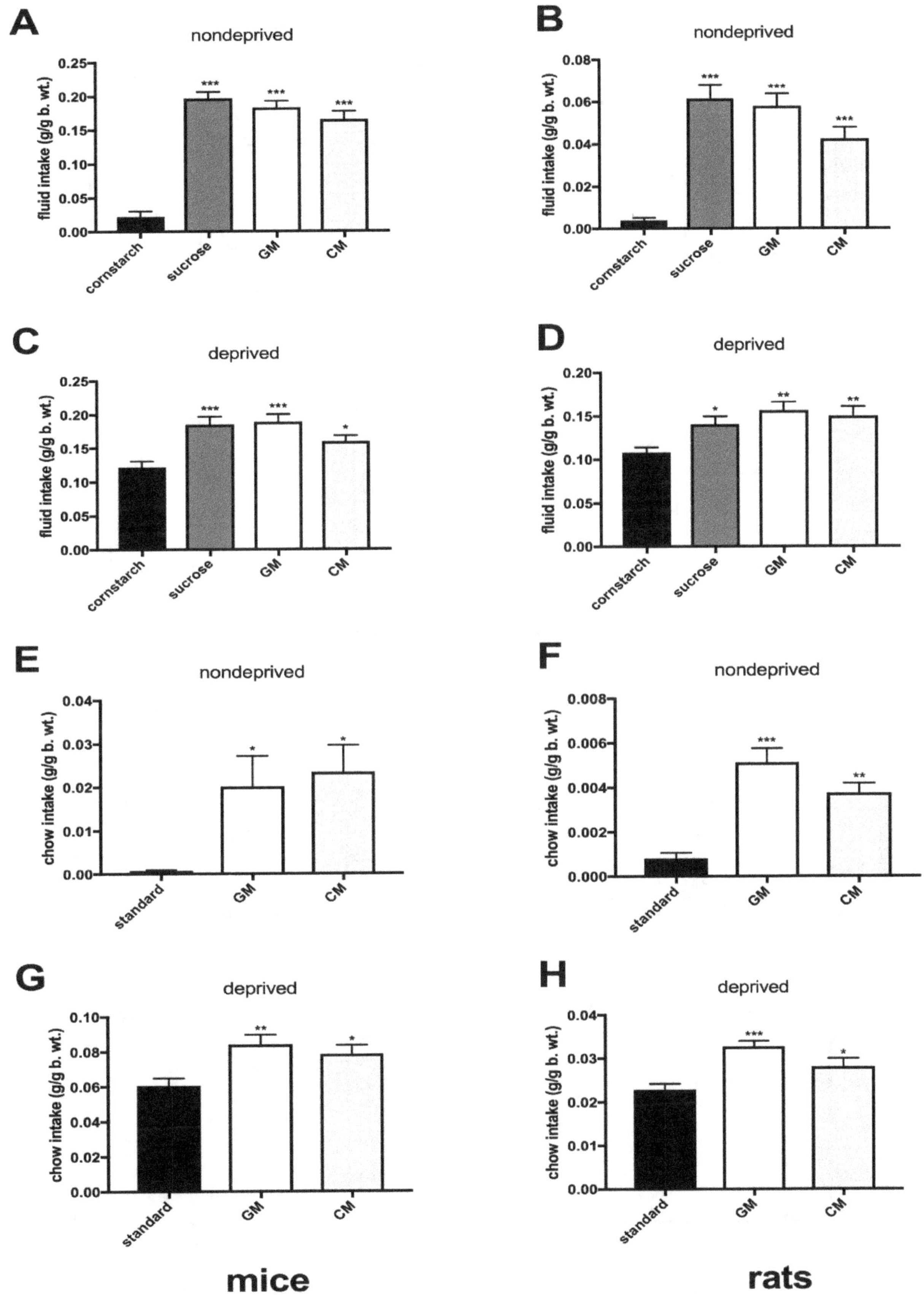

Figure 1. Episodic 2-h consumption of individually presented (acceptance) cornstarch, sucrose, GM, and CM isocaloric solutions (**A–D**), and of standard, GM- and CM-enriched chow (**E–H**) in sated (nondeprived) and energy-deprived mice (left panel) and rats (right panel).*, $p \leq 0.05$; **, $p \leq 0.01$; ***, $p \leq 0.001$.

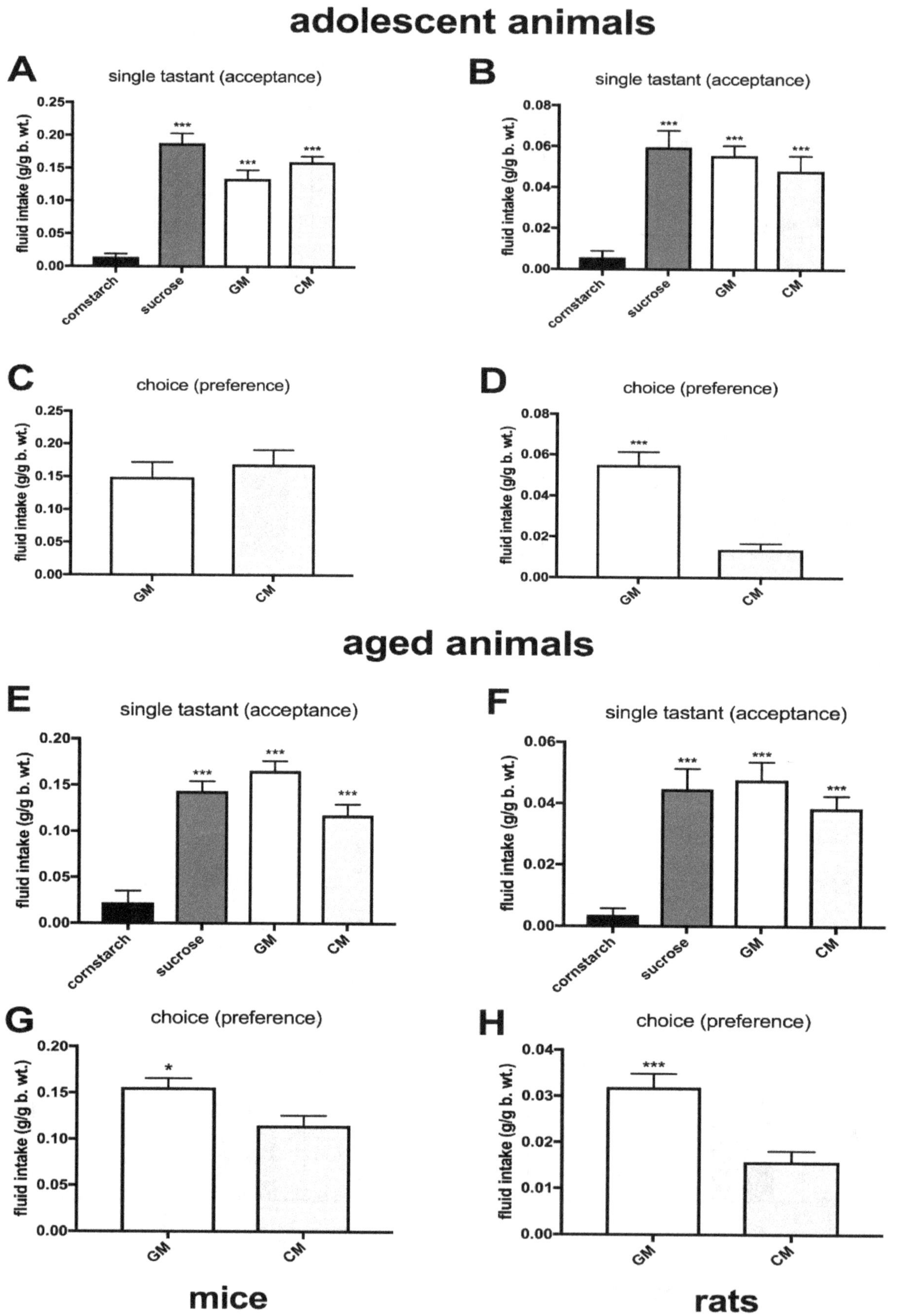

Figure 2. Episodic 2-h consumption of individually presented cornstarch, sucrose, GM, and CM isocaloric solutions (**A**,**B**,**E**,**F**: acceptance) and simultaneously given GM and CM (**C**,**D**,**G**,**H**: preference) in adolescent and aged sated mice (left panel) and rats (right panel). *, $p \leq 0.05$; ***, $p \leq 0.001$.

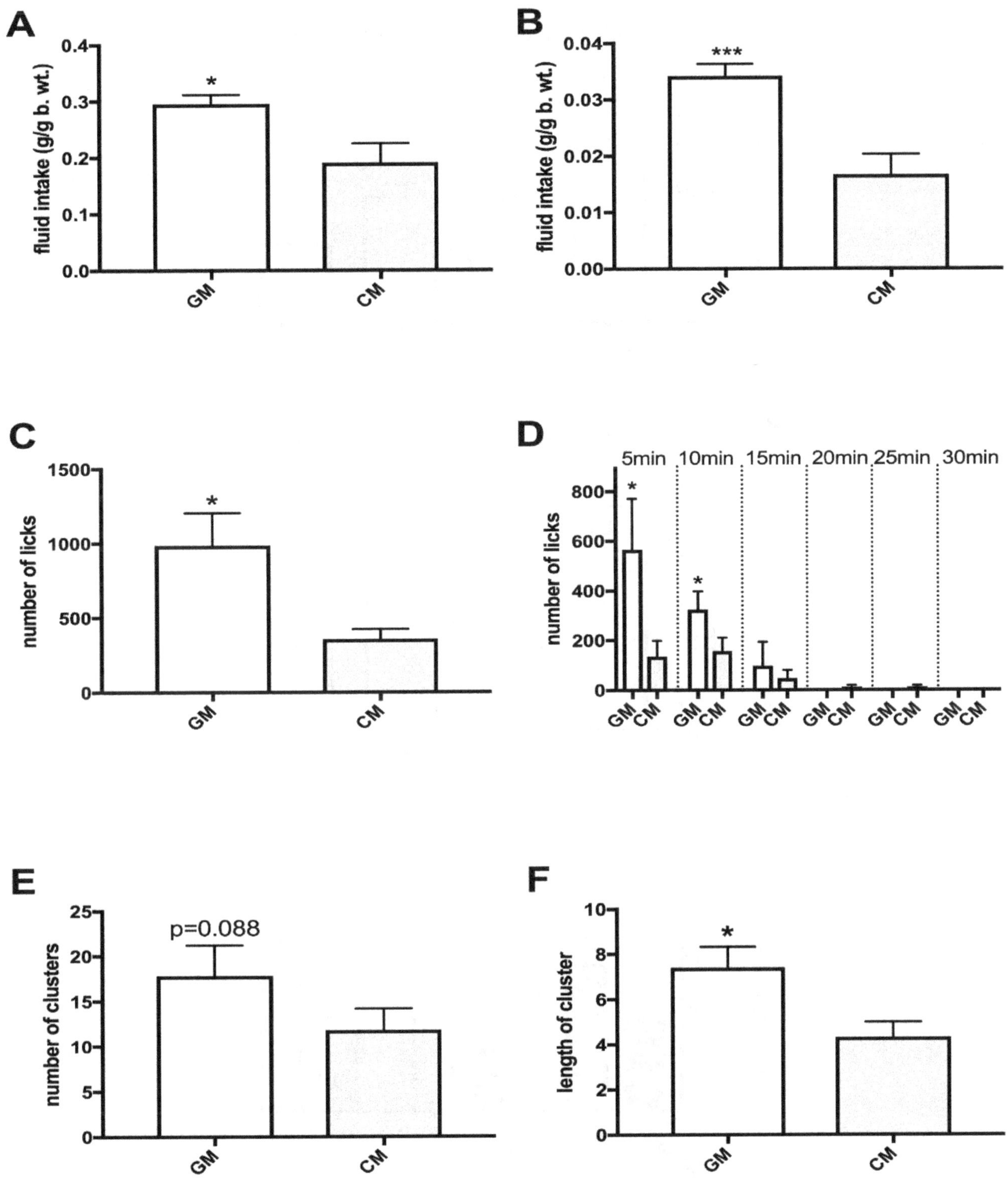

Figure 3. Episodic consumption of simultaneously presented GM and CM over 2-h in sated mice (**A**) and rats (**B**), lickometer activity during a 30-min exposure ((**C**): 0–30 min; (**D**): 5-min intervals), the number of GM over CM licking bouts (cluster number) (**E**), and the cluster length(s) of each GM and CM bout (**F**) in sated rats. *, $p \leq 0.05$; ***, $p \leq 0.001$.

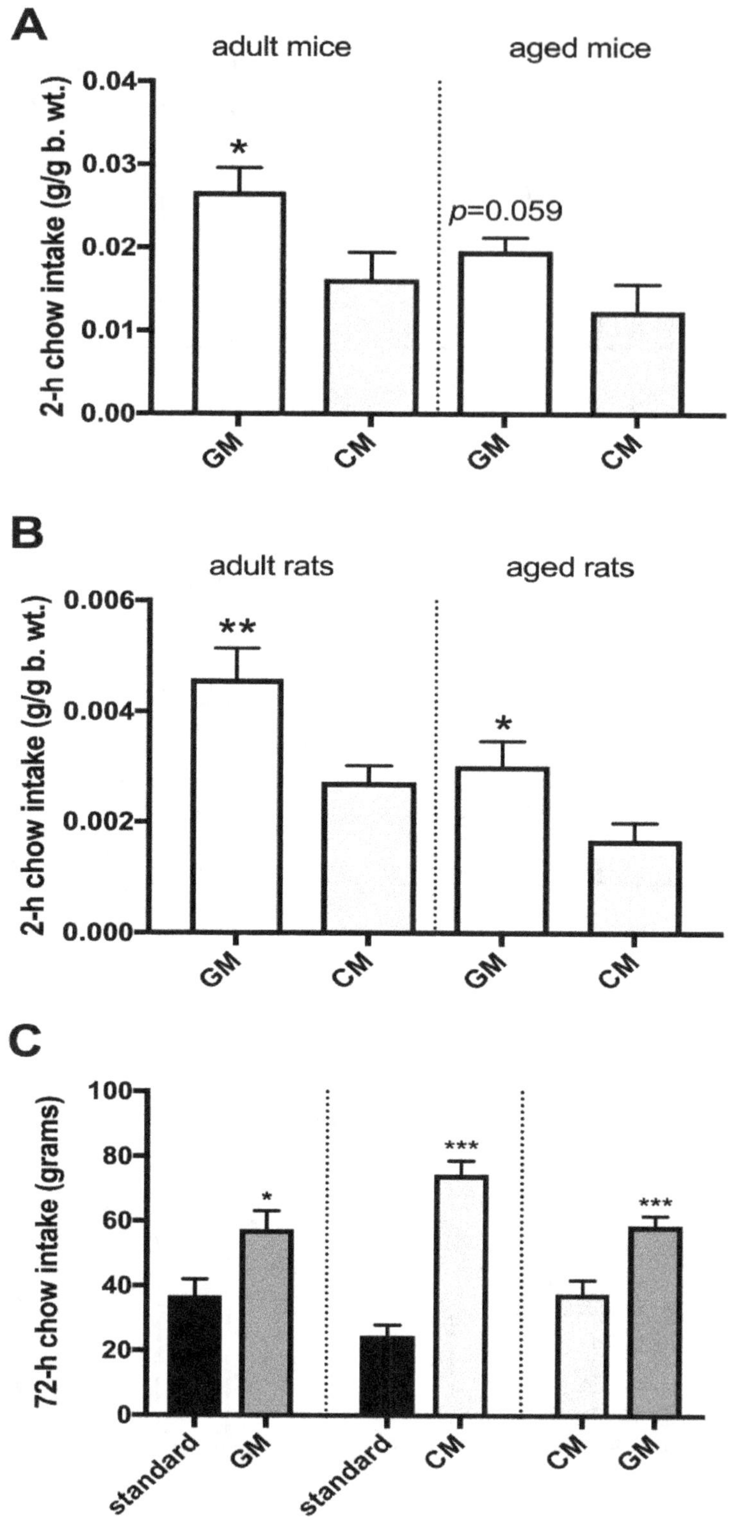

Figure 4. Consumption of simultaneously presented GM- and CM-enriched chow in adult and aged sated mice (**A**) and rats (**B**) over 2 h and simultaneously presented pellets (standard vs. GM; standard vs. CM, and GM vs. CM) over 72 h in adult rats (**C**).*, $p \leq 0.05$; **, $p \leq 0.01$; ***, $p \leq 0.001$.

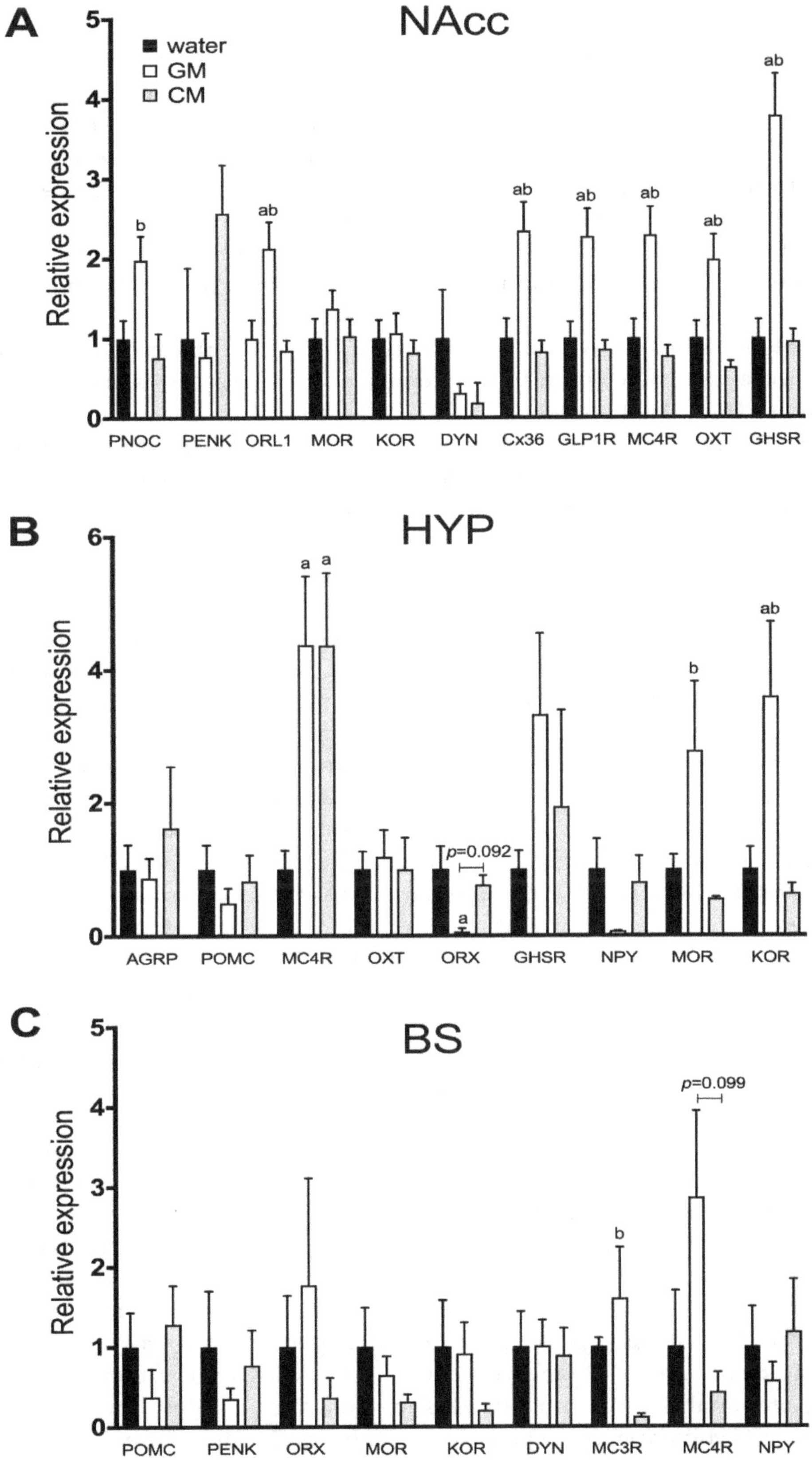

Figure 5. Relative expression of feeding-related genes in the nucleus accumbens (**A**), hypothalamus (**B**), and brain stem (**C**) of mice maintained for 24 h on GM or CM. Water served as a baseline tastant. [a]—significantly different from the water group; [b]—significantly different from the CM group. Analysis performed with ANOVA followed by Bonferroni's test and corrected for multiple comparisons.

4. Discussion

Enhanced motivation to eat in the absence of an immediate need to replenish calories or continuation of a meal beyond levels that restore energy balance typically occur when an individual is given access to food that is highly palatable. In laboratory animal models, similarly to what is observed in humans, a variety of tastants are perceived as palatable. Those include ingestants whose palatability is derived mainly from the flavor and/or postabsorptive effects of either a single macronutrient (e.g., sucrose-sweetened solutions) or from the complex contribution of multiple nutritive components (e.g., in meat rich in protein and fat) [30–32]. Calorie density of food (especially when coupled with high energy needs of an organism) is an additional factor that affects the liking of and preference for a given food [15,33].

The current set of studies show that both GM and CM and milk-enriched solid diets are highly palatable. In no-choice acceptance paradigms, energy non-deprived rats and mice of all age groups (adolescent, adult, and aged) consumed GM and CM as avidly as the calorie-matched 15% sucrose solution (used here as a positive control for a highly palatable tastant in rodents (for review, see [30]), while ingesting only minimal amounts of the 'bland' cornstarch. A similar phenomenon was observed in energy-deprived animals, although the amount by which GM, CM, and sucrose intakes exceeded that of cornstarch was not as pronounced as in sated rodents. That was due to the vigorous energy deficit-driven consumption of cornstarch and a 'ceiling effect' that prevents ingestion of large amounts of the solutions during the brief refeeding period. Importantly, GM and CM enrichment of laboratory chow stimulated intake in both hungry and sated animals well above the level of standard pellets. It indicates that both GM- and CM-derived palatability is a generalized phenomenon, not limited to liquid milks, but extending to solid foods that contain milk powder. This is in concert with the ability of other palatable tastants (including, but not limited to, fat, sucrose, and select amino acids) to have a positive gustatory effect when presented as a component of both liquid and solid foods [34]. The fact that not only adolescent and adult animals, but also the aged ones, readily consume GM and CM suggests that age-related decline in hedonic processing [22,35–37] does not completely abolish a drive to eat milk-based diets. Instead, a slightly depressed intake of GM and CM at an old age parallels that reported for sweet solutions, as shown here and by other authors [38–40]. This finding is particularly relevant from the standpoint of being able to use palatable GM or CM as nutritionally superior alternatives to, e.g., sucrose-sweetened tastants in aged individuals [23]. That adolescent rodents also consume large quantities of both milk types indicates that prolonged dietary habituation is not required to develop the liking of either GM or CM. In fact, the amounts of GM and CM ingested by juveniles were as high as the volume of sucrose (readily consumed in large quantities by young animals, e.g., see [41]) even though the individuals had had only two brief exposures to these solutions prior to the experiment.

The single-tastant scenarios above strongly suggest a high acceptance level for both GM and CM indicating they are palatable, but as these no-choice paradigms produced fairly similar feeding responses, choice studies were needed to define relative preference for these two milk types. Simultaneous 2-h exposure to two bottles containing GM and CM showed that adult and aged mice and rats as well as adolescent rats exhibit a marked preference for GM (adolescent mice were the only cohort in which GM and CM were iso-palatable). The preference for GM did not appear to be related to whether the animals' pre-exposure to the specific diets was simultaneous (such as in adolescents and adults) or sequential (aged rodents). This finding was further expanded by employing the 30-min lickometer analysis in adult rats. It showed approximately four times as many licks at the bottle containing GM compared to CM during the first 5 min of the meal, and twice as many licks at the GM bottle in the subsequent 5-min interval. Overall, the licking activity at both bottles occurred within the same timeframe with neither milk type being ingested in a prolonged fashion. It increases our confidence in that motivation to consume palatable GM rather than maintenance of a meal (due to, e.g., delayed satiation [42]) is the main reason for avid intake of GM. The analysis of the licking bouts provides additional support for this notion. The cluster number (total number of bouts) neared significance for GM, possibly reflecting the incentive motivational properties of the food stimulus; importantly, the relationship of motivation and this measure reflects post-ingestive negative feedback [43–47]. On the other hand, the average cluster length—significantly greater for the GM formulation—typically parallels the hedonic properties (mainly, orosensory pleasure) of ingestive stimuli (as reviewed, e.g., in [45]). In this case, it is the length of clusters that appears to be the main driver for the preference for GM. A good example of the significance of licking bout length versus number in the context of neural regulation of food intake comes from studies on the endogenous opioid system. Ostlund et al. found that mu opioid receptor (MOR) knockout (KO) mice show alterations in sucrose licking: while energy-deprived wild-type mice increased burst length, relative to the nondeprived condition, this aspect of licking was insensitive to changes in food deprivation in MOR KOs. The rate of sucrose and sucralose licking in KOs was lower than in wildtype animals, providing evidence that the MOR was involved in processing palatability [48]. Mendez and colleagues reported that proenkephalin (PENK) KOs given a sucrose solution exhibited fewer bouts of licking (though the length did not differ) than wild type controls, indicating a diminished motivation to eat [46]. Finally, studies on the involvement of nociceptin/orphanin FQ (NOC) revealed that NOC administration initiates new bouts of licking for sweet solutions, which is in line with the notion of its potential relationship to motivational aspects of feeding. Interestingly, energy-deprived NOP KO mice given sucrose showed longer bouts of licking than wild types, suggesting that, under hungry conditions, NOC may also affect hedonics of consumption [49].

The notion that satiety is not delayed by GM intake is supported by the experimental work exploring satiating effects of a CM- versus GM-based meal in humans. In their study, Rubio-Martín et al. presented healthy adults with GM-based or CM-based breakfast after an overnight fast and obtained blood samples and appetite ratings from the subjects just before and up to 5 h after completion of the meal. They found that that the 'desire to eat' rating was significantly lower and hunger rating tended to be lower after the GM breakfast. Interestingly, the area under the curve (AUC) for a satiety hormone GLP-1 was inversely associated with the AUChunger and AUCdesire-to-eat after the GM meal [50].

The aforementioned data obtained in human observations combined with the current results of our experiments in animal models suggest that even though composition differences between GM and CM are relatively minor, they are sufficient to significantly affect appetite-related parameters. It remains to be elucidated whether these effects are produced by a specific macronutrient component, a combination of nutritive components, and/or some physico-chemical characteristics of each milk type (e.g., micelle structures in GM vs. CM differ in diameter, hydration, and mineralization) [51].

The analysis of mRNA levels of feeding-related genes sheds more light on neural processing underlying enhanced preference for GM over CM. One of the most striking outcomes is the fact that, unlike in the NAcc, which showed an increase in multiple mRNA profiles after GM over CM, there are relatively few significant differences in gene expression in the hypothalamus and brain stem. Those two brain areas serve as the foundation for the control of energy homeostasis and consumption-related changes in the internal milieu associated with plasma osmolality, stomach distension, and defense from exposure to food-borne toxins [52]. In this network, the brain stem acts as the relay station between the periphery and the central nervous system, whereas the hypothalamus plays a endocrine role (by releasing, e.g., anorexigenic hormones, such as oxytocin (OXT) via the neurohypophysis) and innervates a number of central target sites (it includes the reciprocal connectivity with the brain stem, as well as multiple pathways with, among others, nigrostriatal and hippocampal structures). It is noteworthy that, despite the same level of intake of GM and CM over the 24-h period, the hypothalamic expression of NPY and orexin (ORX) was lower in the GM group. Both ORX and NPY in the hypothalamus enhance consumption chiefly by increasing hunger and motivating intake of energy-dense tastants [53,54]. Thus, these data suggest that enhanced preference for GM over CM does not stem from the stimulation of neural mechanisms that lead to hunger-driven feeding. In line with the aforementioned conclusion from feeding experiments that the increased preference for GM vs.

CM in choice scenarios is unlikely to be related to suppressed satiety signaling, we found that the brain stem expression of satiation promoting melanocortin receptors [55,56] is elevated after consumption of GM (it remained the same in the hypothalamus). This change in the receptor mRNA level coupled with the lack of a difference in the melanocortin ligand precursor gene expression (proopiomelanocortin, POMC) as well as in the anorexigenic OXT gene [28,57] suggests the lack of impairment in central satiety processing after GM (and, surprisingly, even a somewhat greater sensitivity of the molecular network promoting satiety in response to GM consumption).

Interestingly, the hypothalamic genes whose expression was elevated by GM intake were those encoding the MOR and kappa (KOR) opioid receptors (MOR and KOR brain stem and accumbal mRNA levels were also higher, though the difference did not reach statistical significance). Furthermore, in the NAcc, we found overexpression of genes coding for opioid-related NOC and this peptide's receptor, ORL1. Opioid receptors are directly implicated in the regulation of feeding for reward [14,42]. They are part of a dispersed network that includes the NAcc as one of the key sites mediating hedonic aspects of eating behavior. They are also expressed throughout the 'homeostatic' components of the feeding-related circuit [16], including the hypothalamus and brain stem, where they are theorized to promote excessive consumption of palatable tastants by delaying meal termination. The magnitude at which opioid receptor agonists, such as butorphanol tartrate, dynorphin and beta-endorphin, stimulate consumption parallels the relative palatability of foods [14,58]. Conversely, opioid receptor antagonists, e.g., naltrexone and naloxone, are particularly effective at reducing intake of tasty ingestants [59]. Hence, higher expression of the MOR and KOR mRNA after GM is in line with the observed preference for the GM over CM. Changes in expression of additional NAcc genes that underscore the functional relationship between GM intake and reward processing include upregulation of Cx36 mRNA, as Cx36 ensures proper synchrony of dopaminergic pathways [60], and of the growth hormone secretagogue receptor (GHSR) mRNA, considering that the GHSR in the NAcc has been found to mediate hedonics of ingestive behavior [61]. Again, as in the case of the hypothalamic gene expression analysis, genes encoding molecules that promote satiety—such as OXT, melanocortin receptor 4, and glucagon-like peptide-1 receptor [62]—were upregulated after GM, which points to the heightened reward processing rather than impaired satiation as the factor propelling preference toward GM over CM.

5. Conclusions

We conclude that, in laboratory animal models, GM and CM are highly palatable when presented as liquids and as components of solid diets. Diet choice paradigms reveal preference for GM over CM in mice and rats belonging to different age groups. Feeding studies and analyses of gene expression in the feeding-relevant brain circuit point to feeding reward as the main factor underlying preference for GM. While the current studies draw on the laboratory animal experimental approaches, they have a translational impact relevant to our understanding of the consequences of GM consumption in humans. This outcome is particularly important as, globally, likely more people drink GM than CM. GM owes its popularity to the fact that goats can thrive in diverse and changing environmental conditions, and that GM-based products are regarded as a gourmet food and health benefits of consuming GM have been defined [13]. Here we show that acceptance of GM is high and that GM is even slightly preferred over CM. Therefore, GM can be considered as both a nutritious and palatable choice for individuals at various age groups that incorporate milk in their diets.

Author Contributions: A.K., C.G.P., A.S.L. and P.K.O. designed the studies. A.K., E.L.W., S.N.G. and L.K.M. conducted feeding studies and analyzed the data. A.K. and E.L.W. performed PCR studies and analyzed the results. A.S.L., E.A.C., C.G.P. and P.K.O. aided in interpretation of results. A.K., E.L.W., A.S.L., E.A.C., C.G.P. and P.K.O. co-wrote the manuscript. All authors read and approved the final manuscript.

References

1. Drewnowski, A.; Specter, S.E. Poverty and obesity: The role of energy density and energy costs. *Am. J. Clin. Nutr.* **2004**, *79*, 6–16. [CrossRef] [PubMed]
2. Huth, P.J.; Fulgoni, V.L.; Keast, D.R.; Park, K.; Auestad, N. Major food sources of calories, added sugars, and saturated fat and their contribution to essential nutrient intakes in the U.S. diet: Data from the National Health and Nutrition Examination Survey (2003–2006). *Nutr. J.* **2013**, *12*, 116. [CrossRef] [PubMed]
3. Drewnowski, A. The contribution of milk and milk products to micronutrient density and affordability of the U.S. diet. *J. Am. Coll. Nutr.* **2011**, *30* (Suppl. 1), 422S–428S. [CrossRef]
4. Vissers, P.A.; Streppel, M.T.; Feskens, E.J.; de Groot, L.C. The contribution of dairy products to micronutrient intake in the Netherlands. *J. Am. Coll. Nutr.* **2011**, *30* (Suppl. 1), 415S–421S. [CrossRef]
5. Feskanich, D.; Willett, W.C.; Colditz, G.A. Calcium, vitamin D, milk consumption, and hip fractures: A prospective study among postmenopausal women. *Am. J. Clin. Nutr.* **2003**, *77*, 504–511. [CrossRef]
6. Chevalley, T.; Bonjour, J.P.; Ferrari, S.; Rizzoli, R. High-protein intake enhances the positive impact of physical activity on BMC in prepubertal boys. *J. Bone Miner. Res.* **2008**, *23*, 131–142. [CrossRef] [PubMed]
7. Haenlein, G.F.W. Goat milk in human nutrition. *Small Rumin. Res.* **2007**, *51*, 155–163. [CrossRef]
8. Bellioni-Businco, B.; Paganelli, R.; Lucenti, P.; Giampietro, P.G.; Perborn, H.; Businco, L. Allergenicity of goat's milk in children with cow's milk allergy. *J. Allergy Clin. Immunol.* **1999**, *103*, 1191–1194. [CrossRef]
9. Barrionuevo, M.; Lopez Aliaga, I.; Alferez, M.J.; Mesa, E.; Nestares, T.; Campos, M.S. Beneficial effect of goat milk on bioavailability of copper, zinc and selenium in rats. *J. Physiol. Biochem.* **2003**, *59*, 111–118. [CrossRef]
10. Barrionuevo, M.; Alferez, M.J.; Lopez, A.I.; Sanz, S.M.; Campos, M.S. Beneficial effect of goat milk on nutritive utilization of iron and copper in malabsorption syndrome. *J. Dairy Sci.* **2002**, *85*, 657–664. [CrossRef]
11. Díaz-Castro, J.; López-Frías, M.R.; Campos, M.S.; López-Frías, M.; Alférez, M.J.; Nestares, T.; Ojeda, M.L.; López-Aliaga, I. Severe nutritional iron-deficiency anaemia has a negative effect on some bone turnover biomarkers in rats. *Eur. J. Nutr.* **2012**, *51*, 241–247. [CrossRef] [PubMed]
12. Díaz-Castro, J.; Lopez-Frias, M.R.; Campos, M.S.; Lopez-Frias, M.; Alférez, M.J.; Nestares, T.; Ortega, E.; Lopez-Aliaga, I. Goat milk during iron repletion improves bone turnover impaired by severe iron deficiency. *J. Dairy Sci.* **2011**, *94*, 2752–2761. [CrossRef] [PubMed]
13. Silanikove, N.; Leitner, G.; Merin, U.; Prosser, C.G. Recent advances in exploiting goat's milk: Quality, safety and production aspects. *Small Rumin. Res.* **2010**, *89*, 110–124. [CrossRef]
14. Gosnell, B.A.; Levine, A.S. Reward systems and food intake: Role of opioids. *Int. J. Obes.* **2009**, *33* (Suppl. 2), S54–S58. [CrossRef] [PubMed]
15. Olszewski, P.K.; Alsio, J.; Schioth, H.B.; Levine, A.S. Opioids as facilitators of feeding: Can any food be rewarding? *Physiol. Behav.* **2011**, *104*, 105–110. [CrossRef] [PubMed]
16. Olszewski, P.K.; Cedernaes, J.; Olsson, F.; Levine, A.S.; Schioth, H.B. Analysis of the network of feeding neuroregulators using the Allen Brain Atlas. *Neurosci. Biobehav. Rev.* **2008**, *32*, 945–956. [CrossRef] [PubMed]
17. Agustí, A.; García-Pardo, M.P.; López-Almela, I.; Campillo, I.; Maes, M.; Romaní-Pérez, M.; Sanz, Y. Interplay Between the Gut-Brain Axis, Obesity and Cognitive Function. *Front. Neurosci.* **2018**, *12*, 155. [CrossRef] [PubMed]
18. Schwartz, G.J. Roles for gut vagal sensory signals in determining energy availability and energy expenditure. *Brain Res.* **2018**, *1693*, 151–153. [CrossRef]
19. De Kloet, A.D.; Herman, J.P. Fat-brain connections: Adipocyte glucocorticoid control of stress and metabolism. *Front. Neuroendocrinol.* **2018**, *48*, 50–57. [CrossRef]
20. Olszewski, P.K.; Shaw, T.J.; Grace, M.K.; Höglund, C.E.; Fredriksson, R.; Schiöth, H.B.; Levine, A.S. Complexity of neural mechanisms underlying overconsumption of sugar in scheduled feeding: Involvement of opioids, orexin, oxytocin and NPY. *Peptides* **2009**, *30*, 226–233. [CrossRef]
21. Zink, A.N.; Perez-Leighton, C.E.; Kotz, C.M. The orexin neuropeptide system: Physical activity and hypothalamic function throughout the aging process. *Front. Syst. Neurosci.* **2014**, *8*, 211. [CrossRef] [PubMed]
22. Gosnell, B.A.; Levine, A.S.; Morley, J.E. The effects of aging on opioid modulation of feeding in rats. *Life Sci.* **1983**, *32*, 2793–2799. [CrossRef]
23. Morley, J.E. Pathophysiology of the anorexia of aging. *Curr. Opin. Clin. Nutr. Metab. Care* **2013**, *16*, 27–32. [CrossRef] [PubMed]

24. Van de Heijning, B.J.; Kegler, D.; Schipper, L.; Voogd, E.; Oosting, A.; van der Beek, E.M. Acute and Chronic Effects of Dietary Lactose in Adult Rats Are not Explained by Residual Intestinal Lactase Activity. *Nutrients* **2015**, *7*, 5542–5555. [CrossRef] [PubMed]
25. McCutcheon, J.E.; Marinelli, M. Age matters. *Eur. J. Neurosci.* **2009**, *29*, 997–1014. [CrossRef] [PubMed]
26. Herisson, F.M.; Brooks, L.L.; Waas, J.R.; Levine, A.S.; Olszewski, P.K. Functional relationship between oxytocin and appetite for carbohydrates versus saccharin. *Neuroreport* **2014**, *25*, 909–914. [CrossRef]
27. Herisson, F.M.; Waas, J.R.; Fredriksson, R.; Schioth, H.B.; Levine, A.S.; Olszewski, P.K. Oxytocin Acting in the Nucleus Accumbens Core Decreases Food Intake. *J. Neuroendocrinol.* **2016**, *28*. [CrossRef] [PubMed]
28. Olszewski, P.K.; Klockars, A.; Olszewska, A.M.; Fredriksson, R.; Schioth, H.B.; Levine, A.S. Molecular, immunohistochemical, and pharmacological evidence of oxytocin's role as inhibitor of carbohydrate but not fat intake. *Endocrinology* **2010**, *151*, 4736–4744. [CrossRef] [PubMed]
29. Bonacchi, K.B.; Ackroff, K.; Touzani, K.; Bodnar, R.J.; Sclafani, A. Opioid mediation of starch and sugar preference in the rat. *Pharmacol. Biochem. Behav.* **2010**, *96*, 507–514. [CrossRef] [PubMed]
30. Levine, A.S.; Kotz, C.M.; Gosnell, B.A. Sugars: Hedonic aspects, neuroregulation, and energy balance. *Am. J. Clin. Nutr.* **2003**, *78*, 834S–842S. [CrossRef]
31. Martire, S.I.; Holmes, N.; Westbrook, R.F.; Morris, M.J. Altered feeding patterns in rats exposed to a palatable cafeteria diet: Increased snacking and its implications for development of obesity. *PLoS ONE* **2013**, *8*, e60407. [CrossRef] [PubMed]
32. Martire, S.I.; Maniam, J.; South, T.; Holmes, N.; Westbrook, R.F.; Morris, M.J. Extended exposure to a palatable cafeteria diet alters gene expression in brain regions implicated in reward, and withdrawal from this diet alters gene expression in brain regions associated with stress. *Behav. Brain Res.* **2014**, *265*, 132–141. [CrossRef]
33. Drewnowski, A. Energy density, palatability, and satiety: Implications for weight control. *Nutr. Rev.* **1998**, *56*, 347–353. [CrossRef] [PubMed]
34. Moran, T.H.; Ladenheim, E.E. Physiologic and Neural Controls of Eating. *Gastroenterol. Clin. N. Am.* **2016**, *45*, 581–599. [CrossRef]
35. Landi, F.; Calvani, R.; Tosato, M.; Martone, A.; Ortolani, E.; Savera, G.; Sisto, A.; Marzetti, E. Anorexia of Aging: Risk Factors, Consequences, and Potential Treatments. *Nutrients* **2016**, *8*, 69. [CrossRef] [PubMed]
36. Tenk, J.; Rostás, I.; Füredi, N.; Mikó, A.; Solymár, M.; Soós, S.; Gaszner, B.; Feller, D.; Székely, M.; Pétervári, E.; et al. Age-related changes in central effects of corticotropin-releasing factor (CRF) suggest a role for this mediator in aging anorexia and cachexia. *Geroscience* **2017**, *39*, 61–72. [CrossRef]
37. Tomm, R.J.; Tse, M.T.; Tobiansky, D.J.; Schweitzer, H.R.; Soma, K.K.; Floresco, S.B. Effects of aging on executive functioning and mesocorticolimbic dopamine markers in male Fischer 344 x brown Norway rats. *Neurobiol. Aging* **2018**, *72*, 134–146. [CrossRef]
38. Inui-Yamamoto, C.; Yamamoto, T.; Ueda, K.; Nakatsuka, M.; Kumabe, S.; Inui, T.; Iwai, Y. Taste preference changes throughout different life stages in male rats. *PLoS ONE* **2017**, *12*, e0181650. [CrossRef]
39. Sakai, M.; Kazui, H.; Shigenobu, K.; Komori, K.; Ikeda, M.; Nishikawa, T. Gustatory Dysfunction as an Early Symptom of Semantic Dementia. *Dement. Geriatr. Cogn. Dis. Extra* **2017**, *7*, 395–405. [CrossRef]
40. Shin, Y.K.; Cong, W.N.; Cai, H.; Kim, W.; Maudsley, S.; Egan, J.M.; Martin, B. Age-related changes in mouse taste bud morphology, hormone expression, and taste responsivity. *J. Gerontol. A Biol. Sci. Med. Sci.* **2012**, *67*, 336–344. [CrossRef]
41. Naneix, F.; Darlot, F.; Coutureau, E.; Cador, M. Long-lasting deficits in hedonic and nucleus accumbens reactivity to sweet rewards by sugar overconsumption during adolescence. *Eur. J. Neurosci.* **2016**, *43*, 671–680. [CrossRef]
42. Glass, M.J.; Grace, M.K.; Cleary, J.P.; Billington, C.J.; Levine, A.S. Naloxone's effect on meal microstructure of sucrose and cornstarch diets. *Am. J. Physiol. Regul. Integr. Comp. Physiol.* **2001**, *281*, R1605–R1612. [CrossRef] [PubMed]
43. Higgs, S.; Cooper, S.J. Evidence for early opioid modulation of licking responses to sucrose and intralipid: A microstructural analysis in the rat. *Psychopharmacology* **1998**, *139*, 342–355. [CrossRef] [PubMed]
44. D'Aquila, P.S. Dopamine on D2-like receptors "reboosts" dopamine D1-like receptor-mediated behavioural activation in rats licking for sucrose. *Neuropharmacology* **2010**, *58*, 1085–1096. [CrossRef] [PubMed]
45. Dwyer, D.M. EPS Prize Lecture. Licking and liking: The assessment of hedonic responses in rodents. *Q. J. Exp. Psychol.* **2012**, *65*, 371–394. [CrossRef]

46. Mendez, I.A.; Ostlund, S.B.; Maidment, N.T.; Murphy, N.P. Involvement of Endogenous Enkephalins and beta-Endorphin in Feeding and Diet-Induced Obesity. *Neuropsychopharmacology* **2015**, *40*, 2103–2112. [CrossRef] [PubMed]
47. Davis, J.D.; Smith, G.P. Analysis of the microstructure of the rhythmic tongue movements of rats ingesting maltose and sucrose solutions. *Behav. Neurosci.* **1992**, *106*, 217–228. [CrossRef] [PubMed]
48. Ostlund, S.B.; Kosheleff, A.; Maidment, N.T.; Murphy, N.P. Decreased consumption of sweet fluids in mu opioid receptor knockout mice: A microstructural analysis of licking behavior. *Psychopharmacology* **2013**, *229*, 105–113. [CrossRef] [PubMed]
49. Mendez, I.A.; Maidment, N.T.; Murphy, N.P. Parsing the hedonic and motivational influences of nociceptin on feeding using licking microstructure analysis in mice. *Behav. Pharmacol.* **2016**, *27*, 516–527. [CrossRef]
50. Rubio-Martín, E.; García-Escobar, E.; Ruiz de Adana, M.S.; Lima-Rubio, F.; Peláez, L.; Caracuel, A.M.; Bermúdez-Silva, F.J.; Soriguer, F.; Rojo-Martínez, G.; Olveira, G. Comparison of the Effects of Goat Dairy and Cow Dairy Based Breakfasts on Satiety, Appetite Hormones, and Metabolic Profile. *Nutrients* **2017**, *9*, 877. [CrossRef]
51. Park, Y.W.; Juarez, M.; Ramos, M.; Haenlein, G.F.W. Physico-chemical characteristics of goat and sheep milk. *Small Rumin. Res.* **2007**, *68*, 88–113. [CrossRef]
52. Klockars, A.; Levine, A.S.; Olszewski, P.K. Hypothalamic Integration of the Endocrine Signaling Related to Food Intake. *Curr. Top. Behav. Neurosci.* **2018**. [CrossRef]
53. Levine, A.S.; Jewett, D.C.; Cleary, J.P.; Kotz, C.M.; Billington, C.J. Our journey with neuropeptide Y: Effects on ingestive behaviors and energy expenditure. *Peptides* **2004**, *25*, 505–510. [CrossRef]
54. Nixon, J.P.; Kotz, C.M.; Novak, C.M.; Billington, C.J.; Teske, J.A. Neuropeptides controlling energy balance: Orexins and neuromedins. *Handb. Exp. Pharmacol.* **2012**, *209*, 77–109.
55. Wirth, M.M.; Olszewski, P.K.; Yu, C.; Levine, A.S.; Giraudo, S.Q. Paraventricular hypothalamic alpha-melanocyte-stimulating hormone and MTII reduce feeding without causing aversive effects. *Peptides* **2001**, *22*, 129–134. [CrossRef]
56. Girardet, C.; Butler, A.A. Neural melanocortin receptors in obesity and related metabolic disorders. *Biochim. Biophys. Acta* **2014**, *1842*, 482–494. [CrossRef] [PubMed]
57. Olszewski, P.K.; Klockars, A.; Levine, A.S. Oxytocin: A Conditional Anorexigen whose Effects on Appetite Depend on the Physiological, Behavioural and Social Contexts. *J. Neuroendocrinol.* **2016**, *28*. [CrossRef] [PubMed]
58. Gosnell, B.A.; Levine, A.S.; Morley, J.E. The stimulation of food intake by selective agonists of mu, kappa and delta opioid receptors. *Life Sci.* **1986**, *38*, 1081–1088. [CrossRef]
59. Giraudo, S.Q.; Grace, M.K.; Welch, C.C.; Billington, C.J.; Levine, A.S. Naloxone's anorectic effect is dependent upon the relative palatability of food. *Pharmacol. Biochem. Behav.* **1993**, *46*, 917–921. [CrossRef]
60. Steffensen, S.C.; Bradley, K.D.; Hansen, D.M.; Wilcox, J.D.; Wilcox, R.S.; Allison, D.W.; Merrill, C.B.; Edwards, J.G. The role of connexin-36 gap junctions in alcohol intoxication and consumption. *Synapse* **2011**, *65*, 695–707. [CrossRef] [PubMed]
61. Skibicka, K.P.; Shirazi, R.H.; Rabasa-Papio, C.; Alvarez-Crespo, M.; Neuber, C.; Vogel, H.; Dickson, S.L. Divergent circuitry underlying food reward and intake effects of ghrelin: Dopaminergic VTA-accumbens projection mediates ghrelin's effect on food reward but not food intake. *Neuropharmacology* **2013**, *73*, 274–283. [CrossRef] [PubMed]
62. Kanoski, S.E.; Hayes, M.R.; Skibicka, K.P. GLP-1 and weight loss: Unraveling the diverse neural circuitry. *Am. J. Physiol. Regul. Integr. Comp. Physiol.* **2016**, *310*, R885–R895. [CrossRef] [PubMed]

9

From Probiotics to Psychobiotics: Live Beneficial Bacteria Which Act on the Brain-Gut Axis

Luis G. Bermúdez-Humarán [1,*], Eva Salinas [2], Genaro G. Ortiz [3], Luis J. Ramirez-Jirano [3], J. Alejandro Morales [4] and Oscar K. Bitzer-Quintero [3,*]

1 INRA, Micalis Institute, INRA, AgroParisTech, Université Paris-Saclay, 78352 Jouy-en-Josas, France
2 Department of Microbiology, Center of Basic Science, Universidad Autónoma de Aguascalientes, Aguascalientes 20131, Mexico; emsalin@correo.uaa.mx
3 Neurosciences Division, Centro de Investigación Biomédica de Occidente, Instituto Mexicano del Seguro Social, Guadalajara 44340, Jalisco, Mexico; genarogabriel@yahoo.com (G.G.O.); ramirez_jirano@hotmail.com (L.J.R.-J.)
4 Department of Computer Sciences, Universidad de Guadalajara, Guadalajara 44430, Jalisco, Mexico; jalejandro.morales@academicos.udg.mx
* Correspondence: luis.bermudez@inra.fr (L.G.B.-H.); neuronim26@yahoo.com (O.K.B.-Q.)

Abstract: There is an important relationship between probiotics, psychobiotics and cognitive and behavioral processes, which include neurological, metabolic, hormonal and immunological signaling pathways; the alteration in these systems may cause alterations in behavior (mood) and cognitive level (learning and memory). Psychobiotics have been considered key elements in affective disorders and the immune system, in addition to their effect encompassing the regulation of neuroimmune regulation and control axes (the hypothalamic-pituitary-adrenal axis or HPA, the sympathetic-adrenal-medullary axis or SAM and the inflammatory reflex) in diseases of the nervous system. The aim of this review is to summarize the recent findings about psychobiotics, the brain-gut axis and the immune system. The review focuses on a very new and interesting field that relates the microbiota of the intestine with diseases of the nervous system and its possible treatment, in neuroimmunomodulation area. Indeed, although probiotic bacteria will be concentrated after ingestion, mainly in the intestinal epithelium (where they provide the host with essential nutrients and modulation of the immune system), they may also produce neuroactive substances which act on the brain-gut axis.

Keywords: probiotics; microbiota; beneficial bacteria; psychobiotics; human health

---

1. Introduction

The skin and mucosal surfaces of vertebrates contain a wide collection of microorganisms (collectively named microbiota) which includes bacteria, fungi, parasites and viruses. The human gut harbors one of the most complex and abundant ecosystems composed of up to 10^{13}–10^{14} microorganisms which is between 1 to 10 times more than the number of eukaryotic cells in the body [1,2]. The collective adult human gut microbiota is composed of a maximum of 500–1000 bacterial species [1,3,4].

Hundreds of years of co-evolution have led to a mutual symbiosis between the host and gut microbiome. Indeed, the gut is rich in molecules that can be used as nutrients by the microorganisms, favoring microbiota colonization [1]. Gut colonization begins at birth and is established in the first 3 years of life. The initial interaction between gut microbiota and the host is indispensable for the maturation of the nervous system, the immune system and for the developmental regulation of intestinal physiology [1,5,6]. At this stage, gut microbiota is also able to modulate the process of angiogenesis [7]. Furthermore, microorganisms also display anti-microbial activities, thus maintaining a stable gut ecosystem. Alterations in the process of microbial colonization of the human gut in early life have been shown to influence the risk of disease [8].

Later in life, microbial colonization of the intestine has a significant impact on the host neurophysiology, behavior and function of the nervous system [9–11]. Given the immunomodulatory properties of gut microbiota, it has been shown that different immune pathways, inside and outside the central nervous system (CNS) are involved in important mechanisms like microbial mediation of brain functions and behavior. It has been discovered that neuroimmune modulation by the microbiota is able to contribute to etio-pathogenesis or to display important signs and symptoms in neurodegenerative and behavioral disorders such as autism spectrum disorders (ASD), anxiety, depression, Alzheimer's disease (AD) and Parkinson's disease (PD) [9].

Furthermore, different bacteria, which are commonly present in a large diversity of food products, transit through our gut every day, interacting with the food products themselves, the host microbiota, and our own cells in either a healthy or a pathological context. Many of the latter microorganisms are known as probiotics. Probiotics are defined as "live microorganisms which when administered in adequate amounts confer a health benefit on the host" [12]. This concept is based on the observations made by Élie Metchnikoff in 1907 in which the regular consumption of lactic acid bacteria (LAB) in fermented dairy products, such as yogurt, was associated with enhanced health and longevity in many people living in Bulgarian villages.

In association with probiotics, the concept of prebiotic was firstly introduced by Gibson and Roberfroid in 1995 as a "nondigestible food ingredient that beneficially affects the host by selectively stimulating the growth and/or activity of one or a limited number of bacteria already resident in the colon" [13]. This definition implies their ability to resist host digestion and their unique activity on microbiota intestinal. However, the progress in prebiotic study has forced the evolution of this definition, as they can also be directly administered to other sites of the body that are also colonized by commensal bacteria, such as skin or vagina. Recently, the International Scientific Association for Probiotics and Prebiotics (ISAPP) in a consensus panel proposed a new definition of prebiotics as "a substrate that is selectively utilized by host microorganisms conferring a health benefit", considering that dietary ones must not be degraded by host enzymes [14]. Substrates that fit with this definition include oligosaccharides (OS), polyunsaturated fatty acid, conjugated linoleic acid, plant polyphenols, and certain fermentable fibers. Among prebiotics highlight fructooligosaccharides (FOS), inulin, galactooligosaccharides (GOS), mannanoligosaccharides (MOS), xylooligosaccharides (XOS) and human milk oligosaccharides (HMO), being FOS and GOS the most studied as well as the classically accepted ones [14]. Prebiotics have been demonstrated to exert beneficial effects on the gastrointestinal tract, immune system, bones, lipid and sugar metabolism, and on mental health.

Dinan and coworkers [15] originally defined psychobiotics as probiotics that, upon ingestion in adequate amounts, yield positive influence on mental health. Because prebiotics have demonstrated benefit on mental health and they support the growing of specific commensal bacteria with psychophysiological effects, prebiotics can be included in the definition of psychobiotics [16]. In this sense, most prebiotic substrates analyzed for their neural effects are FOS and GOS, which favorably stimulate the growth of bifidobacteria and lactobacilli.

The effect of psychobiotics is not limited to the regulation of the neuroimmune axes (hypothalamic pituitary adrenal (HPA)-axis, sympatho-adrenal medullary (SAM)-axis and the inflammatory reflex) and in diseases that involve the nervous system, but they are also related to cognitive, memory, learning and behavior. Psychobiotics have thus opened a very broad and interesting panorama that changes the current paradigm of symbiosis between bacteria and humans. From this new point of view, this relationship seems to be more a commensalism, rather than a pure symbiosis.

2. Axes of Neuroimmune Control and Regulation

It has been shown that there is an important neural control of the immune system [17]. A well-known principle of the physiology in mammals is that the nervous system is responsible for achieving homeostasis by modulating of the function of other systems in the body through the HPA axis, the inflammatory reflex, the enteric nervous system (ENS) and finally the brain-gut axis.

Microglia is the resident immune cell in the CNS which represents 5 to 20% of glial cells. It is a myeloid cell, phagocytic, and has the activity of an antigen presenting cell (APC). In addition, it releases cytokines and can activate inflammatory-type responses [18,19]. During the early development stage, the microglia "brand" and "clean" synapses through a process called "synaptic pruning", promotes the "wiring" of neuronal circuits and releases cytokines and chemokines that assist and guide the process of neuronal differentiation [18,20]. The microbiota has a direct influence on the maturation and function of the microglia. In germ-free (GF)-animals, the microglia display a longer development process and with more derivations, with high levels in the expression of receptor-1 of the colony stimulating factor (CSF1R), F4/80 and CD31, factors that decrease in expression during development. This suggests that there is an important effect of the microbiota on the microglia, which depends on the stage of development and/or the time of microbial colonization.

The microglia of adult GF-mice can be functionally damaged when there are alterations caused by lipopolysaccharide (LPS) or by lymphocytic choriomeningitis virus, which in turn causes alterations in the correct activation of the immune system, including an increase in the release of proinflammatory cytokines such as tumor necrosis factor (TNF)-α, interleukin (IL)-1β and IL-6. These functional deficits are consistent with the concept that the naive microglia of adult GF-mice has a significant decrease in the expression of several genes important to interferon (IFN)-mediated responses, in genes for innate immune responses and genes for viral defense response and effector processes [9,21].

The mechanisms through which intestinal microbes exert their influence on microglia in the brain are not clear but it seems that there is a "microglial modulation" according to a specific type of bacteria [9]. This has raised the question of whether the effects of microbiota on microglia are not regulated by bacteria in general, by the microbiome, or if very specific microbial species are required [9]. The alterations in the morphology of the microglia in GF-animals and the alteration in the expression of genes can be normalized thanks to the post-natal supplementation with short-chain fatty acids (SCFAs), which are products of bacterial fermentation [22,23], suggesting that the bacterial species producing SCFAs are able to restore the alterations that occur in the microglia in GF-mice or treated with antibiotics [9].

The coordination of information between neurons, microglia and the responses at the central level with the periphery is carried out through the different axes of regulation and control; the HPA axis, and the inflammatory reflex (Figure 1). The coordination of these defense responses is mediated by signaling pathways related to the hypothalamus, the pituitary gland and the adrenal glands (e.g., HPA-axis), which causes the release of chemical molecules capable of altering behavior, including glucocorticoids, mineralocorticoids, and catecholamines. The activity of the HPA-axis is regulated by multiple sympathetic, parasympathetic and limbic circuits (amygdala, hippocampus and medial prefrontal cortex) that will directly or indirectly activate the hypothalamic paraventricular nucleus (PVN) [24]. Under normal conditions HPA-axis activity exhibits continuous oscillatory activity synchronized with circadian as well as ultradian rhythms [25,26].

The sympathic nervous system (SNS) and HPA-axis activation are the main components of neurotransmitter release and of neuroendocrine molecules of the stress response [27]. To respond to stress, the SNS is responsible for increasing catecholamine levels in the systemic circulation and tissues, with the concomitant release of corticotropin releasing factor (CRF) from hypothalamic paraventricular neurons, then the release of the adrenocorticotropic hormone (ACTH) from the anterior pituitary gland is stimulated, and ACTH travels through the circulation systemic and induces the synthesis and release of glucocorticoids from adrenals, cortisol in humans and corticosterone in animals. The primary function of the SNS and HPA-axis activation is to prepare the body to respond to damage by increasing the level of glucose in the blood through gluconeogenesis, the suppression of the immune system (suppression of cytokines) and increasing the metabolism of fats and proteins [27,28].

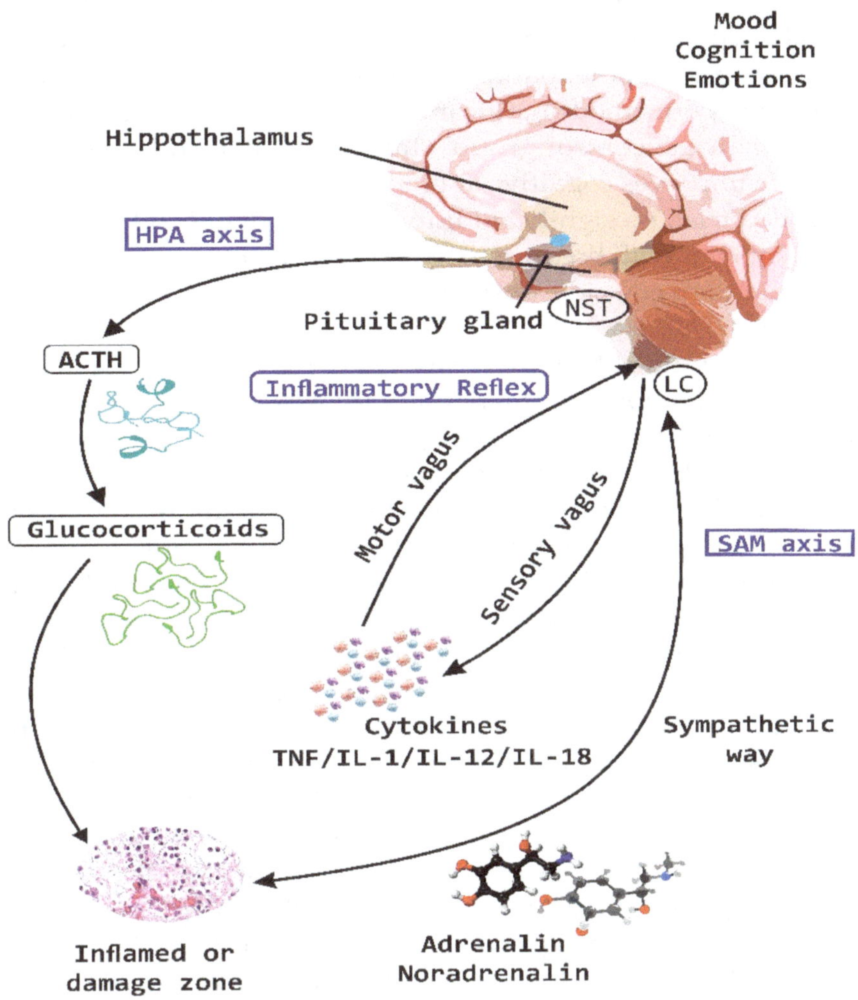

Figure 1. Regulation and control of neuroimmune axes. The three systems of regulation and control of information between the central nervous system (CNS) and the periphery are the hypothalamic pituitary adrenal (HPA)-axis, the sympatho-adrenal medullary (SAM)-axis and the inflammatory reflex. These systems are permanently sensing through nociceptive receptors and send information in real time to the CNS. ACTH, adrenocorticotropic hormone; NST Nucleus of the solitary tract; LC Locus coeruleus; TNF, tumor necrosis factor; IL, interleukin.

The responses of the HPA-axis as well as other variables of the stress response are regulated by exposure to psychological and physical stressors, such as infections [29]. The response of the HPA-axis and the SAM axis to psychological stress is mediated by neurotransmitter systems such as serotonin (5-HT), norepinepherine (NE) and endorphins, which play an important inhibitory role [29].

In addition, the HPA axis is strongly regulated to react efficiently to pathogens such as *Escherichia coli*. This response is mediated by the synthesis of prostanoids induced by the enzyme cyclo-oxygenase (COX). The elevation in corticosterone levels correlates with the increase in prostaglandin (PG) E2 in the circulation [29].

Interestingly, prebiotic intake in early life has been associated with beneficial neurological effects in adulthood. To demonstrate this effect, William and co-workers [30] fed neonatal rats (3 days old) with B-GOS during 19 or 53 days and showed that levels of the *N*-methyl-D-aspartate receptor (NMDAR) N2A subunit, synaptophysin and the brain-derived neurotrophic factor (BDNF) in the hippocampus of adult rats were elevated as compared with control fed animals. As the expression of the microtubule-associated-protein-2 (MAP2) was not affected, authors propose that neonatal B-GOS feeding impacts on neurotransmission, but not on synaptic architecture. Similar results were reported by Oliveros group [31] supplementing rat pups with 2′-fucosyllactose (FL) during the lactation period. When animals were evaluated just after weaning there was no change in behavior, although 2′-FL-feed rats evoked more intense long-term potentiation (LTP) than control ones. Same animals were evaluated at the age of 1 year and they performed significantly better in behavioral tests and still evoked more intense and longer TLP than the control group. Taken together, these results show that prebiotic administration early in life improves cognitive abilities both in childhood and in adulthood. However, in a randomized controlled trial, no significant improvement in neurodevelopmental outcomes was observed in preterm infants fed with breast milk or preterm formula supplemented with short-chain GOS/long-chain FOS/pectin-derived acidic OS between days 3 and 30 of life when they were evaluated at one or two years of age [32,33].

The basic organizational unit of the nervous system is the reflex arc, which is composed of sensory neurons (afferent) that report information to the CNS and motor neurons (efferent) that send "regulatory" signals to "target" tissues in the periphery. Recent advances in both neuroscience and immunology have revealed that there are neural reflexes that can regulate immune function in a wide range of species through evolution, from *Caenorhabditis elegans* to more complex mammals [17,34,35].

Inflammation is a key process of mammals in order to fight against pathogenic microorganisms and in the mechanism of wound healing. The molecular products of a bacterial invasion and of damaged tissue are rapidly detected by pattern recognition receptors (PRRs), which activate the cells of the innate immune system. The early response of these cells starts a cascade of events whose main function is the exclusion of pathogens and the subsequent restoration of homeostasis. This process includes the synthesis and release of proinflammatory cytokines and leukocyte recruitment [17].

It is crucial for the host to regulate and control an inflammatory response. Different mechanisms of regulation and control of inflammatory mediators have been described; for example, the release of inhibitory cytokines and soluble receptors to cytokines, as well as the activation of different subtypes of regulatory lymphocytes [36]. It is interesting to note that PRRs (Toll-like receptors, TLRs, and Nucleotide-binding and oligomerization domain (NOD)-like receptors, NLRs), in addition to the receptors for cytokines and PG are also expressed by sensory neurons [37]. This provides a molecular mechanism by which the CNS acquires information from a process of inflammation localized in the periphery. In addition, sensory nerves can react to the presence of microbial products independently of the activation of the immune system [17]. These nerves form a dense network along the external surfaces of the organism, and it has been suggested that this type of innervation provides the anatomical basis for a very precise "sensing" by the CNS against a potential infection with a pathogen, a tissue damage or an inflammatory process [17,37]. Reciprocally, many of the cells of the immune system express receptors for neurotransmitters such as dopamine (DA), acetylcholine (Ach) and norepinephrine (NE), all of which in turn regulate the differentiation and activity of leukocytes [17,38–40].

In this phenomenon, afferent signals are transmitted through the "vagus nerve", which are processed at the central level (CNS) and return to the periphery via the vagus efferent nerve, a process by which the release of cytokines is regulated by splenic macrophages [17,41]. Spleen is the major organ where TNF-α is synthesized and released systematically during an endotoxic process (endotoxemia). It has been shown that electrical stimulation of the vagus nerve significantly reduces the release of TNF-α in the spleen. However, the vagus nerve does not directly supply the spleen, the signal travels to the celiac ganglion, where the splenic adrenergic nerve also flows. The electrical stimulation of the latter also reduces the synthesis of TNF-α in the spleen. For this inhibition to occur, activation of the α7 subunit of the nicotinic acetylcholine receptor (α7nAchR) in splenic macrophages is necessary. The adrenergic nerve terminals are very close to a sub-type of T lymphocytes in the spleen that expresses the enzyme choline acetyltransferase (AchT), which has the ability to synthesize Ach, a neurotransmitter that is necessary to inhibit the synthesis and release of TNF-α in the spleen [42].

The vagus nerve, in addition to the splenic and splanchnic nerves, provide an important line of communication with the HPA-axis [29]. For instances, 2 h after vagal stimulation in rodents there is an increase in the expression of the mRNA of CRF in the hypothalamus and corticotropin-releasing hormone (CRH) which in turn increases the levels of ACTH and plasma corticosterone levels. The clinical relevance is the fact that vagal stimulation is associated with clinical benefits (signs and symptoms) antidepressants, together with the "normalization" of HPA-axis parameters in patients with refractory depression [43].

The impact of other prebiotics on brain physiology and biochemistry has also been experimentally studied. Rats that received a diet for 5 weeks supplemented with 2′-FL, the most abundant HMO, experienced increased BNDF levels in the striatum and hippocampus [44]. The expression of other two brain functional markers involved in the LTP process, the postsynaptic density protein (PSD)-95 and phosphorylated calcium/calmodulin-dependent kinase II (pCaMKII), was also augmented at frontal cortex and hippocampus, and at hippocampus, respectively. In accordance, authors reported an enhancement of synaptic plasticity in rats with that feeding regimen and in mice with a 2′-FL long-term feeding (12 weeks) protocol. Both species improved input/output curves and LPT experimentally evoked at hippocampal synapses, with a better performance of the animals in different applied tests of learning behavior.

Finally, some studies have addressed the impact of prebiotics in experimental models of neural dysfunctions. The first one was focused on analyzing the effect of GOS intake in a mouse model of amyotrophic lateral sclerosis (ALS) [45]. Animals started to receive the prebiotic at the age of 8 weeks on a daily basis until the end of the protocol. Mice orally fed with GOS experienced delayed onset of the disease, extended lifespan, improved muscle atrophy, attenuated oxidative stress of skeletal muscles, suppressed astrocyte and microglia activation, inflammatory response and apoptosis in spinal cord tissue. Authors attributed neuroprotective effects of GOS on ALS-sick mice to the amelioration on homocysteine serum levels, an amino acid related to neurotoxic effects in the pathogenesis of ALS, and to the increases in the amount of VitB12 and folato, both of which are involved in homocysteine metabolism [46]. Besides, beneficial effects of GOS have been also described in neuropsychiatric disorders where anxiety and neuroinflammation are clinically involved [47]. In this sense, the supplementation of 8 weeks-old mice standard diet with B-GOS incorporated to drink water during 3 weeks reduced LPS-induced anxiety. B-GOS intake also decreased elevated cortical IL-1β and 5-HT2A receptor expression mediated by LPS in the frontal cortex, in the absence of altered 5-HT metabolism. Thus, the anti-inflammatory effect of the prebiotic is probably modulating its anxiolytic activity. A similar link between anti-inflammation and neuroprotection was reported for chitosan oligosaccharides (CHO) [48] and FOS [49] in a rat model of AD. When CHO was orally administered to amyloid-$\beta_{1\text{-}42}$-induced rats during 2 weeks, the learning and memory deficits were reduced, and the hippocampal cell death decreased. At the same time, CHO treatment inhibited oxidative stress together with a reduction in proinflammatory cytokines expression at the hippocampus, particularly IL-1β and TNF-α [48]. In the case of a study done with FOS, it was orally and daily administered to amyloid-$\beta_{1\text{-}42}$-induced rats for 4 weeks or to D-Galactose-induced rats for 8 weeks, with similar outcomes. FOS intake improves inflammation and oxidative stress disorder, ameliorates learning and memory difficulties, and regulates the synthesis and secretion of neurotransmitters such as NE, DA, 5-HT, and 5-hydroxyindole acetic acid (5-HIAA) [49]. All these FOS-induced effects on AD are mediated by the regulation of the gut microbiota.

3. The Interaction of Microbiota with Enteric Nervous System and Brain-Gut Axes

In the last 10 years the importance of the brain-gut axis has been highlighted [50–52]. A connection has been established between the gut and the CNS, which is essential to achieve host homeostasis. It has been called the "brain-gut axis" or "GB axis" [53] (Figure 2). The brain-gut axis includes: the CNS, neuroendocrine and neuroimmune systems, the sympathetic and parasympathetic "arms" of the autonomic nervous system (ANS), the enteric nervous system (ENS) and noticeably the intestinal microbiota [29]. All these components interact and form a very complex network of reflexes, with afferent fibers (input) that project towards integrative structures of the CNS and efferent fibers (output) with projections towards the smooth muscle. This bi-directional communication network enables the sending of signals from the brain and influences the motor, sensory and secretory part of the gut, and conversely, visceral messages from the intestine can influence brain functions, especially in areas dedicated to the regulation of stress at the hypothalamic level [29].

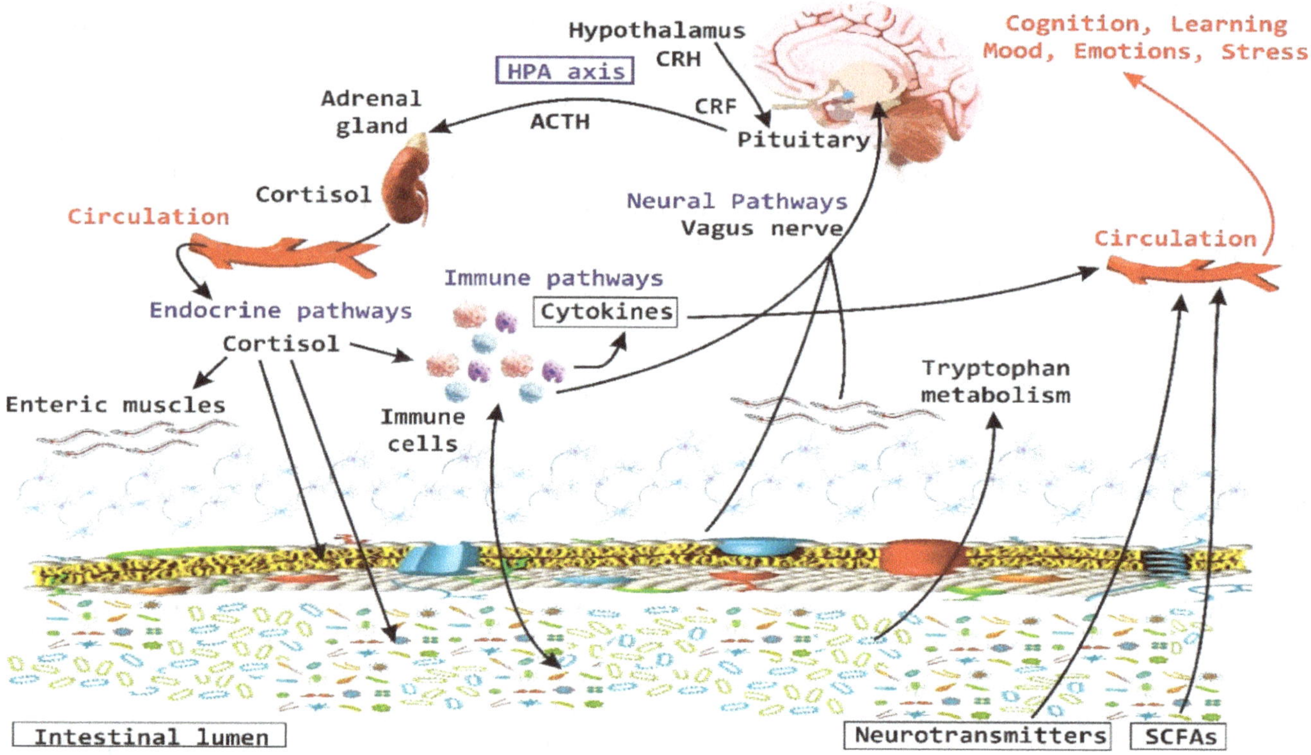

Figure 2. Brain-Gut Axis. The brain-gut axis is essential for the regulation established between the intestine and the brain. It includes the central nervous system and the endocrine and neuroimmune systems; as well as the enteric nervous system. CRH, corticotropin-releasing hormone; CRF, corticotropin releasing factor; SCFAs, short chain fatty acids; ACTH, adrenocorticitropic hormone; HPA, hypothalamic pituitary adrenal.

The sympathetic nervous system (SNP) enables the selective presentation of enteric bacteria to the mucosal immune system. Nerve fibers containing NE have been identified very close to the epithelium surrounding the lymphoid follicles in the jejunum of pigs; the administration of NE increases the reception of pathogenic bacteria inside the follicles [7]. In this sense, it has been suggested that the release of biogenic amines, such as NE, can influence the composition of the intestinal microbiota. For instance, it has been observed that this neurotransmitter stimulates the growth of both pathogenic and nonpathogenic *Escherichia coli in vitro*, in addition to influencing its adherence to the mucous membranes [48,54,55]. Changes in the physiology of the host that originated within the gut or from signals from the CNS, produce changes in the bacterial composition of the gut [7].

The ENS is a complex neuronal network that involves multiple neurotransmitters such as 5-HT, Ach and CRF, where a prominent role is given to the CRF that is mediating changes at the level of gastrointestinal function. At the ENS level, this CRF demonstrates that peripheral pathways also play a preponderant role in the local regulation of the intestine and its function in states of stress [56]. The activation of CRF-1 receptor (CRFR1) in the intestine induced by stress increases the motility of the colon, defecation, permeability of the intestine and the sensation of visceral pain [57]. The activation of CRFR2 inhibits gastric emptying, suppresses the motor function of stimulating the colon and prevents hypersensitivity generated by colorectal distension. It has been proposed that CRFR2 may have a key role in stress-induced patency dysfunction and in mucosal immune modulation and in inflammatory responses in the colon [58]. CRF can directly activate mesenteric neurons to increase motility, permeability and stimulate diarrhea in rodents [59].

The contrasting actions of CRFR1 and CRFR2 are associated with differential expression patterns. CRFR2 is present in anterior regions of the intestinal tract [60], whereas CRFR1 is mostly distributed in the colon, and is expressed in a very important way in the cells of the colon mucosa [56]. The presence of CRFR2 in the colonic mucus has been demonstrated and it has been proposed that in this area it may also have an important role in the stress-induced patency dysfunction in the modulation of immune and inflammatory responses within the colon mucosa [61]. The evidence shows that stress causes the recruitment and activation of CRF receptors in the colon, which induces changes related to the same stress in the intestinal function and in turn causes an increase in sensitivity to stress that results in an altered expression of receptors to CRF [29].

5-HT is recognized as the most important biological substrate in the pathogenesis of mood disorders [62]. There is evidence of the role of serotonergic signaling in the neurobiology of anxiety [63,64]. In GF-mice, altered levels of 5-HT have been reported in the striatum and in the hippocampus, which suggest an association between the microbiota and serotonergic signaling [62]. In addition to its role as a neurotransmitter in the brain, monoamine 5-HT is a potent regulator in the gut. More than 90% of all 5-HT in the body is synthesized in the intestine, where it activates 14 different types of receptors located in enterocytes [65,66], in enteric neurons [67] and in cells of the immune system [68]. In addition, circulating platelets sequester 5-HT from the gut and release it for the purpose of distributing it in different parts of the body [69]. 5-HT derived from the intestine regulates various functions including motor and secretory reflexes, platelet aggregation, regulation of immune responses, bone development, and cardiac function [69]. A dysregulation of peripheral 5-HT levels is implicated in the pathogenesis of diseases such as irritable bowel syndrome (IBS), cardiovascular diseases [70] and in osteoporosis processes. The molecular mechanisms that control the metabolism of 5-HT at the intestinal level are still unclear, but it has been shown to be synthesized by specialized endocrine cells called enterochromaffin cells (ECs), as well as by mast cells of the mucosa and by mesenteric neurons (Figure 3) [69].

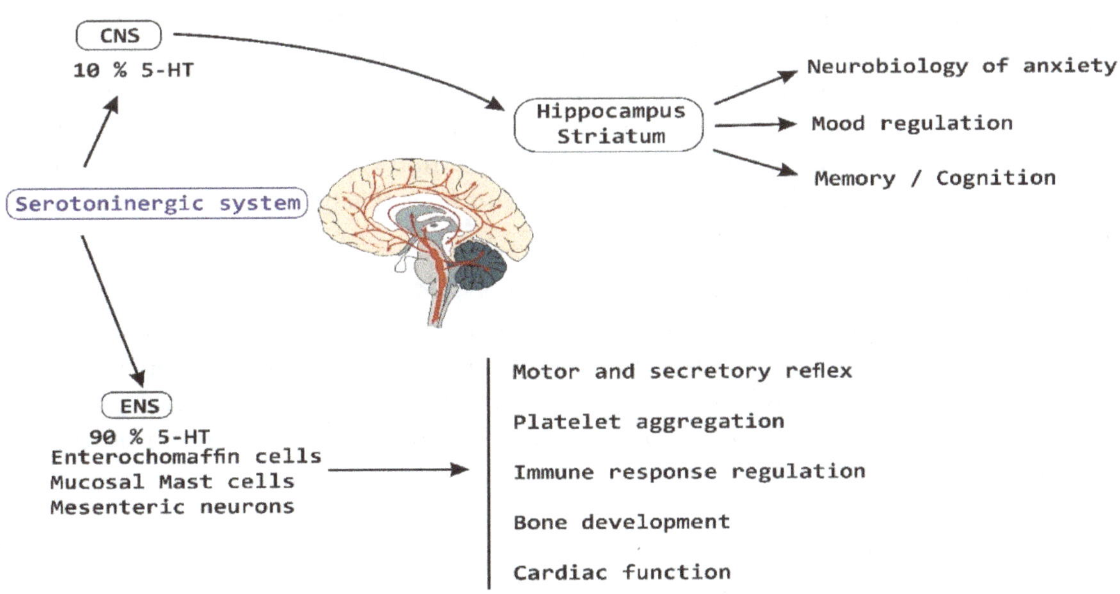

Figure 3. Serotoninergic system. The serotoninergic system is involved in the pathogenesis of diseases at the intestinal level, as well as in the regulation of different functions at a systemic level, which includes the regulation of memory processes, cognition and humor, among others. CNS, central nervous system; 5-HT, serotonin; ENS, enteric nervous system.

Exposure to chronic psychosocial stress decreases the levels of *Bacteroides* spp. and increases the levels of *Clostridium* spp. in the caecum, while increasing circulating levels of IL-6 and CCL2 chemokine (monocyte chemoattractant protein, MCP-1), which is indicative of an immune activation. The levels of IL-6 and CCL2 correlate with changes in the levels of *Coprococcus* spp., *Pseudobutyrivibrio* spp. and *Dorea* spp. induced by stressors directly in the intestine [53].

Some types of bacteria, such as lactobacilli, are able to convert nitrate to nitric oxide (NO), a potent regulator of responses to different levels of immune and nervous system. Lactobacilli also increase the activity of the enzyme indol-amine-2,3-dioxygenase (IDO), involved in the catabolism of tryptophan (TRP) and in formation of neuroactive compounds of kinuric and quinolinic acid [71]. Modification of the intestinal microbiota in adult mice causes changes in behavior, which may be related to immune, neural and hormonal mechanisms. In relation to immune mechanisms, it is known that TLR-2, 4 and 5 are over-regulated in the gut during colonization, which implies that there is interaction between these receptors and the microbiota [72,73]. The dendritic cells (DCs) of the gut break the epithelial layer and interact with commensal bacteria to induce the production of immunoglobulin-A (IgA) by B-lymphocytes and plasma cells. The secreted IgA confines penetration of the microbiota through the epithelium. This mechanism hampers an inflammatory response to commensal bacteria under normal conditions. The DCs are very close to nerve areas of the gut, the neuropeptide sensor calcitonin gene-related peptide (CGRP) modulates the function of these DCs [74] and can send signals about the presence of commensal bacteria to the brain via the vagus nerve [75]. The vagus nerve plays an important role in signaling the gut to the brain and can be stimulated by bacterial products such as endotoxins or inflammatory cytokines such as IL-1β and TNF-α [75]. The vagal response to stimulation by peripheral inflammatory events is the suppression in the release of pro-inflammatory cytokines from intestinal macrophages mediated by α7nAchR [76,77].

Dai, et al. [78] showed that certain probiotics are able to trigger IL-10 mediated anti-inflammatory responses by downregulating the proinflammatory cytokines TNF-α and IL-6. Both of these proinflammatory cytokines, along with IL-2 and IL-1β, are key participants in depressive states and other affective disorders (78). Several other microbe associated molecular patterns (MAMPs) are able to trigger or block inflammatory responses that are associated with different bacterial genera, e.g., bifidobacteria inhibits TLR activation, preventing the inflammatory response [79,80]. Other MAMPs-TLR interactions include OS and the intestinal epithelium. The inflammatory response is directly responsible for the intestinal barrier permeability, nutrient absorption, and microbiome translocation. That is the case in acute stress, that initiates inflammation and secondary dysbiosis, due to aberrant translocation, where the probiotic *Lactobacillus helveticus R0052* has been shown to be able to restore the intestinal barrier [16,79,81,82].

Colonization with *Bacteroides thetaiotaomicron* induces a 2- to 5-fold increase in the expression of mRNA that codes for the synaptic protein-33 associated with vesicles, which is involved in synaptic neurotransmission. This finding confirms that commensal bacteria can influence nervous system functions [7,50]. The intestinal microbiota is essential for the normal development of the immune and mucosal systems, which are intimately associated with the impact of the same microbiota on brain development and function [50].

4. Behavior, Cognition, and Emotion

It has been demonstrated that bi-directional communication exists between the intestine and the brain and that it involves neurological, metabolic, hormonal and immunological signaling pathways; and that disturbance or alteration in these systems can result in altered behavior [83]. A clear example is intestinal inflammation, which has been associated with changes in bowel-brain interactions, as well as a high morbidity between inflammatory bowel disorder and anxiety states (Figure 4) [84].

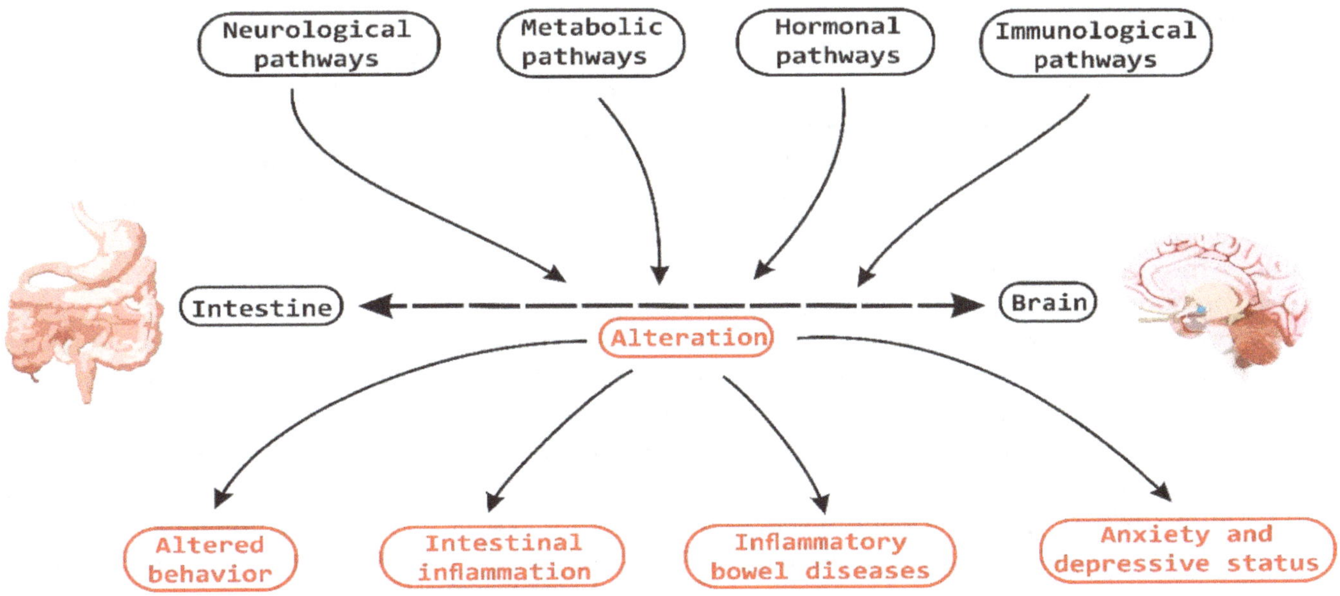

Figure 4. Brain-Gut Homeostasis. The relationship between the intestine and the brain involves signaling pathways at a neural, metabolic, hormonal and immune system levels. The alteration in these pathways is capable of causing changes in cognitive and behavioral processes, as well as inducing inflammatory processes at the periphery level.

The role of microbiota has not only focused on the impact it exerts on the brain and central nervous function but also on how it is intimately related to the constitutive modulation of nerve function at the peripheral central level [71].

Stress has been defined as a very complex dynamic condition in which homeostasis or the internal "resting state" is altered or threatened [85,86]. Throughout life all organisms are exposed to factors that exceed the homeostatic threshold, which results in a stress response, which may be physical, psychological or immunological. Evolution has armed most organisms with the necessary biological machinery to mount a defense response to acute stressors and restore the homeostatic balance once the stress or damage has subsided [85].

A significant number of animal studies provide abundant evidence that the medial prefrontal cortex (MPFC) plays an important role in the regulation of stress circuitry [28]. While the ventral part of the MPFC has been augmented with a stimulatory role, the more dorsal part in contrast has been described to possess an activity of HPA-axis inhibition. It has been also described that this negative feedback mechanism is mediated by the inhibition of glucocorticoid receptors (GRs) in the MPFC [28]. The amygdala is a key region in the process of stress responses in addition to being an important target for the inhibitory feedback system by the MPFC [87]. In humans, the MPFC area is involved in the modulation of amygdala activity during emotional conflicts and in the regulation of autonomic and affective responses [28,88].

Stress, particularly in the early stages of life, is one of the major predictors of the onset of major depression disorder (MDD) [89]. Early exposure to stress and MDD is associated with a significant de-regularization of the HPA-axis and the stress/cortisol response system. Exposure to stressors, HPA-axis deregulation, elevated corticosteroid levels and major depression states are related to structural alterations in the hippocampus and amygdala, key regions in the regulation of the HPA-axis [90,91].

In one study of early life maternal separation, a group of male rats were submitted to stress tests [79]. They all showed the typical pattern: poor forced swim performance while the group that was separated also showed records of high IL-6 blood levels, low NE levels in brain and higher expression of CRF gene in the amygdala [92]. By administering *L. rhamnosus R011* plus *L. helveticus R0052*, the rats downregulated their HPA axis and normalized their corticosterone levels [16,92].

Psychobiotics are now considered key elements in affective disorders. In one experiment with mice that were administered with *L. rhamnosus*, they featured lesser signs of anxiety and depression in forced swim and plus elevated maze respectively than their control counterparts, even at the same levels of corticosterone [16,93]. This suggests that the probiotic had a downregulation effect over HPA axis [93]. In the presence of *L. rhamnosus*, mice showed a lower hippocampal expression of the $GABA_{B1b}$ receptor gene and a higher expression of it in the cingulated cortex and limbic regions. Since GABA is the main inhibitory neurotransmitter of the nervous system, it would appear that psycobiotics are able to modulate the local balance of inhibition/exciting in order to control the systemic responses to stress, anxiety and depression [93].

As previously described, GF-mice exhibit an exaggerated response to stressors, with the presentation of anxious-type behaviors and cognitive deficits [94,95]. This behavior is influenced by the amygdala and the hippocampus. The signaling between the basolateral amygdala (BLA) and the ventral hippocampus modulates anxiety behaviors and social behaviors [96]. Tune changes (structural changes) in the amygdala and hippocampus are associated with anxiety disorders in humans and in rodents in early stages of development. There is evidence of hypertrophy of the dendrites of excitatory neurons in the BLA area under a state of repeated (repetitive) stress that induces atrophy of the dendrites in hippocampal neurons [94].

The "germ-free" status induces dendritic hypertrophy in inhibitory interneurons, and the excitatory pyramidal neurons of the BLA area show increased density of spines type: "thin", "stubby" and "mushroom". The absence of intestinal microbiota induces dendritic atrophy in other areas of the CNS, as is the case of hippocampal pyramidal neurons and granular cells of the dentate gyrus. In GF-animals, there is a significant loss of "stubby" and "mushroom" spines in hippocampal pyramidal neurons [94].

It has been estimated that there are 32% fewer synaptic connections in hippocampal pyramidal neurons of GF-animals when the dendrite size decreases and this is combined with a smaller size in the same dendritic spines [94].

A characteristic shared by the animal models of autism and GF-mice is an important alteration in the processes of social behavior. This type of alterations is in turn associated with alterations in the volume of the hippocampus and the amygdala. Changes in the size of these structures have been well documented in experiments with rodents, subject to severe stressors. Prenatally stressed rats experience an increase in the volume of the lateral amygdala [97,98] whereas chronic stress or treatment with corticosteroids induces hippocampal atrophy [98]. Changes in these structures of the CNS are frequently observed in human patients with anxiety disorders or with autism, clearly indicating that the volumetric alterations of the limbic structures can in turn be the result of a maladaptive response to stress [94]. In chronically stressed mice, dendrite hypertrophy is observed in inhibitory GABAergic neurons of the prefrontal cortex area [99].

The amygdala has different "target" areas that are responsible for modulating neuroendocrine responses to stress. The BLA area is activated by psychological stressors, and lesions in this area significantly reduce the HPA-axis response efficiency [94]. While, on the other hand, the area of the central nucleus of the amygdala (CeA) is not involved in the signaling of the HPA-axis induced by stressors, it is an area that also regulates autonomic responses to stress [94]. GF-mice have a lower degree of anxiety and social cognitive deficit, and it has been mentioned previously that there is an important relationship between anxiety and social behavior; the amygdala and the area of the ventral hypothalamus are directly involved in the regulation of this type of behavior [100]. In addition to having a preponderant role in the regulation of anxiety, the ventral hypothalamus is also involved in processes of sociability, and an alteration or damage in this area leads to the appearance of abnormal responses to social situations [101]. Besides, this ventral hippocampus exhibits a very important reciprocal connection with the amygdala, another area involved in anxiety and sociability [100].

The different tonsillar sub-regions have different roles in the regulation of anxiety and social behavior. The areas of the lateral amygdala (LA) and the BLA area integrate sensory information and adverse situations and then send their projections to the CeA area [100]. The stimulation of the projections from the BLA to the CeA area induces an anxiolytic phenotype in mice [102]. This is in contrast to direct stimulation of the entire BLA area, where an opposite effect is generated, suggesting that most of the BLA neurons project towards areas that regulate anxiogenic effects [102].

It has been mentioned that chronic stress in the adult stage is also capable of affecting the composition of the gut microbiota [11]. It is clear that alterations in the brain-gut axis interactions are associated with intestinal inflammatory processes, syndromes of chronic abdominal pain, and with eating disorders [11,103]. This altered modulation of the brain-gut axis is associated with alterations in the regulation of stress responses and behavioral alterations. The high co-morbidity that exists between stress and some symptoms of psychiatric illnesses such as high anxiety, gastrointestinal disorders (included in irritable bowel syndrome, IBS) is clear evidence of the importance of this axis in the pathophysiology of certain types of diseases [11].

Chronic stress on the other hand breaks the intestinal barrier, causes filtrations and alters the ability of the HPA-axis to reverse the deleterious effects of stress (Figure 5) [93,94].

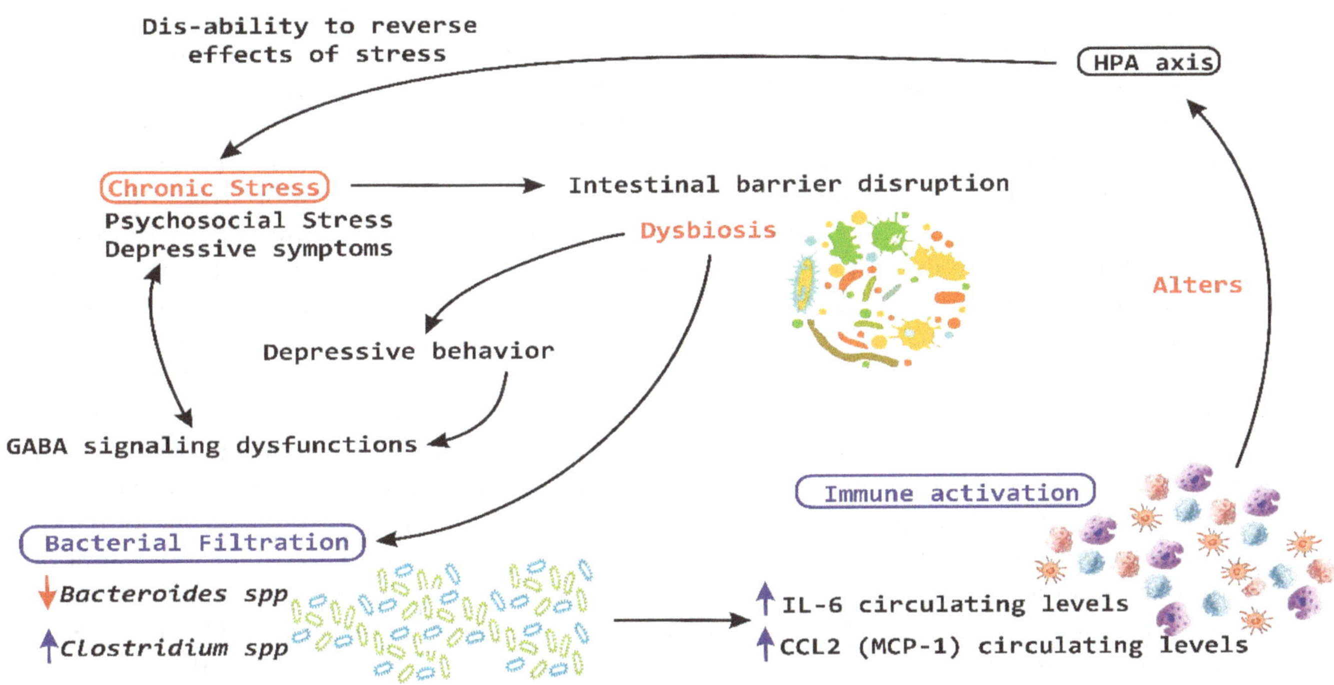

Figure 5. Chronic stress and HPA axis. A chronic stress process is capable of causing disruption at a level of the intestinal barrier and cause dysbiosis, which in turn induces the leakage of bacteria and the activation of the local immune system, leading to a significant alteration of the hypothalamic pituitary adrenal (HPA)-axis. IL, interleukin; MCP-1, monocyte chemoattractant protein; red arrow down mean decrease levels; blue arrow up mean increase levels.

GABA is the major inhibitory neurotransmitter in the CNS. Dysfunctions in GABA signaling are associated with anxiety and depression [104]. Lactobacilli and bifidobacteria are able to metabolize glutamate to produce GABA *in vitro* [62,104,105]. In an *in vivo* experiment in mice, a strain of *Lactobacillus rhamnosus* shows an effect and influence on depressive and ancestral behavior, and it can also alter the central expression of GABA receptors in key brain regions for stress management [62].

In 2006, Kamiya et al. [106] demonstrated that oral administration of *Lactobacillus* species for anesthetized rats is capable of completely suppressing colonic distension induced by pseudo-affective cardiac responses, which is reflected in the inhibition of visceral pain perception. This treatment is also effective in reducing electrical charges in fibers of the dorsal root of the ganglia [71]. The administration of these same strains of *Lactobacillus* to healthy adult rats is enough to activate calcium (Ca^{2+}) and potassium (K^+) channels in neurons-AH (after hyperpolarization) of the ENS in mesenteric plexus of the colon [71].

It has been shown that the oral administration of specific strains of *Lactobacillus* induces the expression of opioids-μ receptors and cannabinoids and promotes analgesic functions similar to effects of morphine. This suggests that intestinal microbiota can influence our visceral perception [107]. Altogether, these findings indicate that probiotics are able to modulate the function responsible for the visceral and somatic perception of pain [71].

Currently, there is evidence that supports the influence of intestinal microbiota on the behavior and health of SNC [1]. Patients with depressive symptoms show a significant improvement in the symptoms of depression accompanied by a reduction in plasma TRP after a fructose-restricted diet. Furthermore, fructose malabsorption provides the substrate for a rapid bacterial fermentation, which results in changes in gut motility [72]. The administration of a strain of *Bifidobacterium infantis* for 14 days increases the levels of plasma TRP, suggesting that commensal bacteria have the ability to influence the metabolism of TRP [93].

Intestinal bacteria are potent regulators of systemic and local immune responses such as that related to mucous membranes, in addition to contributing to the development of inflammatory disorders in the CNS. GF-animals or animals treated with antibiotics with an experimental autoimmune encephalomyelitis (EAE) process present reduced inflammation and a lower degree of disease compared to conventional mice, which suggest the existence of complex interactions between commensal bacteria and the inflammatory process in CNS [9,97,98]. For example, segmented filamentous bacteria (frequently associated with the intestinal epithelium) promote the development of Th17 helper T cells, which produce IL-17. They have been termed as Th17 cells in the small intestine of mice [99,108].

There is important evidence that the brain-gut axis can influence brain chemistry and is able to modulate behavior in adult mice [43]. A transient disturbance in the microbiota is able to increase the levels of BDNF in the hippocampus, as well as increase the exploratory behavior of animals. In the hippocampus, BDNF is associated with memory and learning processes and recent evidence indicates that this increase is associated with anxiolytic and antidepressant-like behavior [43]. On the other hand, the amygdala is also associated with memory and disorders in the mood and there has been an increase in the expression of BDNF in the amygdala during processes of "learning fear" [109]. Low levels of BDNF in the amygdala increase the exploratory behavior of the animals (Figure 6) [9,43].

Some other molecules with psychobiotic potential are SCFAs. These are macronutrients from non-digestible metabolites e.g., microbiome secondary degradation products of plant polysaccharides, and their production and release can be enhanced by prebiotic consumption [110,111]. These SCFAs include butyrate, acetate and propionate. It has been shown that butyrate crosses the blood-brain barrier and exhibits important neuroprotective, cognitive and anti-depressive effects [112]. Some mechanisms related to SCFAs include epigenomic histone-deacetylase gene expression regulation and HPA axis regulation [79,113,114].

Other secondary products of the psychobiotic-mediated metabolism of non-digestible fiber is DA and NE from bacilli, GABA from bifidobacteria, serotonin from enteroccocci and streptoccocci, NE and serotonin from *E. coli* and acetylcholine from lactobacilli. It is not entirely clear how much these neurotransmitters modulate the synaptic activity of the ENS [115–117].

The SCFAs regulate the metabolism of free fatty acids, glucose and cholesterol through various signaling cascades involving receptors linked to G-proteins [1,48]. It has also been found that acetylation of histones and SCFAs can improve cognitive function in animal models of neurodevelopment and neurodegenerative diseases, however, another group of researchers showed that the administration of a specific SCFAs, the propionic acid (PPA), can induce altered behavior traits in patients with ASD in addition to neurochemical changes [118]. These changes include neuroinflammation, elevation in levels of oxidative stress, and an important depletion in the efficiency of the antioxidant system; and all together can cause mitochondrial dysfunction, which is common in patients with ASD and in other neurodegenerative diseases such as AD and PD [119,120]. The PPA also exhibits neurotransmitter effects, effects on tight junctions and on immune function. SCFAs are associated with high levels of phosphorylated cAMP response element-binding (CREB), which induces a significant increase in catecholamine levels [121].

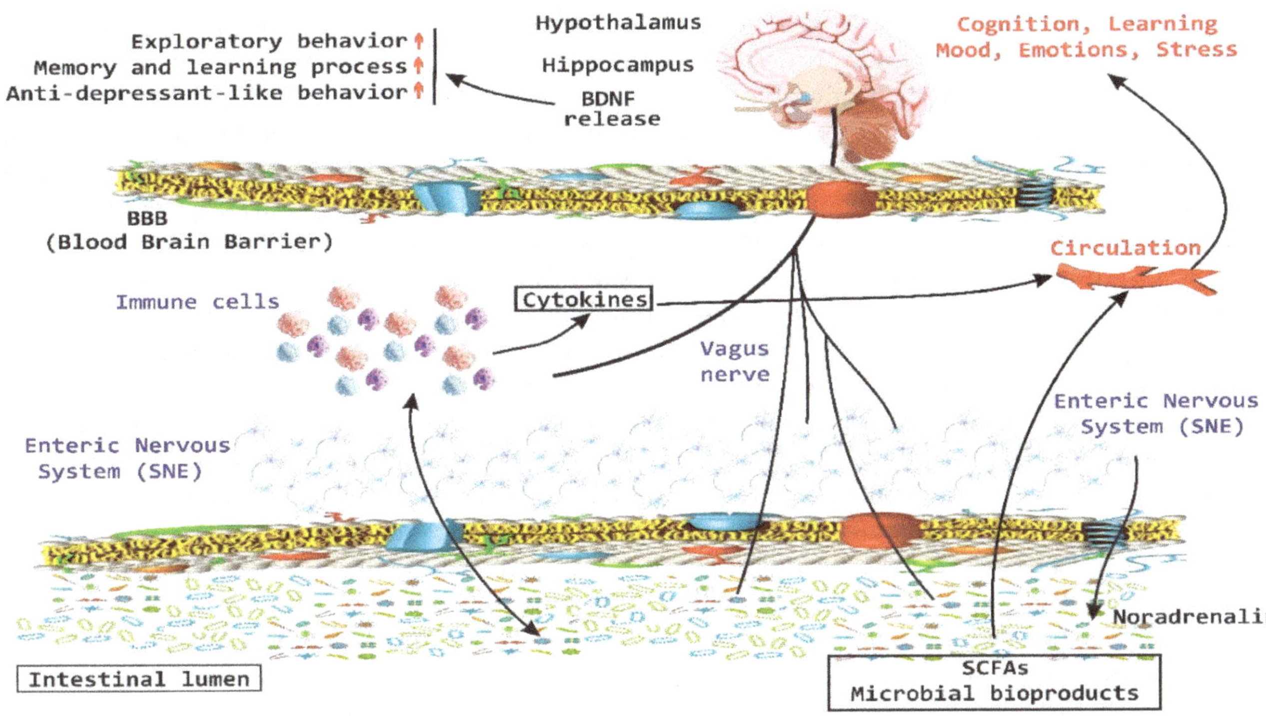

Figure 6. BDNF release system. The brain-derived neurotrophic factor (BDNF) released via the activation of the brain-gut axis has been associated with cognitive and behavioral processes, as well as with anxiolytic and antidepressive effects. SCFAs, short chain fatty acids; red arrow up mean increase levels.

A first experimental study developed in rats orally administered with FOS or GOS for 5 weeks showed that both prebiotics augmented the amount of hippocampal BDNF and NR1 subunit of glutamate *N*-methyl-D-aspartate receptor (NMDAR) [122]. Besides, oral administration of GOS induced an increase in NR2A subunit expression in hippocampus, NR1 subunit and D-serine expression in frontal cortex, and plasma D-alanine. Brain levels of other amino acids related with glutamate neurotransmission were not modified by either prebiotic. Authors demonstrated that both prebiotics increased the number of fecal *Bifidobacteria*, with the effect being greater with GOS intake. However, OG may be modulating brain chemistry independently of its prebiotic activity, as gut hormones such as peptide YY (PYY) were increased in plasma of GOS-fed rats in relation with BDNF increase, suggesting a direct interaction between GOS and gut mucosa that may inclusive influence the immune system. Based in these experimental results, the same research group developed a clinical study in healthy human volunteers that received FOS, Bimuno® GOS (B-GOS) or placebo daily during 3 weeks [123]. Although no effects in cortisol secretion and emotional processing were observed in relation to FOS consumption, the intake of B-GOS decreased salivary cortisol awakening response and attentional bias in participants as compared to those receiving placebo. Recently, Burokas and co-workers developed a protocol in mice supplemented with FOS, GOS or a FOS-GOS combination during 3 weeks to analyze endocrine response to stress, neurotransmitters and their receptor brain expression, gut microbiota composition, and SCFAs levels [124]. FOS-GOS treatment exhibited both antidepressant and anxiolytic effects and reduced stress-induced corticosterone release. The same decrease on corticosterone level was achieved with GOS intake, however FOS had no effect. Prebiotics also modified specific gene expression of neurotransmitters and involved-receptors in hippocampus and hypothalamus. Notably, cecal acetate and propionate concentrations were increased and that of isobutyrate was diminished by prebiotics, changes that correlated significantly with the positive effects seen on behavior. When FOS-GOS-treated mice were exposed to chronic psychosocial stress, elevations in corticosterone and proinflammatory cytokine levels, and depression- and anxiety-like behavior were reduced, as well as changes on microbiota were normalized. Thus, as previously demonstrated with probiotics, specific prebiotics may also modulate HPA axis activity and attention to emotional stimuli, suggesting a beneficial role of prebiotic treatment for stress-related behaviors.

Another path through which microbiota is able to affect functions in the CNS is by the alteration of hippocampal neurogenesis (AHN) in adults. Indeed, it has been described that the adult brain has the capacity to generate new neurons within the hippocampus and the lateral ventricles [125]. AHN is involved in memory and learning processes and can be affected by an important variety of neurological disorders such as epilepsy, major depression, AD and PD, among others [126,127]. A decrease in the number of neural stem cells and in the AHN process is observed in old age, with the concomitant cognitive decline [127]. Since metabolic and immune system pathways are involved in this process, dysbiosis of the intestinal microbiota due to diseases in the early stages of development may have long-term effects on behavior and cognitive function.

During an episode of medium stress, they observed an increase in ACTH and corticosterone release in young GF-mice, compared to young conventional specific pathogen free (SPF) mice [128]. The increases in ACTH and corticosterone levels induced by stress were completely reversed in GF mice when colonized with *B. infantis*, but only partially reversed when the mice were colonized with the microbiota of SPF mice. These findings suggest that within the microbiota of SPF mice there are bacteria that contribute to the suppression of the ACTH response.

Microbiome studies in autoimmune diseases have shown important alterations in the levels of certain bacterial groups such as *Bifidobacteria* spp. and *Lactobacillus* spp., as well as elevated levels of *Clostridia* spp., *Staphilococcus* spp. and *E. coli* [129–131], which are capable of alter the immune response, proinflammatory cytokine (TNF-α and IL-1-β) and anti-inflammatory (IL-10) levels, and generate feedback loops of dysbiosis while altering the immune responses. Celiac disease is a chronic inflammatory bowel disease caused by an autoimmune response to gluten [129]; in patients with celiac disease, the persistence of GABA has been suggested by mediating intracortical dysfunction despite dietary restriction. This hyperexcitability can be the result of a regulation in the GABAergic inhibitory interneurons mediated in the immune system or by a cortical reorganization mediated by glutamate, an excitatory neurotransmitter, which tries to compensate for the illness of the gluten disease [132]. In celiac disease, autoreactive clones of anti-tissue transglutaminase (anti-tTG)2 and anti-tTG6 antibodies have been found in intestine and areas of the nervous system (cerebellum, pons, bone marrow and blood vessels), addition to possible injury to the integrity of the BBB by infiltration of activated Th1 cell-exposing the brain parenchyma to the action of auto-antibodies [133]. This process leads to synaptic hyper-excitation and low inhibition at the cortical level [132,133], promoting the typical neurological signs of this disease.

Another important finding made by Sudo et al. [128] was a severe reduction in BDNF expression, at mRNA and protein levels, in the cortex and hippocampus of GF-mice, compared with SPF-mice. BDNF regulates important aspects of brain activity, including mood and cognitive functions [128]. Other reports have shown the influence of gut microbiota on the development of brain responses to stress and on cognitive functions in young mice [7,128].

5. Conclusions and Future Research

Nowadays, we recognize the need to study the human microbiota and probiotics as a whole ecosystem to better understand the relation between microbiota and host health or disease. One of the major limitations in using psychobiotics in humans is the lack of its possible interaction with sex hormones (estrogen and/or testosterone) and its long-term effect. Preliminary findings on how probiotic treatments, called psychobiotics, may help improve your mood, decrease your anxiety, and strengthen your memory suggest that in the near future these probiotics could be prescribed to treat depression, anxiety, and other mental health issues, by using them in the form of food or supplements to alter the gut microbiome and treat psychiatric conditions.

Author Contributions: Conceptualization, O.K.B.-Q., L.G.B.-H., J.A.M.; Compiling and curation of the state-of-the-art, O.K.B.-Q., L.G.B.-H., E.S., L.J.R.-J., G.G.O., J.A.M.; Project administration, OKB; Visualization, O.K.B.-Q., L.J.R.-J., J.A.M.; Writing—original draft, O.K.B.-Q., L.G.B.-H., E.S., L.J.R.-J., G.G.O., J.A.M.; Writing—review & editing, O.K.B.-Q., L.G.B.-H., E.S., L.J.R.-J., J.A.M.; Supervision, O.K.B.-Q., L.G.B.-H.

References

1. Leung, K.; Thuret, S. Gut Microbiota: A Modulator of Brain Plasticity and Cognitive Function in Ageing. *Healthcare* **2015**, *3*, 898–916. [CrossRef]
2. Qin, J.; Li, R.; Raes, J.; Arumugam, M.; Burgdorf, K.S.; Manichanh, C.; Nielsen, T.; Pons, N.; Levenez, F.; Yamada, T.; et al. A human gut microbial gene catalogue established by metagenomic sequencing. *Nature* **2010**, *464*, 59–65. [CrossRef]
3. Palmer, C.; Bik, E.M.; DiGiulio, D.B.; Relman, D.A.; Brown, P.O. Development of the human infant intestinal microbiota. *PLoS Biol.* **2007**, *5*, e177. [CrossRef]
4. Jasarevic, E.; Howerton, C.L.; Howard, C.D.; Bale, T.L. Alterations in the Vaginal Microbiome by Maternal Stress Are Associated with Metabolic Reprogramming of the Offspring Gut and Brain. *Endocrinology* **2015**, *156*, 3265–3276. [CrossRef] [PubMed]
5. Bercik, P.; Collins, S.M.; Verdu, E.F. Microbes and the gut-brain axis. *Neurogastroenterol. Motil.* **2012**, *24*, 405–413. [CrossRef]
6. Kamada, N.; Seo, S.U.; Chen, G.Y.; Nunez, G. Role of the gut microbiota in immunity and inflammatory disease. *Nat. Rev. Immunol.* **2013**, *13*, 321–335. [CrossRef] [PubMed]
7. Collins, S.M.; Bercik, P. The relationship between intestinal microbiota and the central nervous system in normal gastrointestinal function and disease. *Gastroenterology* **2009**, *136*, 2003–2014. [CrossRef] [PubMed]
8. Moustafa, A.; Li, W.; Anderson, E.L.; Wong, E.H.M.; Dulai, P.S.; Sandborn, W.J.; Biggs, W.; Yooseph, S.; Jones, M.B.; Venter, J.C.; et al. Genetic risk, dysbiosis, and treatment stratification using host genome and gut microbiome in inflammatory bowel disease. *Clin. Transl. Gastroenterol.* **2018**, *9*, e132. [CrossRef] [PubMed]
9. Fung, T.C.; Olson, C.A.; Hsiao, E.Y. Interactions between the microbiota, immune and nervous systems in health and disease. *Nat. Neurosci.* **2017**, *20*, 145–155. [CrossRef]
10. Collins, S.M.; Surette, M.; Bercik, P. The interplay between the intestinal microbiota and the brain. *Nat. Rev. Microbiol.* **2012**, *10*, 735–742. [CrossRef]
11. Cryan, J.F.; Dinan, T.G. Mind-altering microorganisms: The impact of the gut microbiota on brain and behaviour. *Nat. Rev. Neurosci.* **2012**, *13*, 701–712. [CrossRef]
12. Hill, C.; Guarner, F.; Reid, G.; Gibson, G.R.; Merenstein, D.J.; Pot, B.; Morelli, L.; Canani, R.B.; Flint, H.J.; Salminen, S.; et al. Expert consensus document. The International Scientific Association for Probiotics and Prebiotics consensus statement on the scope and appropriate use of the term probiotic. *Nat. Rev. Gastroenterol. Hepatol.* **2014**, *11*, 506–514. [CrossRef]
13. Gibson, G.R.; Roberfroid, M.B. Dietary modulation of the human colonic microbiota: Introducing the concept of prebiotics. *J. Nutr.* **1995**, *125*, 1401–1412. [CrossRef] [PubMed]
14. Gibson, G.R.; Hutkins, R.; Sanders, M.E.; Prescott, S.L.; Reimer, R.A.; Salminen, S.J.; Scott, K.; Stanton, C.; Swanson, K.S.; Cani, P.D.; et al. Expert consensus document: The International Scientific Association for Probiotics and Prebiotics (ISAPP) consensus statement on the definition and scope of prebiotics. *Nat. Rev. Gastroenterol. Hepatol.* **2017**, *14*, 491–502. [CrossRef]
15. Dinan, T.G.; Stanton, C.; Cryan, J.F. Psychobiotics: A novel class of psychotropic. *Biol. Psychiatry* **2013**, *74*, 720–726. [CrossRef] [PubMed]
16. Sarkar, A.; Lehto, S.M.; Harty, S.; Dinan, T.G.; Cryan, J.F.; Burnet, P.W.J. Psychobiotics and the Manipulation of Bacteria-Gut-Brain Signals. *Trends Neurosci.* **2016**, *39*, 763–781. [CrossRef]
17. Sundman, E.; Olofsson, P.S. Neural control of the immune system. *Adv. Physiol. Educ.* **2014**, *38*, 135–139. [CrossRef]

18. Nayak, D.; Roth, T.L.; McGavern, D.B. Microglia development and function. *Annu. Rev. Immunol.* **2014**, *32*, 367–402. [CrossRef] [PubMed]
19. Nayak, D.; Zinselmeyer, B.H.; Corps, K.N.; McGavern, D.B. In vivo dynamics of innate immune sentinels in the CNS. *Intravital* **2012**, *1*, 95–106. [CrossRef] [PubMed]
20. Hu, X.; Leak, R.K.; Shi, Y.; Suenaga, J.; Gao, Y.; Zheng, P.; Chen, J. Microglial and macrophage polarization-new prospects for brain repair. *Nat. Rev. Neurol.* **2015**, *11*, 56–64. [CrossRef]
21. Matcovitch-Natan, O.; Winter, D.R.; Giladi, A.; Vargas Aguilar, S.; Spinrad, A.; Sarrazin, S.; Ben-Yehuda, H.; David, E.; Zelada González, F.; Perrin, P.; et al. Microglia development follows a stepwise program to regulate brain homeostasis. *Science* **2016**, *353*, aad8670. [CrossRef]
22. Erny, D.; Hrabe de Angelis, A.L.; Jaitin, D.; Wieghofer, P.; Staszewski, O.; David, E.; Keren-Shaul, H.; Mahlakoiv, T.; Jakobshagen, K.; Buch, T.; et al. Host microbiota constantly control maturation and function of microglia in the CNS. *Nat. Neurosci.* **2015**, *18*, 965–977. [CrossRef] [PubMed]
23. Borre, Y.E.; O'Keeffe, G.W.; Clarke, G.; Stanton, C.; Dinan, T.G.; Cryan, J.F. Microbiota and neurodevelopmental windows: Implications for brain disorders. *Trends Mol. Med.* **2014**, *20*, 509–518. [CrossRef] [PubMed]
24. Smith, S.M.; Vale, W.W. The role of the hypothalamic-pituitary-adrenal axis in neuroendocrine responses to stress. *Dialogues Clin. Neurosci.* **2006**, *8*, 383–395.
25. Dallman, M.F.; Akana, S.F.; Levin, N.; Walker, C.D.; Bradbury, M.J.; Suemaru, S.; Scribner, K.S. Corticosteroids and the control of function in the hypothalamo-pituitary-adrenal (HPA) axis. *Ann. N. Y. Acad. Sci.* **1994**, *746*, 22–31; discussion 31–32, 64–67. [CrossRef]
26. Dickmeis, T.; Weger, B.D.; Weger, M. The circadian clock and glucocorticoids—Interactions across many time scales. *Mol. Cell Endocrinol.* **2013**, *380*, 2–15. [CrossRef]
27. Mayer, E.A. The neurobiology of stress and gastrointestinal disease. *Gut* **2000**, *47*, 861–869. [CrossRef] [PubMed]
28. Ma, S.T.; Abelson, J.L.; Okada, G.; Taylor, S.F.; Liberzon, I. Neural circuitry of emotion regulation: Effects of appraisal, attention, and cortisol administration. *Cogn. Affect. Behav. Neurosci.* **2017**, *17*, 437–451. [CrossRef] [PubMed]
29. Dinan, T.G.; Cryan, J.F. Regulation of the stress response by the gut microbiota: Implications for psychoneuroendocrinology. *Psychoneuroendocrinology* **2012**, *37*, 1369–1378. [CrossRef]
30. Williams, S.; Chen, L.; Savignac, H.M.; Tzortzis, G.; Anthony, D.C.; Burnet, P.W. Neonatal prebiotic (BGOS) supplementation increases the levels of synaptophysin, GluN2A-subunits and BDNF proteins in the adult rat hippocampus. *Synapse* **2016**, *70*, 121–124. [CrossRef] [PubMed]
31. Oliveros, E.; Ramirez, M.; Vazquez, E.; Barranco, A.; Gruart, A.; Delgado-Garcia, J.M.; Buck, R.; Rueda, R.; Martin, M.J. Oral supplementation of 2′-fucosyllactose during lactation improves memory and learning in rats. *J. Nutr. Biochem.* **2016**, *31*, 20–27. [CrossRef] [PubMed]
32. Van den Berg, J.P.; Westerbeek, E.A.; Broring-Starre, T.; Garssen, J.; van Elburg, R.M. Neurodevelopment of Preterm Infants at 24 Months After Neonatal Supplementation of a Prebiotic Mix: A Randomized Trial. *J. Pediatr. Gastroenterol. Nutr.* **2016**, *63*, 270–276. [CrossRef] [PubMed]
33. LeCouffe, N.E.; Westerbeek, E.A.; van Schie, P.E.; Schaaf, V.A.; Lafeber, H.N.; van Elburg, R.M. Neurodevelopmental outcome during the first year of life in preterm infants after supplementation of a prebiotic mixture in the neonatal period: A follow-up study. *Neuropediatrics* **2014**, *45*, 22–29. [CrossRef]
34. Olofsson, P.S.; Rosas-Ballina, M.; Levine, Y.A.; Tracey, K.J. Rethinking inflammation: Neural circuits in the regulation of immunity. *Immunol. Rev.* **2012**, *248*, 188–204. [CrossRef] [PubMed]
35. Sun, J.; Singh, V.; Kajino-Sakamoto, R.; Aballay, A. Neuronal GPCR controls innate immunity by regulating noncanonical unfolded protein response genes. *Science* **2011**, *332*, 729–732. [CrossRef]
36. Nathan, C. Points of control in inflammation. *Nature* **2002**, *420*, 846–852. [CrossRef] [PubMed]
37. Chiu, I.M.; von Hehn, C.A.; Woolf, C.J. Neurogenic inflammation and the peripheral nervous system in host defense and immunopathology. *Nat. Neurosci.* **2012**, *15*, 1063–1067. [CrossRef] [PubMed]
38. Elenkov, I.J.; Wilder, R.L.; Chrousos, G.P.; Vizi, E.S. The sympathetic nerve—An integrative interface between two supersystems: The brain and the immune system. *Pharmacol. Rev.* **2000**, *52*, 595–638. [PubMed]
39. Kipnis, J.; Cardon, M.; Avidan, H.; Lewitus, G.M.; Mordechay, S.; Rolls, A.; Shani, Y.; Schwartz, M. Dopamine, through the extracellular signal-regulated kinase pathway, downregulates CD4+CD25+ regulatory T-cell activity: Implications for neurodegeneration. *J. Neurosci.* **2004**, *24*, 6133–6143. [CrossRef]

40. Prado, C.; Contreras, F.; Gonzalez, H.; Diaz, P.; Elgueta, D.; Barrientos, M.; Herrada, A.A.; Lladser, Á.; Bernales, S.; Pacheco, R. Stimulation of dopamine receptor D5 expressed on dendritic cells potentiates Th17-mediated immunity. *J. Immunol.* **2012**, *188*, 3062–3070. [CrossRef]
41. Tracey, K.J. The inflammatory reflex. *Nature* **2002**, *420*, 853–859. [CrossRef] [PubMed]
42. Rosas-Ballina, M.; Olofsson, P.S.; Ochani, M.; Valdes-Ferrer, S.I.; Levine, Y.A.; Reardon, C.; Tusche, M.W.; Pavlov, V.A.; Andersson, U.; Chavan, S.; et al. Acetylcholine-synthesizing T cells relay neural signals in a vagus nerve circuit. *Science* **2011**, *334*, 98–101. [CrossRef]
43. Bercik, P.; Denou, E.; Collins, J.; Jackson, W.; Lu, J.; Jury, J.; Deng, Y.; Blennerhassett, P.; Macri, J.; McCoy, K.D.; et al. The intestinal microbiota affect central levels of brain-derived neurotropic factor and behavior in mice. *Gastroenterology* **2011**, *141*, 599–609, 609.e1-3. [CrossRef] [PubMed]
44. Vazquez, E.; Barranco, A.; Ramirez, M.; Gruart, A.; Delgado-Garcia, J.M.; Martinez-Lara, E.; Blanco, S.; Martín, M.J.; Castanys, E.; Buck, R.; et al. Effects of a human milk oligosaccharide, 2′-fucosyllactose, on hippocampal long-term potentiation and learning capabilities in rodents. *J. Nutr. Biochem.* **2015**, *26*, 455–465. [CrossRef] [PubMed]
45. Song, L.; Gao, Y.; Zhang, X.; Le, W. Galactooligosaccharide improves the animal survival and alleviates motor neuron death in SOD1G93A mouse model of amyotrophic lateral sclerosis. *Neuroscience* **2013**, *246*, 281–290. [CrossRef] [PubMed]
46. Castro, R.; Rivera, I.; Blom, H.J.; Jakobs, C.; Tavares de Almeida, I. Homocysteine metabolism, hyperhomocysteinaemia and vascular disease: An overview. *J. Inherit. Metab Dis.* **2006**, *29*, 3–20. [CrossRef] [PubMed]
47. Savignac, H.M.; Couch, Y.; Stratford, M.; Bannerman, D.M.; Tzortzis, G.; Anthony, D.C.; Burnet, P.W.J. Prebiotic administration normalizes lipopolysaccharide (LPS)-induced anxiety and cortical 5-HT2A receptor and IL1-beta levels in male mice. *Brain Behav. Immun.* **2016**, *52*, 120–131. [CrossRef]
48. Jia, S.; Lu, Z.; Gao, Z.; An, J.; Wu, X.; Li, X.; Dai, X.; Zheng, Q.; Sun, Y. Chitosan oligosaccharides alleviate cognitive deficits in an amyloid-beta1-42-induced rat model of Alzheimer's disease. *Int. J. Biol. Macromol.* **2016**, *83*, 416–425. [CrossRef] [PubMed]
49. Chen, D.; Yang, X.; Yang, J.; Lai, G.; Yong, T.; Tang, X.; Shuai, O.; Zhou, G.; Xie, Y.; Wu, Q. Prebiotic Effect of Fructooligosaccharides from Morinda officinalis on Alzheimer's Disease in Rodent Models by Targeting the Microbiota-Gut-Brain Axis. *Front. Aging Neurosci.* **2017**, *9*, 403. [CrossRef]
50. Neufeld, K.A.; Foster, J.A. Effects of gut microbiota on the brain: Implications for psychiatry. *J. Psychiatry Neurosci.* **2009**, *34*, 230–231.
51. Carabotti, M.; Scirocco, A.; Maselli, M.A.; Severi, C. The gut-brain axis: Interactions between enteric microbiota, central and enteric nervous systems. *Ann. Gastroenterol.* **2015**, *28*, 203–209. [PubMed]
52. Ogbonnaya, E.S.; Clarke, G.; Shanahan, F.; Dinan, T.G.; Cryan, J.F.; O'Leary, O.F. Adult Hippocampal Neurogenesis Is Regulated by the Microbiome. *Biol. Psychiatry* **2015**, *78*, e7–e9. [CrossRef] [PubMed]
53. Bailey, M.T.; Dowd, S.E.; Galley, J.D.; Hufnagle, A.R.; Allen, R.G.; Lyte, M. Exposure to a social stressor alters the structure of the intestinal microbiota: Implications for stressor-induced immunomodulation. *Brain Behav. Immun.* **2011**, *25*, 397–407. [CrossRef] [PubMed]
54. Chen, C.; Brown, D.R.; Xie, Y.; Green, B.T.; Lyte, M. Catecholamines modulate Escherichia coli O157:H7 adherence to murine cecal mucosa. *Shock* **2003**, *20*, 183–188. [CrossRef] [PubMed]
55. Freestone, P.P.; Williams, P.H.; Haigh, R.D.; Maggs, A.F.; Neal, C.P.; Lyte, M. Growth stimulation of intestinal commensal Escherichia coli by catecholamines: A possible contributory factor in trauma-induced sepsis. *Shock* **2002**, *18*, 465–470. [CrossRef] [PubMed]
56. O'malley, D.; Julio-Pieper, M.; Gibney, S.M.; Gosselin, R.D.; Dinan, T.G.; Cryan, J.F. Differential stress-induced alterations of colonic corticotropin-releasing factor receptors in the Wistar Kyoto rat. *Neurogastroenterol. Motil.* **2010**, *22*, 301–311. [CrossRef] [PubMed]
57. Larauche, M.; Gourcerol, G.; Wang, L.; Pambukchian, K.; Brunnhuber, S.; Adelson, D.W.; Rivier, J.; Million, M.; Taché, Y. Cortagine, a CRF1 agonist, induces stresslike alterations of colonic function and visceral hypersensitivity in rodents primarily through peripheral pathways. *Am. J. Physiol. Gastrointest. Liver Physiol.* **2009**, *297*, G215–G227. [CrossRef]
58. Gareau, M.G.; Silva, M.A.; Perdue, M.H. Pathophysiological mechanisms of stress-induced intestinal damage. *Curr. Mol. Med.* **2008**, *8*, 274–281. [CrossRef] [PubMed]

59. Tache, Y. Corticotropin releasing factor receptor antagonists: Potential future therapy in gastroenterology? *Gut* **2004**, *53*, 919–921. [CrossRef]
60. Wu, Y.; Hu, J.; Zhang, R.; Zhou, C.; Xu, Y.; Guan, X.; Li, S. Enhanced intracellular calcium induced by urocortin is involved in degranulation of rat lung mast cells. *Cell Physiol. Biochem.* **2008**, *21*, 173–182. [CrossRef] [PubMed]
61. Teitelbaum, A.A.; Gareau, M.G.; Jury, J.; Yang, P.C.; Perdue, M.H. Chronic peripheral administration of corticotropin-releasing factor causes colonic barrier dysfunction similar to psychological stress. *Am. J. Physiol. Gastrointest. Liver Physiol.* **2008**, *295*, G452–G459. [CrossRef]
62. Foster, J.A.; McVey Neufeld, K.A. Gut-brain axis: How the microbiome influences anxiety and depression. *Trends Neurosci.* **2013**, *36*, 305–312. [CrossRef] [PubMed]
63. Leonardo, E.D.; Hen, R. Anxiety as a developmental disorder. *Neuropsychopharmacology* **2008**, *33*, 134–140. [CrossRef] [PubMed]
64. Stein, M.B.; Seedat, S.; Gelernter, J. Serotonin transporter gene promoter polymorphism predicts SSRI response in generalized social anxiety disorder. *Psychopharmacology* **2006**, *187*, 68–72. [CrossRef] [PubMed]
65. Gershon, M.D.; Tack, J. The serotonin signaling system: From basic understanding to drug development for functional GI disorders. *Gastroenterology* **2007**, *132*, 397–414. [CrossRef] [PubMed]
66. Hoffman, J.M.; Tyler, K.; MacEachern, S.J.; Balemba, O.B.; Johnson, A.C.; Brooks, E.M.; Zhao, H.; Swain, G.M.; Moses, P.L.; Galligan, J.J.; et al. Activation of colonic mucosal 5-HT(4) receptors accelerates propulsive motility and inhibits visceral hypersensitivity. *Gastroenterology* **2012**, *142*, 844-854.e4. [CrossRef]
67. Mawe, G.M.; Hoffman, J.M. Serotonin signalling in the gut–functions, dysfunctions and therapeutic targets. *Nat. Rev. Gastroenterol. Hepatol.* **2013**, *10*, 473–486. [CrossRef]
68. Baganz, N.L.; Blakely, R.D. A dialogue between the immune system and brain, spoken in the language of serotonin. *ACS Chem. Neurosci.* **2013**, *4*, 48–63. [CrossRef]
69. Yano, J.M.; Yu, K.; Donaldson, G.P.; Shastri, G.G.; Ann, P.; Ma, L.; Nagler, C.R.; Ismagilov, R.F.; Mazmanian, S.K.; Hsiao, E.Y. Indigenous bacteria from the gut microbiota regulate host serotonin biosynthesis. *Cell* **2015**, *161*, 264–276. [CrossRef] [PubMed]
70. Stasi, C.; Bellini, M.; Bassotti, G.; Blandizzi, C.; Milani, S. Serotonin receptors and their role in the pathophysiology and therapy of irritable bowel syndrome. *Tech. Coloproctol.* **2014**, *18*, 613–621. [CrossRef]
71. Forsythe, P.; Sudo, N.; Dinan, T.; Taylor, V.H.; Bienenstock, J. Mood and gut feelings. *Brain Behav. Immun.* **2010**, *24*, 9–16. [CrossRef]
72. Gibson, P.R.; Newnham, E.; Barrett, J.S.; Shepherd, S.J.; Muir, J.G. Review article: Fructose malabsorption and the bigger picture. *Aliment Pharmacol. Ther.* **2007**, *25*, 349–363. [CrossRef] [PubMed]
73. Lundin, A.; Bok, C.M.; Aronsson, L.; Bjorkholm, B.; Gustafsson, J.A.; Pott, S.; Arulampalam, V.; Hibberd, M.; Rafter, J.; Pettersson, S. Gut flora, Toll-like receptors and nuclear receptors: A tripartite communication that tunes innate immunity in large intestine. *Cell Microbiol.* **2008**, *10*, 1093–1103. [CrossRef]
74. Hosoi, J.; Murphy, G.F.; Egan, C.L.; Lerner, E.A.; Grabbe, S.; Asahina, A.; Granstein, R.D. Regulation of Langerhans cell function by nerves containing calcitonin gene-related peptide. *Nature* **1993**, *363*, 159–163. [CrossRef] [PubMed]
75. Goehler, L.E.; Gaykema, R.P.; Nguyen, K.T.; Lee, J.E.; Tilders, F.J.; Maier, S.F.; Watkins, L.R. Interleukin-1beta in immune cells of the abdominal vagus nerve: A link between the immune and nervous systems? *J. Neurosci.* **1999**, *19*, 2799–2806. [CrossRef]
76. Borovikova, L.V.; Ivanova, S.; Zhang, M.; Yang, H.; Botchkina, G.I.; Watkins, L.R.; Wang, H.; Abumrad, N.; Eaton, J.W.; Tracey, K.J. Vagus nerve stimulation attenuates the systemic inflammatory response to endotoxin. *Nature* **2000**, *405*, 458–462. [CrossRef] [PubMed]
77. Ghia, J.E.; Blennerhassett, P.; Kumar-Ondiveeran, H.; Verdu, E.F.; Collins, S.M. The vagus nerve: A tonic inhibitory influence associated with inflammatory bowel disease in a murine model. *Gastroenterology* **2006**, *131*, 1122–1130. [CrossRef]
78. Dai, C.; Zheng, C.Q.; Meng, F.J.; Zhou, Z.; Sang, L.X.; Jiang, M. VSL#3 probiotics exerts the anti-inflammatory activity via PI3k/Akt and NF-kappaB pathway in rat model of DSS-induced colitis. *Mol. Cell Biochem.* **2013**, *374*, 1–11.
79. Bambury, A.; Sandhu, K.; Cryan, J.F.; Dinan, T.G. Finding the needle in the haystack: Systematic identification of psychobiotics. *Br. J. Pharmacol.* **2018**, *175*, 4430–4438. [CrossRef]

80. Chu, H.; Mazmanian, S.K. Innate immune recognition of the microbiota promotes host-microbial symbiosis. *Nat. Immunol.* **2013**, *14*, 668–675. [CrossRef] [PubMed]
81. Takeda, K.; Akira, S. Toll-like receptors in innate immunity. *Int. Immunol.* **2005**, *17*, 1–14. [CrossRef]
82. Moussaoui, N.; Braniste, V.; Ait-Belgnaoui, A.; Gabanou, M.; Sekkal, S.; Olier, M.; Théodorou, V.; Martin, P.G.; Houdeau, E. Changes in intestinal glucocorticoid sensitivity in early life shape the risk of epithelial barrier defect in maternal-deprived rats. *PLoS ONE* **2014**, *9*, e88382. [CrossRef] [PubMed]
83. Rhee, S.H.; Pothoulakis, C.; Mayer, E.A. Principles and clinical implications of the brain-gut-enteric microbiota axis. *Nat. Rev. Gastroenterol. Hepatol.* **2009**, *6*, 306–314. [CrossRef]
84. Bercik, P.; Verdu, E.F.; Foster, J.A.; Macri, J.; Potter, M.; Huang, X.; Malinowski, P.; Jackson, W.; Blennerhassett, P.; Neufeld, K.A.; et al. Chronic gastrointestinal inflammation induces anxiety-like behavior and alters central nervous system biochemistry in mice. *Gastroenterology* **2010**, *139*, 2102-2112.e1. [CrossRef] [PubMed]
85. Rea, K.; Dinan, T.G.; Cryan, J.F. The microbiome: A key regulator of stress and neuroinflammation. *Neurobiol. Stress.* **2016**, *4*, 23–33. [CrossRef]
86. McEwen, B.S.; Gray, J.D.; Nasca, C. 60 YEARS OF NEUROENDOCRINOLOGY: Redefining neuroendocrinology: Stress, sex and cognitive and emotional regulation. *J. Endocrinol.* **2015**, *226*, T67–T83. [CrossRef]
87. Herman, J.P.; Ostrander, M.M.; Mueller, N.K.; Figueiredo, H. Limbic system mechanisms of stress regulation: Hypothalamo-pituitary-adrenocortical axis. *Prog. Neuropsychopharmacol. Biol. Psychiatry* **2005**, *29*, 1201–1213. [CrossRef]
88. De Voogd, L.D.; Klumpers, F.; Fernandez, G.; Hermans, E.J. Intrinsic functional connectivity between amygdala and hippocampus during rest predicts enhanced memory under stress. *Psychoneuroendocrinology* **2017**, *75*, 192–202. [CrossRef]
89. Pagliaccio, D.; Luby, J.L.; Bogdan, R.; Agrawal, A.; Gaffrey, M.S.; Belden, A.C.; Botteron, K.N.; Harms, M.P.; Barch, D.M. Stress-system genes and life stress predict cortisol levels and amygdala and hippocampal volumes in children. *Neuropsychopharmacology* **2014**, *39*, 1245–1253. [CrossRef]
90. Lupien, S.J.; McEwen, B.S.; Gunnar, M.R.; Heim, C. Effects of stress throughout the lifespan on the brain, behaviour and cognition. *Nat. Rev. Neurosci.* **2009**, *10*, 434–445. [CrossRef] [PubMed]
91. Montiel-Castro, A.J.; Gonzalez-Cervantes, R.M.; Bravo-Ruiseco, G.; Pacheco-Lopez, G. The microbiota-gut-brain axis: Neurobehavioral correlates, health and sociality. *Front. Integr. Neurosci.* **2013**, *7*, 70. [CrossRef] [PubMed]
92. Gareau, M.G.; Jury, J.; MacQueen, G.; Sherman, P.M.; Perdue, M.H. Probiotic treatment of rat pups normalises corticosterone release and ameliorates colonic dysfunction induced by maternal separation. *Gut* **2007**, *56*, 1522–1528. [CrossRef] [PubMed]
93. Bravo, J.A.; Forsythe, P.; Chew, M.V.; Escaravage, E.; Savignac, H.M.; Dinan, T.G.; Bienenstock, J.; Cryan, J.F. Ingestion of Lactobacillus strain regulates emotional behavior and central GABA receptor expression in a mouse via the vagus nerve. *Proc. Natl. Acad. Sci. USA* **2011**, *108*, 16050–16055. [CrossRef] [PubMed]
94. Luczynski, P.; Whelan, S.O.; O'Sullivan, C.; Clarke, G.; Shanahan, F.; Dinan, T.G.; Cryan, J.F. Adult microbiota-deficient mice have distinct dendritic morphological changes: Differential effects in the amygdala and hippocampus. *Eur. J. Neurosci.* **2016**, *44*, 2654–2666. [CrossRef]
95. Arentsen, T.; Raith, H.; Qian, Y.; Forssberg, H.; Diaz Heijtz, R. Host microbiota modulates development of social preference in mice. *Microb. Ecol. Health Dis.* **2015**, *26*, 29719. [CrossRef] [PubMed]
96. Felix-Ortiz, A.C.; Tye, K.M. Amygdala inputs to the ventral hippocampus bidirectionally modulate social behavior. *J. Neurosci.* **2014**, *34*, 586–595. [CrossRef]
97. Lee, Y.K.; Menezes, J.S.; Umesaki, Y.; Mazmanian, S.K. Proinflammatory T-cell responses to gut microbiota promote experimental autoimmune encephalomyelitis. *Proc. Natl. Acad. Sci. USA* **2011**, *108* (Suppl. 1), 4615–4622. [CrossRef] [PubMed]
98. Ochoa-Reparaz, J.; Mielcarz, D.W.; Ditrio, L.E.; Burroughs, A.R.; Foureau, D.M.; Haque-Begum, S.; Kasper, L.H. Role of gut commensal microflora in the development of experimental autoimmune encephalomyelitis. *J. Immunol.* **2009**, *183*, 6041–6050. [CrossRef]
99. Gaboriau-Routhiau, V.; Rakotobe, S.; Lecuyer, E.; Mulder, I.; Lan, A.; Bridonneau, C.; Rochet, V.; Pisi, A.; De Paepe, M.; Brandi, G.; et al. The key role of segmented filamentous bacteria in the coordinated maturation of gut helper T cell responses. *Immunity* **2009**, *31*, 677–689. [CrossRef]

100. Allsop, S.A.; Vander Weele, C.M.; Wichmann, R.; Tye, K.M. Optogenetic insights on the relationship between anxiety-related behaviors and social deficits. *Front. Behav. Neurosci.* **2014**, *8*, 241. [CrossRef]
101. Kheirbek, M.A.; Drew, L.J.; Burghardt, N.S.; Costantini, D.O.; Tannenholz, L.; Ahmari, S.E.; Zeng, H.; Fenton, A.A.; Hen, R. Differential control of learning and anxiety along the dorsoventral axis of the dentate gyrus. *Neuron* **2013**, *77*, 955–968. [CrossRef]
102. Tye, K.M.; Prakash, R.; Kim, S.Y.; Fenno, L.E.; Grosenick, L.; Zarabi, H.; Thompson, K.R.; Gradinaru, V.; Ramakrishnan, C.; Deisseroth, K. Amygdala circuitry mediating reversible and bidirectional control of anxiety. *Nature* **2011**, *471*, 358–362. [CrossRef] [PubMed]
103. Mayer, E.A. Gut feelings: The emerging biology of gut-brain communication. *Nat. Rev. Neurosci.* **2011**, *12*, 453–466. [CrossRef]
104. Cryan, J.F.; Kaupmann, K. Don't worry 'B' happy!: A role for GABA(B) receptors in anxiety and depression. *Trends Pharmacol. Sci.* **2005**, *26*, 36–43. [CrossRef]
105. Higuchi, T.; Hayashi, H.; Abe, K. Exchange of glutamate and gamma-aminobutyrate in a Lactobacillus strain. *J. Bacteriol.* **1997**, *179*, 3362–3364. [CrossRef] [PubMed]
106. Kamiya, T.; Wang, L.; Forsythe, P.; Goettsche, G.; Mao, Y.; Wang, Y.; Tougas, G.; Bienenstock, J. Inhibitory effects of Lactobacillus reuteri on visceral pain induced by colorectal distension in Sprague-Dawley rats. *Gut* **2006**, *55*, 191–196. [CrossRef] [PubMed]
107. Amaral, F.A.; Sachs, D.; Costa, V.V.; Fagundes, C.T.; Cisalpino, D.; Cunha, T.M.; Ferreira, S.H.; Cunha, F.Q.; Silva, T.A.; Nicoli, J.R.; et al. Commensal microbiota is fundamental for the development of inflammatory pain. *Proc. Natl. Acad. Sci. USA* **2008**, *105*, 2193–2197. [CrossRef] [PubMed]
108. Ivanov, I.I.; Atarashi, K.; Manel, N.; Brodie, E.L.; Shima, T.; Karaoz, U.; Wei, D.; Goldfarb, K.C.; Santee, C.A.; Lynch, S.V.; et al. Induction of intestinal Th17 cells by segmented filamentous bacteria. *Cell* **2009**, *139*, 485–498. [CrossRef]
109. Drevets, W.C. Neuroimaging studies of mood disorders. *Biol. Psychiatry* **2000**, *48*, 813–829. [CrossRef]
110. Roy, C.C.; Kien, C.L.; Bouthillier, L.; Levy, E. Short-chain fatty acids: Ready for prime time? *Nutr. Clin. Pract.* **2006**, *21*, 351–366. [CrossRef]
111. Psichas, A.; Sleeth, M.L.; Murphy, K.G.; Brooks, L.; Bewick, G.A.; Hanyaloglu, A.C.; Ghatei, M.A.; Bloom, S.R.; Frost, G. The short chain fatty acid propionate stimulates GLP-1 and PYY secretion via free fatty acid receptor 2 in rodents. *Int. J. Obes. (Lond.)* **2015**, *39*, 424–429. [CrossRef]
112. Han, A.; Sung, Y.B.; Chung, S.Y.; Kwon, M.S. Possible additional antidepressant-like mechanism of sodium butyrate: Targeting the hippocampus. *Neuropharmacology* **2014**, *81*, 292–302. [CrossRef] [PubMed]
113. Stilling, R.M.; Dinan, T.G.; Cryan, J.F. Microbial genes, brain & behavior—Epigenetic regulation of the gut-brain axis. *Genes Brain Behav.* **2014**, *13*, 69–86. [PubMed]
114. Perry, R.J.; Peng, L.; Barry, N.A.; Cline, G.W.; Zhang, D.; Cardone, R.L.; Petersen, K.F.; Kibbey, R.G.; Goodman, A.L.; Shulman, G.I. Acetate mediates a microbiome-brain-beta-cell axis to promote metabolic syndrome. *Nature* **2016**, *534*, 213–217. [CrossRef]
115. Barrett, E.; Ross, R.P.; O'Toole, P.W.; Fitzgerald, G.F.; Stanton, C. gamma-Aminobutyric acid production by culturable bacteria from the human intestine. *J. Appl. Microbiol.* **2012**, *113*, 411–417. [CrossRef]
116. Dinan, T.G.; Stilling, R.M.; Stanton, C.; Cryan, J.F. Collective unconscious: How gut microbes shape human behavior. *J. Psychiatr. Res.* **2015**, *63*, 1–9. [CrossRef] [PubMed]
117. Lyte, M. Probiotics function mechanistically as delivery vehicles for neuroactive compounds: Microbial endocrinology in the design and use of probiotics. *Bioessays* **2011**, *33*, 574–581. [CrossRef] [PubMed]
118. Macfabe, D.F. Short-chain fatty acid fermentation products of the gut microbiome: Implications in autism spectrum disorders. *Microb. Ecol. Health Dis.* **2012**, *23*. [CrossRef] [PubMed]
119. Rossignol, D.A.; Frye, R.E. Mitochondrial dysfunction in autism spectrum disorders: A systematic review and meta-analysis. *Mol. Psychiatry* **2012**, *17*, 290–314. [CrossRef]
120. Coskun, P.; Wyrembak, J.; Schriner, S.E.; Chen, H.W.; Marciniack, C.; Laferla, F.; Wallace, D.C. A mitochondrial etiology of Alzheimer and Parkinson disease. *Biochim. Biophys. Acta* **2012**, *1820*, 553–564. [CrossRef]
121. Shah, P.; Nankova, B.B.; Parab, S.; La Gamma, E.F. Short chain fatty acids induce TH gene expression via ERK-dependent phosphorylation of CREB protein. *Brain Res.* **2006**, *1107*, 13–23. [CrossRef]
122. Savignac, H.M.; Corona, G.; Mills, H.; Chen, L.; Spencer, J.P.; Tzortzis, G.; Burnet, P.W. Prebiotic feeding elevates central brain derived neurotrophic factor, *N*-methyl-D-aspartate receptor subunits and D-serine. *Neurochem. Int.* **2013**, *63*, 756–764. [CrossRef]

123. Schmidt, K.; Cowen, P.J.; Harmer, C.J.; Tzortzis, G.; Errington, S.; Burnet, P.W. Prebiotic intake reduces the waking cortisol response and alters emotional bias in healthy volunteers. *Psychopharmacology* **2015**, *232*, 1793–1801. [CrossRef]
124. Burokas, A.; Arboleya, S.; Moloney, R.D.; Peterson, V.L.; Murphy, K.; Clarke, G.; Stanton, C.; Dinan, T.G.; Cryan, J.F. Targeting the Microbiota-Gut-Brain Axis: Prebiotics Have Anxiolytic and Antidepressant-like Effects and Reverse the Impact of Chronic Stress in Mice. *Biol. Psychiatry* **2017**, *82*, 472–487. [CrossRef] [PubMed]
125. Gage, F.H. Mammalian neural stem cells. *Science* **2000**, *287*, 1433–1438. [CrossRef] [PubMed]
126. Zhao, C.; Deng, W.; Gage, F.H. Mechanisms and functional implications of adult neurogenesis. *Cell* **2008**, *132*, 645–660. [CrossRef] [PubMed]
127. Villeda, S.A.; Luo, J.; Mosher, K.I.; Zou, B.; Britschgi, M.; Bieri, G.; Stan, T.M.; Fainberg, N.; Ding, Z.; Eggel, A.; et al. The ageing systemic milieu negatively regulates neurogenesis and cognitive function. *Nature* **2011**, *477*, 90–94. [CrossRef]
128. Sudo, N.; Chida, Y.; Aiba, Y.; Sonoda, J.; Oyama, N.; Yu, X.N.; Kubo, C.; Koga, Y. Postnatal microbial colonization programs the hypothalamic-pituitary-adrenal system for stress response in mice. *J. Physiol.* **2004**, *558 Pt 1*, 263–275. [CrossRef]
129. Brown, K.; DeCoffe, D.; Molcan, E.; Gibson, D.L. Diet-induced dysbiosis of the intestinal microbiota and the effects on immunity and disease. *Nutrients* **2012**, *4*, 1095–1119. [CrossRef] [PubMed]
130. Cristofori, F.; Indrio, F.; Miniello, V.L.; De Angelis, M.; Francavilla, R. Probiotics in Celiac Disease. *Nutrients* **2018**, *10*, 1824. [CrossRef]
131. Ou, G.; Hedberg, M.; Horstedt, P.; Baranov, V.; Forsberg, G.; Drobni, M.; Sandström, O.; Wai, S.N.; Johansson, I.; Hammarström, M.L.; et al. Proximal small intestinal microbiota and identification of rod-shaped bacteria associated with childhood celiac disease. *Am. J. Gastroenterol.* **2009**, *104*, 3058–3067. [CrossRef] [PubMed]
132. Bella, R.; Lanza, G.; Cantone, M.; Giuffrida, S.; Puglisi, V.; Vinciguerra, L.; Pennisi, M.; Ricceri, R.; D'Agate, C.C.; Malaguarnera, G.; et al. Effect of a Gluten-Free Diet on Cortical Excitability in Adults with Celiac Disease. *PLoS ONE* **2015**, *10*, e0129218. [CrossRef] [PubMed]
133. Pennisi, M.; Bramanti, A.; Cantone, M.; Pennisi, G.; Bella, R.; Lanza, G. Neurophysiology of the "Celiac Brain": Disentangling Gut-Brain Connections. *Front. Neurosci.* **2017**, *11*, 498. [CrossRef] [PubMed]

10

Early-Life Iron Deficiency Reduces Brain Iron Content and Alters Brain Tissue Composition Despite Iron Repletion: A Neuroimaging Assessment

Austin T. Mudd [1,2,*], Joanne E. Fil [1,2], Laura C. Knight [1,3], Fan Lam [4], Zhi-Pei Liang [4,5] and Ryan N. Dilger [1,2,3,4,6,*]

1 Piglet Nutrition & Cognition Laboratory, University of Illinois Urbana-Champaign, Urbana, IL 61801, USA; jfil2@illinois.edu (J.E.F.); knight24@illinois.edu (L.C.K.)
2 Neuroscience Program, University of Illinois Urbana-Champaign, Urbana, IL 61801, USA
3 Division of Nutrition Sciences, University of Illinois Urbana-Champaign, Urbana, IL 61801, USA
4 Beckman Institute for Advanced Science & Technology, University of Illinois Urbana-Champaign, Urbana, IL 61801, USA; fanlam1@illinois.edu (F.L.); z-liang@illinois.edu (Z.-P.L.)
5 Department of Electrical & Computer Engineering, University of Illinois Urbana-Champaign, Urbana, IL 61801, USA
6 Department of Animal Sciences, University of Illinois Urbana-Champaign, Urbana, IL 61801, USA
* Correspondence: amudd2@illinois.edu (A.T.M.); rdilger2@illinois.edu (R.N.D.)

Abstract: Early-life iron deficiency has lifelong influences on brain structure and cognitive function, however characterization of these changes often requires invasive techniques. There is a need for non-invasive assessment of early-life iron deficiency with potential to translate findings to the human clinical setting. In this study, 28 male pigs were provided either a control diet (CONT; n = 14; 23.5 mg Fe/L milk replacer) or an iron-deficient diet (ID; n = 14; 1.56 mg Fe/L milk replacer) for phase 1 of the study, from postnatal day (PND) 2 until 32. Twenty pigs (n = 10/diet from phase 1 were used in phase 2 of the study from PND 33 to 61, where all pigs were provided a common iron-sufficient diet, regardless of their phase 1 dietary iron status. All pigs were subjected to magnetic resonance imaging at PND 32 and again at PND 61, and quantitative susceptibility mapping was used to assess brain iron content at both imaging time-points. Data collected on PND 61 were analyzed using voxel-based morphometry and tract-based spatial statistics to determine tissue concentration difference and white matter tract integrity, respectively. Quantitative susceptibility mapping outcomes indicated reduced iron content in the pons, medulla, cerebellum, left cortex, and left hippocampus of ID pigs compared with CONT pigs, regardless of imaging time-point. In contrast, iron contents were increased in the olfactory bulbs of ID pigs compared with CONT pigs. Voxel-based morphometric analysis indicated increased grey and white matter concentrations in CONT pigs compared with ID pigs that were evident at PND 61. Differences in tissue concentrations were predominately located in cortical tissue as well as the cerebellum, thalamus, caudate, internal capsule, and hippocampi. Tract-based spatial statistics indicated increased fractional anisotropy values along subcortical white matter tracts in CONT pigs compared with ID pigs that were evident on PND 61. All described differences were significant at $p \leq 0.05$. Results from this study indicate that neuroimaging can sensitively detect structural and physiological changes due to early-life iron deficiency, including grey and white matter volumes, iron contents, as well as reduced subcortical white matter integrity, despite a subsequent period of dietary iron repletion.

Keywords: neurodevelopment; iron deficiency; pig; iron repletion; myelination; pediatric nutrition; brain iron

---

1. Introduction

Iron deficiency is the most common micronutrient deficiency worldwide [1,2] and a deficiency during the perinatal period has lifelong implications. Infants are at an increased risk for iron deficiency [3] and the developing brain is highly vulnerable to alterations in iron status [4–7]. Research in humans has shown that iron deficiency early in life results in delayed motor development by ten months of age [8], delayed cognitive processing by ten years of age [9], altered recognition memory and executive functions at 19 years of age [10], and poorer emotional health in the mid-twenties [11]. It is clear that early-life iron deficiency has lasting effects on cognitive performance, yet it remains to be elucidated what structural differences in brain development might underlie these persistent cognitive changes. Some studies in humans have used other non-invasive techniques such as evoked potential recordings [12], electrophysiological recording and processing [9] and electroencephalography [13] to explain structural alterations in brain development related to iron deficiency. While these methods may potentially explain a mechanism for altered brain development, more sensitive assessments are needed to non-invasively characterize the brain regions influenced by iron deficiency.

The presence of iron in the brain is necessary for proper vascular development [14], myelination [15], neurotransmitter synthesis [16,17], and neuron morphology [18,19]. To date, many of the mechanisms for iron's involvement in brain development have been determined using invasive techniques in animal models. While necessary and informative, these methods are not feasible in clinical populations, thus there is a need to characterize similar findings using non-invasive techniques. Magnetic resonance imaging (MRI) is one method that may bridge the gap between invasive techniques used in animal models and cognitive and surface recording assessments used in humans. A recent study indicated maternal iron status and cord blood ferritin measures related to markers of infant brain development, which were assessed using diffusion tensor imaging [20]. While this finding is informative, hematological indices of iron status often do not predict brain iron content, as the brain tends to deplete prior to blood tissue [5]. Thus, a non-invasive assessment of brain iron is needed to quantify iron levels throughout development, thereby illuminating differences that may not be predicted by hematological indices. Quantitative susceptibility mapping (QSM) is an MRI method that has been used to quantify altered iron status in clinical cases of restless leg syndrome [21] and β-thalassemia [22]; thus, it is possible that these methods may be able to sensitively detect altered brain iron status in cases of dietary iron deficiency. In fact, a recent neuroimaging study that used QSM in children found that brain iron content in the caudate nucleus related to performance on spatial intelligence quotient tests [23], thereby offering insight into brain regions that may underlie cognitive differences due to iron status. Moreover, neuroimaging allows for assessment of structural brain development such as myelination, and grey matter and white matter tissue distributions, and may prove useful in sensitively characterizing structural differences later in life.

We previously reported that early-life iron deficiency resulted in decreased relative brain volumes of specific regions and region-specific reductions in diffusion tensor measures, which persisted in developing pig brains even after a subsequent period of dietary iron repletion [24]. Interestingly, these differences in microstructural brain development were present at postnatal day (PND) 61 despite a lack of difference in absolute brain volume between iron-deficient (ID) and control (CONT) pigs at that time-point. These findings suggest comprehensively assessing the effects of iron deficiency is necessary to elucidate region-specific, rather than whole brain, implications of altered nutrient status. To further expand upon our previous findings, herein we analyzed differences between early-life ID and control CONT pigs in concentrations of brain grey matter, white matter, and measures of white matter tract development at PND 61. Due to the highly dynamic nature of the developing brain and the influence of iron on myelin and neuron morphology, we hypothesized that grey and white matter tissue concentrations would be altered by early life iron status and remain evident at PND 61. Thus, the aim of this study was to identify specific regions of the brain that remained structurally different in ID pigs after a subsequent period of iron repletion Additionally we used, a non-invasive neuroimaging technique, QSM, to characterize changes in brain iron content. Using this method, we hypothesized that piglets provided an ID diet early in life would exhibit decreased iron content in the brain, as measured through QSM.

2. Materials and Methods

2.1. Animal Care and Housing

Twenty-eight, naturally-farrowed, intact male pigs were obtained from Carthage Veterinary Services and transferred to the University of Illinois Piglet Nutrition and Cognition Laboratory (PNCL) at PND 2. Per standard agricultural protocol, pigs were provided an intramuscular injection of a prophylactic antibiotic (0.1 mL of ceftiofur crystalline free acid (Exceed, Zoetis, Parsippany, NJ, USA)) within 24 h of birth. Contrary to typical agricultural procedures, pigs on this study were not administered an intramuscular injection of iron dextran because iron was the nutrient being manipulated as per the experimental design. Recent pig studies observed hippocampal transcriptome changes [25] and possible effects of iron overload [26] after a bolus administration of iron dextran in the first few days of life, which further justifies our decision to not provide iron dextran to any pigs. Upon arrival to PNCL on PND 2, pigs were stratified into one of two experimental diets, described below. Pigs were randomly allocated into treatment groups to account for initial bodyweight and maternal genetics, with no bodyweight or iron status differences between the groups at the start of the study. Pigs were provided experimental milk replacer diets from PND 2 until PND 32 (phase 1), at which point both treatment groups were weaned onto a series of nutritionally-adequate diets from PND 33 until PND 61 (phase 2). A detailed description of phase 1 and phase 2 rearing environments has been previously described [24]. All animal and experimental procedures were in accordance with the National Research Council Guide for the Care and Use of Laboratory Animals and approved by the University of Illinois at Urbana-Champaign Institutional Animal Care and Use Committee. Approval for this research project was confirmed on 3 March 2015 and is identified as IACUC 15034 at the University of Illinois Urbana-Champaign.

2.2. Dietary Treatments

For phase 1 of this study, pigs ($N = 28$; $n = 14$ per diet) were provided one of two dietary treatments with varying iron content. The CONT diet was formulated to meet all of the nutrient requirements of the growing pig and was formulated to contain 117.5 mg Fe/kg milk replacer powder. The ID diet was similar to the CONT diet, however iron was only formulated to be supplemented at 7.8 mg Fe/kg milk replacer powder. Additionally, both diets were formulated to contain arachidonic acid (ARA) (2.08 g ARA/kg milk replacer powder) and docosahexanoeic acid (DHA) (1.04 g DHA/kg milk replacer powder). Milk replacer was reconstituted fresh daily with 200 g of milk replacer powder per 800 g water. Thus, formulated iron concentrations in reconstituted pig milk replacers were: CONT, 23.5 mg Fe/L milk replacer, and ID, 1.56 mg Fe/L milk replacer. All pigs were provided ad libitum access to liquid diets from PND 2 until PND 32.

For phase 2 of this study, all pigs ($N = 20$, $n = 10$/phase 1 diet) were weaned onto the same series of age-appropriate, nutritionally-adequate solid diets, regardless of their phase 1 dietary iron status. Pigs were provided ad libitum access to water and standard complex diets (major ingredients including corn, whey, and soybean meal) and standard agricultural feeding practices were followed by sequentially switching from stage 1 diets, to stage 2 diets, to stage 3 diets, on PND 33, 41, and 50 respectively. During this phase of the study, all diets were formulated to meet all nutrient requirements of the growing pig [27], including iron. No zinc oxide, copper sulfate, or in-feed antibiotics were included in any diets.

2.3. Magnetic Resonance Imaging

All pigs remaining in each phase underwent MRI procedures on PND 32 or 33 for phase 1 and again at PND 61 or 62 for phase 2, at the Beckman Institute for Advanced Science and Technology

Biomedical Imaging Center. For phase 1, 28 pigs (n = 14 per diet) were subjected to neuroimaging procedures and for phase 2, 20 pigs (n = 10 per phase 1 diet) were subjected to neuroimaging procedures. Imaging procedures were performed using a Siemens MAGNETOM Trio 3T scanner (Siemens, Erlangen, Germany), with a custom pig-specific 8-channel head coil at PND 32 and a human 8-channel head coil at PND 61. Upon arrival to the imaging facility, anesthesia was induced using an intramuscular injection of telazol: ketamine: xylazine solution [50.0 mg tiletamine plus 50.0 mg of zolazepam reconstituted with 2.50 mL ketamine (100 g/L) and 2.50 mL xylazine (100 g/L); Fort Dodge Animal Health] administered at 0.03 mL/kg body weight, and maintained with inhalation of isoflurane (98% O_2, 2% isoflurane). Pigs were immobilized during all MRI procedures. Visual observation of each pig's well-being, as well as observations of heart rate, PO_2 and percent of isoflurane were recorded every 5 min. during the procedure. Total scan time for each pig was approximately 60 min. Upon completion of the scan, pig respiration and heart rate were monitored every 15 min. until complete recovery from anesthesia. Imaging techniques are briefly described below.

2.3.1. Structural MRI Acquisition & Analysis

A T_1-weighted magnetization-prepared rapid gradient echo (MPRAGE) sequence was used to obtain anatomic images of the pig brain, with a 0.7 mm isotropic voxel size. The following specific parameters were used for the MPRAGE sequence: repetition time (TR) = 1900 ms; echo time (TE) = 2.49 ms; inversion time (TI) = 900 ms; 224 slices; field of view (FOV) = 180 × 180 mm^2; flip angle = 9°. Pig brains were manually extracted as previously described [28]. All toolboxes described herein were available in SPM12 (Wellcome Department of Clinical Neurology, London, UK) and Matlab R2015a was used for data processing. Once extracted, the 'Coregister: Estimate & Reslice' toolbox was used to coregister individual brains to the Pig MRI Atlas [29]. Next, the 'Old Normalize: Estimate & Reslice' toolbox was used to transform individual pig brains into atlas space. The following parameters in Old Normalize were used for pig specific data processing: template image (Pig MRI Atlas), bounding box (−30.1 −35 −28/30.1 44.8 31.5), voxel size (0.7). The "Segment" function of SPM12 and pig-specific prior probability tissue maps were then used to segment the brains into grey matter and white matter. Voxel-based morphometry (VBM) analysis was performed to assess grey and white matter tissue concentrations using SPM12 software. The Diffeomorphic Anatomical Registration using Exponentiated Lie Algebra (DARTEL) toolbox was used with pig-specific specifications that included changing the bounding box of −30.1 to 30.1, −35 to 44.8, −28 to 31.5; and a voxel size of 0.7 mm^3. After the nonlinear transformation of the data in the DARTEL procedure, flow fields were created and converted to warp files. The warp files generated were then applied to the subject's grey and white matter. The modulated data were smoothed with a 4 mm full-width half maximum, and were subjected to VBM procedures using the SPM12 toolbox.

2.3.2. Quantitative Susceptibility Mapping

Brain tissue susceptibility was obtained to access the iron content change due to iron-deficiency. To this end, whole brain ^1H magnetic resonance spectroscopic imaging (MRSI) data without water suppression were acquired using the recently proposed spectroscopic imaging by exploiting spatiospectral correlation SPICE-based acquisition [30,31]. Without water suppression, QSM of brain tissues can be extracted from the phase information encoded in the water spectroscopic signals [31,32]. The detailed acquisition parameters are as follows: TR/TE = 310/4 ms, FOV = 200 × 160 × 64 mm^3, matrix size = 100 × 120 × 26, flip angle = 37°, readout bandwidth = 167 kHz, number of echoes acquired each TR = 200, and echo spacing = 850 ms. Susceptibility maps were extracted from the water spectroscopic data using the following algorithm (see Peng et al., 2017 [31] for more details): (1) total B_0 field inhomogeneity maps were estimated by using a voxel-by-voxel least-squares fitting of the multi-echo data; (2) the tissue susceptibility induced field inhomogeneity was extracted from the total field by solving the Laplacian boundary value problem [33]; (3) susceptibility maps were then determined by solving the tissue field to susceptibility dipole inversion [32]; and (4) regional susceptibility values were obtained by averaging the susceptibility values in different regions of interest ROIs, using the University of Illinois Piglet Brain Atlas [29] (http://pigmri.illinois.edu/).

2.3.3. Tract-Based Spatial Statistics

Diffusion tensor imaging was used to assess white matter maturation and axonal tract integrity using a b-value = 1000 s/mm^2 across 30 directions and a 2 mm isotropic voxel. Diffusion-weighted echoplanar imaging EPI images were assessed in FMRIB Software Library (FSL) for fractional anisotropy (FA), mean diffusivity (MD), axial diffusivity (AD), and radial diffusivity (RD) using methods previously described [28]. The FSL 5.0 toolbox was used for tract-based spatial statistics (TBSS) assessment of FA data [34,35]. Fractional anisotropy images, previously generated from diffusion data, were manually extracted, and all FA data from individual subjects were aligned using the FSL nonlinear registration tool FNIRT. Upon alignment, the study-specific mean FA image was created and a mean FA skeleton representing the center of all common tracts was established. A threshold of 0.2 was determined to be sensitive for mean FA tract delineation. Once the study-specific mean FA skeleton was created, each subjects' aligned FA data were projected onto the mean FA skeleton and the resulting voxel-wise cross-subject data were used for statistical analyses [34,35]. For all TBSS analyses involving registration to an atlas, the University of Illinois Piglet Brain Atlas (http://pigmri.illinois.edu/) was used in place of human brain templates [29].

2.4. Statistical Analysis

All researchers involved in this study (i.e., those performing daily procedures, data collection, and data analysis steps) remained blinded to dietary treatment identity until final data analyses had been completed. Data were analyzed by using the MIXED procedure of SAS 9.4 (SAS Institute, Cary, NC, USA). Quantitative susceptibility measures were analyzed from data generated at PND 32 and 61, thus all data were analyzed using a 2-way repeated measures analysis of variance (ANOVA) (i.e., dietary iron status with postnatal day at time of neuroimaging acquisition as the repeated measure). Interactive effects were defined as an interaction between diet (CONT vs. ID) and MRI day (PND 32 vs. 61). The number of animals per treatment group was based on a power analysis using the variability estimates from previous studies to detect differences with sufficient power of 80% and at a significance of 0.05. Data were analyzed for outliers (defined as having a studentized residual with an absolute value greater than 3) and outliers were removed prior to statistical analysis. Significance was accepted at $p \leq 0.05$. Data are presented as least-squares means with pooled standard errors of the mean (SEM).

2.4.1. Voxel-Based Morphometry Statistics

Voxel-based morphometry analyses were performed on data acquired at PND 61. As such, two-sample permutation t-tests were performed on a voxel-by-voxel basis for grey and white matter volume differences between animals on the early-life CONT and ID diets, with an uncorrected $p < 0.001$. An additional threshold criterion of at least 20 edge-connected voxels was used.

2.4.2. Tract-Based Spatial Statistics

For TBSS analysis, only data acquired at PND 61 was analyzed. A nonparametric permutation inference function called 'randomise' was used within the FSL toolbox and run as a two-sample t-test with 500 permutations to compare the effects of early-life CONT and ID diets. Multiple comparisons were also accounted for within the randomize function. The resulting statistical analysis was then presented as heat maps indicating brain areas where FA values differed between dietary treatments.

3. Results

3.1. Quantitative Susceptibility Mapping

Interactive effects of diet and MRI day were not observed for region-specific QSM measures. A main effect of dietary treatment (i.e., independent of MRI day) ($p < 0.05$) was observed in the pons, medulla, cerebellum, left cortex, olfactory bulb, and left hippocampus, Figure 1 and Table 1. Regardless of imaging time-point, pigs receiving the ID diet exhibited lower QSM values in the pons ($p < 0.001$), medulla ($p = 0.02$), cerebellum ($p < 0.01$), left cortex ($p < 0.01$), and left hippocampus ($p < 0.001$) when compared with CONT pigs. Conversely, pigs on the ID diet exhibited higher ($p = 0.04$) QSM values in the olfactory bulb when compared with CONT pigs, regardless of imaging time-point.

A main effect of MRI day (i.e., independent of early-life iron status) ($p < 0.05$) was observed for corpus callosum, hypothalamus, and right cortex. The QSM measures in the corpus callosum ($p = 0.03$) increased from 0.26 ± 1.36 ppb on PND 32 to 4.89 ± 1.36 ppb at PND 61. In the right cortex, QSM measures increased ($p = 0.03$) from -1.83 ± 0.42 ppb on PND 32 to -0.21 ± 0.42 ppb at PND 61. Conversely, the QSM measures in hypothalamus decreased ($p = 0.04$) from -3.65 ± 1.70 ppb on PND 32 to -8.62 ± 1.70 ppb on PND 61. Notably, as iron content increases, QSM measures change from negative (i.e., indicating diamagnetic tissue properties) to positive (i.e., indicating paramagnetic tissue properties). Note, no interactive effects were observed, but means for both dietary treatments at both imaging time points are presented in Table 1. Accordingly, a main effect of diet can be determined by averaging the measures within dietary treatment group for each brain region and a main effect of time can be determined by averaging the two treatment groups at each imaging time point.

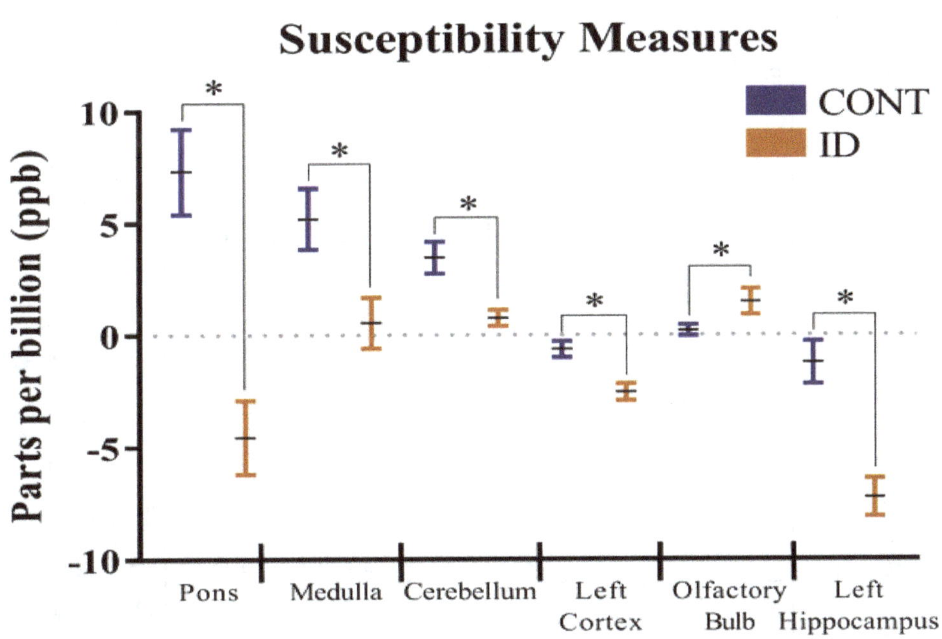

Figure 1. Measures of average iron content in brain regions were influenced by dietary iron status, regardless of imaging time-point. Because there was no significant interaction between diet and magnetic resonance imaging (MRI) day, this figure only shows the significant main effects of diet, regardless of time. Reduced iron content in the pons ($p < 0.001$), medulla ($p = 0.018$), cerebellum ($p = 0.005$), left cortex ($p = 0.004$), and left hippocampus ($p < 0.001$) was observed in ID pigs compared with CONT pigs. Iron content of the olfactory bulb was increased ($p = 0.043$) in ID pigs compared with CONT pigs. Note that as iron content increases, quantitative susceptibility measures values change from diamagnetic (negative values) to paramagnetic (positive values). Abbreviations: control (CONT); iron deficient (ID). * Main effect of early-life dietary iron status, differs by $p < 0.05$.

Table 1. Quantitative susceptibility measures indicating iron concentrations (ppb) in defined brain regions of pigs differing in early-life iron status [1].

Title	CONT		ID			*p*-Value		
Region of interest	PND 32	PND 61	PND 32	PND 61	SEM	Diet	Day	Diet × Day
Caudate	−6.3	−3.4	−2.1	−2.4	1.51	0.103	0.318	0.217
Cerebellum	4.6	1.6	0.9	0.5	0.91	0.005	0.069	0.144
Cerebral Aqueduct	−9.0	−15.8	−13.3	−9.2	3.14	0.723	0.609	0.065
Corpus Callosum	0.6	5.3	−0.1	4.5	2.04	0.676	0.029	0.994
Fourth Ventricle	−1.1	−9.8	−3.6	−7.5	3.59	0.985	0.057	0.428
Hypothalamus	−4.7	−11.0	−2.6	−6.3	2.48	0.161	0.044	0.550
Internal Capsule	−8.6	−8.0	−9.5	−7.5	1.04	0.760	0.303	0.560
Lateral Ventricle	−3.8	−1.3	−4.3	−2.4	1.48	0.542	0.110	0.834
Left Cortex	−0.6	−0.5	−2.2	−2.8	0.60	0.004	0.614	0.470
Left Hippocampus	−0.5	−1.9	−7.6	−6.9	1.53	<0.001	0.811	0.447
Medulla	5.1	5.3	−0.2	1.5	2.09	0.018	0.666	0.729
Midbrain	−6.5	−6.0	−8.8	−7.8	2.15	0.351	0.684	0.867
Olfactory Bulb	0.4	−0.2	1.6	1.5	0.77	0.043	0.601	0.715
Pons	4.7	10.9	−6.5	−2.2	2.83	<0.001	0.064	0.702
Putamen-Globus Pallidus	−6.3	−3.9	−5.1	−4.5	1.22	0.786	0.175	0.392
Right Cortex	−1.0	0.0	−2.7	−0.5	0.72	0.083	0.033	0.383
Right Hippocampus	−3.2	−0.6	−7.0	−4.2	2.29	0.141	0.127	0.979
Thalamus	−7.7	−11.0	−7.0	−7.6	1.88	0.322	0.166	0.319
Third Ventricle	−4.1	−4.8	−1.8	0.9	2.49	0.105	0.663	0.433

[1] Data presented as least square means and pooled standard errors of the mean (SEM) for each treatment group. Statistical significance of the main effects of early-life dietary treatment (Diet; CONT vs. ID) and postnatal magnetic resonance imaging (MRI) day (Day; PND 32 vs. 61) and the interaction between Diet and Day are presented. Number of pigs per treatment group that were subjected to MRI are as follows: PND 32 (CONT, n = 9–11; ID, n = 8–10), PND 61 (CONT, n = 5–7; ID, n = 7–9). In general susceptibility measures increase from negative (diamagnetic) to positive (paramagnetic) as iron accumulates in tissues. Abbreviations: control (CONT), iron deficient (ID), parts per billion (ppb), postnatal day (PND).

3.2. Voxel-Based Morphometry

Voxel-based morphometry is an analytical technique used to compare grey or white matter tissue distribution between two treatment groups. Accordingly, each treatment group may have more or less grey matter or white matter, resulting in clusters of voxels that indicate differences in tissue composition. Analysis of grey and white matter tissue segmentations from the PND 61 imaging time-point indicated region-specific differences ($p < 0.001$) between CONT and ID pigs, Table 2. A comparison of grey matter voxels where CONT pigs exhibited more ($p < 0.001$) grey matter voxels than ID pigs indicated differences in the left cortex, right cortex, cerebellum, hippocampus, thalamus, and caudate (CONT > ID), Figure 2 (red comparisons). The opposite comparison, in which ID pigs exhibited increased grey matter ($p < 0.001$) compared with CONT pigs (ID > CONT) indicated small grey matter clusters, in each of the left and right cortex, Figure 2 (blue comparisons). Comparison of white matter voxels where CONT pigs exhibited more ($p < 0.001$) white matter voxels than ID pigs indicated differences in the internal capsule, left cortex, right cortex, left hippocampus, and right hippocampus (CONT > ID), Figure 3 (red comparisons) and Table 2. There were no instances in which ID pigs exhibited more white matter compared with CONT pigs (ID > CONT). Table 2 lists clusters of edge-connected voxels where a statistical difference between the two dietary treatments was observed. The anatomical regions described were determined from *X*, *Y*, *Z* coordinates that corresponded to peak maximum differences within the clusters, thus it is possible to have multiple peaks per cluster.

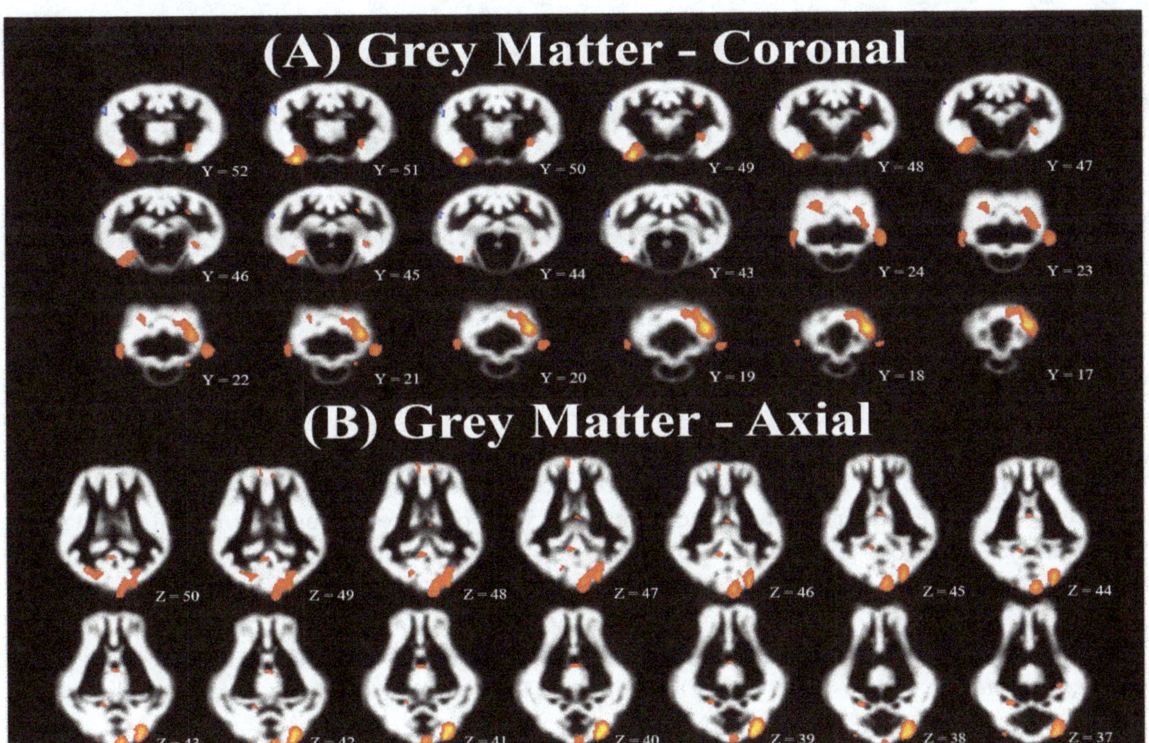

Figure 2. Pictured here is a population-averaged pig brain, with a statistical heat map indicating differences in grey matter between dietary treatment groups. The range of red-to-yellow indicates the degree of statistical difference from significant pseudo-*t* values of 3.80 to 7.35, respectively, in voxels where CONT pigs exhibited increased grey matter concentrations compared with ID pigs (i.e., CONT grey matter > ID grey matter). Clusters that range from dark-to-light blue indicate increasing significance from significant pseudo-*t* values of 4.30 to 5.55, respectively, in voxels where ID pigs exhibit increased grey matter compared with CONT pigs (i.e., ID grey matter > CONT grey matter). (**A**) Brain images in coronal orientation and (**B**) Brain images in axial orientation. Abbreviations: control (CONT); iron deficient (ID).

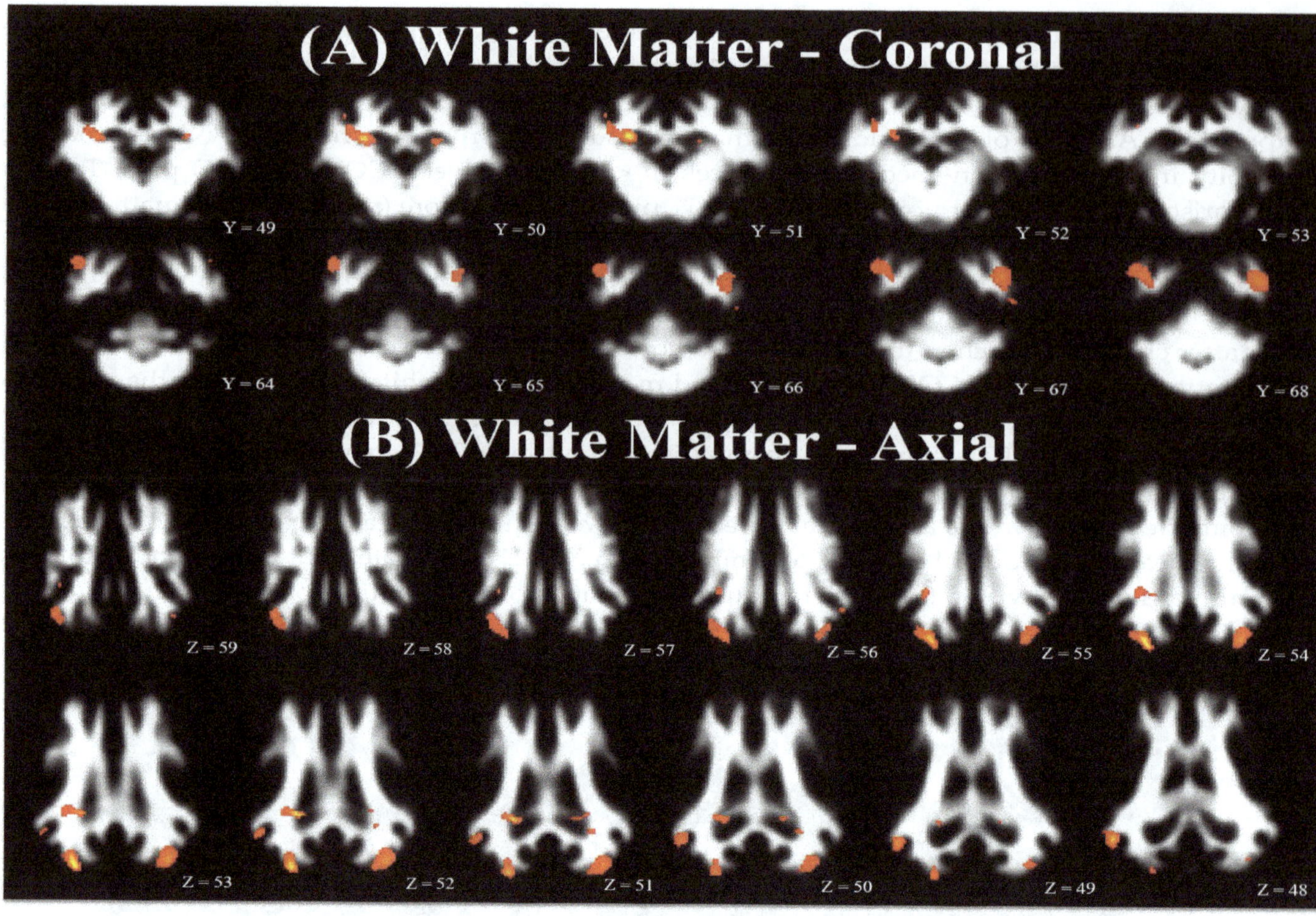

Figure 3. Pictured here is a population-averaged pig brain, with a statistical heat map indicating differences in white matter between dietary treatment groups. The range of red-to-yellow indicates the degree of statistical difference from significant pseudo-*t* values of 4.00 to 6.40, respectively, in voxels where CONT pigs exhibited increased white matter concentrations compared with ID pigs (i.e., CONT white matter > ID white matter). Notably, no differences were observed where ID pigs exhibited increased white matter concentrations compared with CONT pigs. (**A**) Brain images in coronal orientation and (**B**) Brain images in axial orientation. Abbreviations: control (CONT); iron deficient (ID).

3.3. Tract-Based Spatial Statistics

Tract-based spatial statistics allows assessment of differences due to diet in FA values along predetermined white matter tracts from data acquired at the PND 61 time-point. Analysis of FA values indicated subcortical areas in which CONT pigs exhibited greater ($p < 0.05$) FA values compared with ID pigs, Figure 4. Upon visual inspection, the greatest FA value differences appear to be in the white matter tracts located in the caudate and thalamus. Analysis of the opposite comparison, where FA values were greater in ID pigs compared with CONT pigs, revealed no differences ($p > 0.05$).

Table 2. Voxel-based morphometry assessment of grey and white matter at PND 61 comparing pigs from differing early-life iron status [1].

			Cluster Level		Peak Level		Local Maxima Coordinates [3]		
Tissue	Comparison	Anatomic Region [2]	Number of Voxels	*p*-Value	*p*-Value	Pseudo-*t*	X	Y	Z
		Right Cortex	2045	<0.001	<0.001	7.31	14.0	0.0	−12.6
		Right Cortex			<0.001	5.32	18.9	−13.3	−8.4
		Cerebellum	2772	<0.001	<0.001	6.92	−10.5	−25.2	0.0
		Cerebellum			<0.001	5.98	−2.8	−27.3	2.8
		Left Cortex			<0.001	5.16	−10.5	−16.8	5.6
		Right Cortex	443	0.004	<0.001	5.98	11.9	−15.4	7.7
		Cerebellum	997	<0.001	<0.001	5.55	−18.9	−18.9	−7.7
		Cerebellum	251	0.023	<0.001	5.54	9.1	−9.8	−2.1
Grey	CONT > ID	Right Hippocampus			<0.001	5.12	2.1	−9.1	6.3
		Left Cortex	242	0.025	<0.001	5.27	−14.0	−1.4	−3.5
		Left Cortex	204	0.037	<0.001	5.01	−13.3	−7.0	13.3
		Cerebellum	47	0.291	<0.001	4.83	11.9	−25.9	−2.8
		Thalamus	160	0.061	<0.001	4.36	0.0	10.5	0.7
		Right Cortex	79	0.175	<0.001	4.35	3.5	36.4	4.9
		Right Cortex	72	0.194	<0.001	4.15	13.3	−9.8	11.2
		Left Cortex	24	0.455	0.001	3.97	−5.6	−20.3	11.9
		Left Cortex	42	0.318	0.001	3.97	−2.1	33.6	5.6
		Caudate	21	0.486	0.001	3.81	2.1	18.2	2.8
		Right Cortex	419	0.005	<0.001	5.51	22.4	0.7	10.5
Grey	CONT <ID	Left Cortex	57	0.246	<0.001	4.45	−19.6	4.2	7.0
		Right Cortex	35	0.363	<0.001	4.34	18.2	16.1	12.6
		Right Hippocampus	234	0.022	<0.001	6.37	8.4	−2.1	8.4
		Right Cortex	629	0.001	<0.001	6.19	10.5	−16.8	9.1
		Right Cortex			<0.001	4.61	15.4	−9.8	13.3
		Right Cortex	378	0.005	<0.001	5.85	20.3	−7.0	4.2
		Left Cortex	653	0.001	<0.001	5.26	−14.0	−15.4	9.1
White	CONT > ID	Cerebellum			<0.001	4.26	−18.9	−16.1	0.7
		Internal Capsule	51	0.252	<0.001	4.48	−11.2	−5.6	7.7
		Left Hippocampus	61	0.212	<0.001	4.42	−7.0	−1.4	7.0
		Left Cortex	26	0.415	<0.001	4.07	−18.9	−7.7	11.2
		Internal Capsule	40	0.310	0.001	4.00	−8.4	20.3	3.5
White	CONT < ID	None	-	-	-	-	-	-	-

[1] Voxel-based morphometry analysis of gray and white matter differences in the CONT and ID pig brains at PND 61. A threshold of $p < 0.001$ and minimum cluster size of 20 voxels were used to determine *p*-uncorrected values listed in the table. Abbreviations: control (CONT), iron deficient (ID). [2] Brain regions based on visual inspection of the cluster location and cross-referenced with the Piglet Brain Atlas [29]. [3] Local maxima coordinates: *X* increases from left (−) to right (+), *Y* increases from posterior (−) to anterior (+), and Z increases from inferior (−) to superior (+).

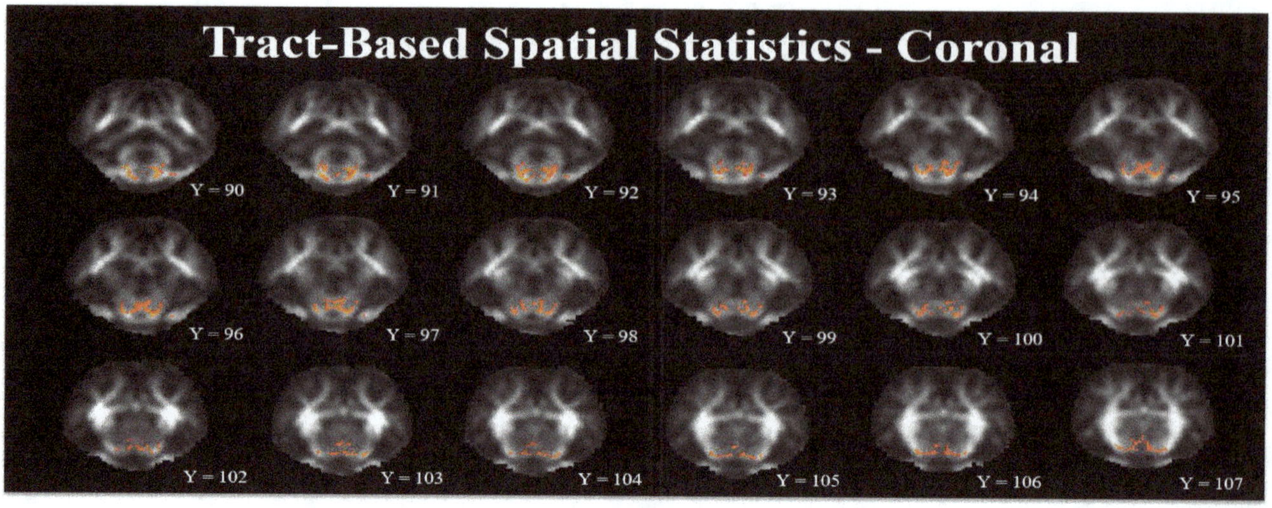

Figure 4. Pictured here is a population-averaged pig brain, with a statistical heat map indicating differences in white matter tract development between dietary treatment groups. Fractional anisotropy (FA) differences along predetermined white matter tracts where CONT pigs exhibited higher ($p < 0.05$) FA values compared with ID pigs. Representative slices were chosen to highlight areas in which FA values in CONT pigs were higher than in ID pigs. The range of red-to-yellow indicates degree of statistical difference from $p = 0.05$ to $p = 0.001$, respectively. Brain images in coronal orientation. Abbreviations: control (CONT); fractional anisotropy (FA); iron deficient (ID).

4. Discussion

Iron is pivotal for proper brain development, and alterations in both prenatal and postnatal iron status severely influence brain structure and function [4,6,16,36]. Moreover, brain development is a dynamic and heterogeneous process, thus the effects of iron deficiency are highly dependent on the timing and severity of the altered iron status [6]. In our study, pigs were provided either an ID or CONT diet from PND 2 until PND 32, at which point all pigs were switched to iron-replete diets until PND 61. The aim of this study was to determine what microstructural differences persisted in the brain at PND 61, despite all pigs being provided iron-replete diets from PND 33 to PND 61. In doing so, our study was designed to mimic postnatal dietary iron deficiency in human infants from birth up until four to six months of age when iron-fortified foods tend to be introduced into the diet. We previously published results indicating that total brain volumes are different between ID and CONT pigs at PND 32 but are not different at PND 61 [24]. Despite the observed compensatory brain volume growth during the period of dietary iron repletion, results from our analyses indicated tissue microstructural differences remained at PND 61. Therefore, to further elucidate how dietary iron status influenced brain development, we used voxel-based morphometry and tract-based spatial statistics to provide visual characterizations of neurodevelopment at PND 61. Herein we provide evidence that structural differences in grey and white matter are present in specific regions of the brain, even after 30 days of iron repletion. We also utilized quantitative susceptibility mapping to non-invasively characterize differences in brain iron content due to early-life dietary iron deficiency. These results are poised to have clinical relevance as we show neuroimaging can sensitively quantify differences in brain iron content due to dietary iron status.

4.1. *Quantitative Susceptibility Measures*

Iron is essential throughout early-life brain development to facilitate proper myelination [15], neurotransmitter synthesis [16,17], and neuron morphology [18,19]. Accordingly, the concentration of iron varies by brain region [37,38] and its presence is critical to ensure proper development throughout the brain. To date, many animal studies have focused on quantification of brain iron using invasive techniques to analyze samples of brain tissue [14,26,39]. Importantly, assessment of iron status through blood biomarkers is not always a reliable predictor of brain iron content. As evidence of this, a recent study where pigs were provided with ID diets early in life followed by iron replete diets indicated hematocrit and hemoglobin measures were not different between CONT and ID pigs at 12 weeks of age, but hippocampal iron content remained lower in ID pigs [26]. Provided the ethical limitations of collecting brain samples from human infants and the unreliable relationship between blood and brain iron concentrations, there is a need for a non-invasive assessment of brain iron content early in life. Quantitative susceptibility mapping is a non-invasive neuroimaging technique which can be used to sensitively characterize brain iron content [32]. This technique quantifies magnetic properties of tissue, and as iron is deposited into tissue, the tissue becomes increasingly paramagnetic. Thus, as development occurs and iron is accreted, it is expected that QSM values will increase (indicating stronger paramagnetic tissue properties). A previous report, where QSM methods were used in children, indicates that increased brain iron concentrations in the caudate related to increased spatial IQ [23]. Accordingly, this method may prove to be a sensitive non-invasive biomarker for quantifying brain iron content, and may help to explain differences in brain structural and functional development. To our knowledge, there do not appear to be any studies using QSM to determine the iron status of infant brains, however this method has been shown to sensitively characterize altered iron content in clinical cases of restless leg syndrome [21] and β-thalassemia [22].

In the present analysis, we used QSM to assess whether differences in brain iron could be detected non-invasively after a period of early-life iron deficiency. Our results indicate that pigs provided an early-life ID diet exhibited decreased brain iron concentrations in the cerebellum, pons, medulla, left cortex, and right cortex compared with CONT pigs at PND 32 and after receiving iron replete diets (i.e., at PND 61). Interestingly, ID pigs exhibited increased iron content in the olfactory bulb compared with CONT pigs. Previous analysis of brain volumes and diffusion tensor measures in this group of pigs indicated decreased relative brain volumes in the left hippocampus and the cerebellum of ID pigs [24]. Iron is needed for growth and expansion of neurons as well as dendrite morphogenesis in rodents [40] and pigs [41]. Thus, our QSM data may suggest a mechanism whereby decreased brain iron content attenuated neuron growth in the left hippocampus and cerebellum, thereby resulting in reduced relative volumes of these regions. The suggestion that iron is necessary for neuron growth is also supported by our findings of increased brain iron content in the olfactory bulbs of ID pigs and our previous report of increased relative volumes of the olfactory bulbs in ID pigs [24]. It remains to be elucidated why the olfactory bulb exhibits opposite growth trends during an ID state, however this finding of increased brain iron content in the olfactory bulb adds to evidence that this is likely not a spurious finding. We previously reported decreased FA values in the left cortex and the cerebellum of ID pigs. Fractional anisotropy is often used as a non-invasive marker of myelination and fiber coherence in the brain and increases throughout development [42,43]. It is also known that iron is an essential co-factor in myelinating events [15,44,45]. Thus, the decreased iron concentrations in the cerebellum and left cortex further support our hypothesis of decreased myelination in these two brain regions in young pigs.

Interestingly, a study of brain iron content in adults ranging from 22 to 78 years of age indicated increased iron content in left hemisphere brain regions compared with right hemisphere regions [46]. Xu and colleagues [46] suggest that this hemispheric difference in iron content may be due to lateralization of motor control, which is largely controlled by the dopaminergic system and is dependent on iron for neurotransmitter synthesis. Although handedness in our pigs was not assessed, our data of decreased iron in the left hippocampus and left cortex in ID pigs compared with CONT pigs may suggest an apparent hemispheric sensitivity of brain iron accumulation due to dietary iron status. In a rodent model of chronic early-life iron deficiency followed by iron repletion into adulthood, concentrations of brain iron restored to levels not different than in CONT animals in all regions except the thalamus [17]. Results from our study assessed brain iron at PND 32 and 61 and only a main effect of dietary treatment was noted for the brain regions discussed. Thus, future research should seek to non-invasively characterize brain iron content after a longer period of repletion to identify if iron content in ID pig brains is able to recover to levels observed in CONT pigs. In doing so, researchers will be able to better define the extent of dietary iron adequacy that is necessary to restore brain iron content back to baseline levels within an individual. It should be noted, however, that Felt and colleagues [17] observed altered monoamine metabolism and behavior in adult rodents that were previously ID, indicating that restoring brain iron to normal levels may not be sufficient to counteract the alterations in brain development due to early life iron deficiency. Our QSM findings of altered brain iron content stand to have clinical relevance, as we were able to use a non-invasive neuroimaging technique to sensitively quantify differences in brain iron content between ID and CONT pigs. Knowing that brain iron tends to decrease prior to hematological decreases in iron [5], neuroimaging of at-risk infants may help to identify and correct alterations in brain iron before overt signs of clinical iron deficiency are observed.

It is also worth mentioning that three brain regions indicated a change of iron content over time that was independent of dietary treatment. Notably, we observed an increase in QSM values in the corpus callosum and right cortex from PND 31 to PND 62, whereas a decrease in values was observed in the hypothalamus. Because these findings did not indicate sensitivity to dietary treatment, it suggests that these regions might be more resilient or less affected by alterations in dietary iron status when accumulating iron-containing compounds. We previously reported no differences due to dietary iron status in diffusion tensor fractional anisotropy, a measure indicating myelin and fiber tract development, in the corpus callosum [24]. Despite the lack of dietary effect in the corpus callosum FA values [24], we did observe an increase in corpus callosum FA values over time, which is consistent with the QSM values we report herein. Notably, our analysis of FA values in the right cortex did indicate a dietary effect [24], whereas our QSM values did not exhibit an effect of diet. This might suggest that the presence of iron-containing compounds is not solely responsible for changes in brain structure. As this is one of the first studies to assess QSM over time in early development, it is unclear if the decrease in hypothalamus values is of physiological relevance. Thus, future work should seek to better characterize changes in QSM across multiple time points to elucidate the trajectory of QSM changes from birth until adulthood. Doing so in the context of a longer period of iron deficiency might illuminate brain regions that are susceptible to alterations in QSM at different time points throughout the developmental process.

4.2. Voxel-Based Morphometry

We previously reported a reduction of approximately 10% in total brain volume at PND 32 in ID pigs compared with CONT pigs. However, after a period of dietary iron repletion from PND 33 to 61, brain volumes were not statistically different between early life ID and CONT pigs [24]. Despite this finding of similar brain volume, we observed microstructural differences in diffusion tensor measures between the two groups at PND 61, indicating that dietary iron repletion did not recover all aspects of brain development. Therefore, to further explore these microstructural differences we used voxel-based morphometry to visually assess differences in grey and white matter tissue concentrations that remained present at PND 61. Assessment of grey matter tissue differences between CONT and ID pigs indicated more voxels in which CONT pigs had greater concentrations of grey matter compared with ID pigs. Interestingly, these clusters of increased grey matter in CONT pigs were located in the left cortex, right cortex, cerebellum, thalamus, caudate, and right hippocampus. A previous study of iron deficiency in 30-day-old pigs indicated differences in cortical grey matter in CONT pigs compared with ID pigs [47]. In our study and the study by Leyshon and colleagues, the most abundant differences in grey matter appeared to be localized to cortical brain regions. However, the differences that were observed by Leyshon and colleagues between CONT and ID pigs at 30 d of age contained more voxels and larger clusters than what we observed in our pigs after a period of iron repletion on PND 61. Thus, it is possible that a period of iron repletion may be able to compensate for some alterations in tissue grey matter, yet it is clear that structural differences are present after 30 days of iron repletion.

In a rodent model of perinatal iron deficiency, ID rodents exhibited decreased branching complexity of cortical apical and basal dendrites, but no difference in dendrite length when compared with CONT rodents [19]. Pigs that were provided ID diets from birth until 4 weeks of life and iron replete diets from 4 until 12 weeks of life exhibited no difference in brain-derived neurotrophic factor (BDNF) expression in the prefrontal cortex [48]. In pigs, cortical brain tissue is just reaching its maximal growth rate at 4 weeks of age [49], corresponding to the age at which our study and the study by Nelissen and colleagues [48] switched ID pigs to iron replete diets. Thus, the lack of difference in BDNF in the prefrontal cortex of 12-week-old pigs and our observation of similar brain volumes at 8 weeks of age between ID and CONT pigs may suggest neuron outgrowth was not drastically influenced by early-life iron deficiency. However, the persistent differences in localized grey matter concentrations in the cortex may suggest altered neuron morphology, thus corroborating the findings by Greminger and colleagues [19]. The observed reductions in right hippocampal grey matter in ID pigs may also be a result of altered dendritic arborization, as this has previously been observed in ID hippocampal cell cultures from rodents [18]. These findings may suggest a non-invasive technique for characterizing altered cortical neuronal complexity in pigs that were ID early in life.

When assessing white matter, CONT pigs exhibited localized increases in both hippocampi, both cortices, the cerebellum, and the internal capsule when compared with ID pigs. In contrast, assessment of regions in which ID pigs exhibited increased white matter compared with CONT pigs yielded no significant results. This finding substantiates previous findings in 30-day-old pigs in which ID pigs did not have any voxels containing more white matter when compared with CONT pigs [47]. Together, these findings indicate that once detriments in white matter maturation have occurred early in life, recovery may not be possible, even after a subsequent period of dietary iron repletion. This observation of decreased white matter also aligns with our previous results of decreased FA values in the whole brain, cortex, cerebellum, and internal capsule due to early-life iron deficiency in pigs [24]. Previous research indicates reduced cerebellar myelination in rodents [45], thus suggesting that our observed reductions in cerebellar white matter may be due to reduced myelination. A previous study of 30-day-old ID pigs also indicated reduced white matter concentrations in the internal capsule [47]. It is known that the internal capsule and cerebellum are critical for coordinating motor skills and previous research in ID and ID anemic infants indicates delayed motor development [8], thus our findings of reduced white matter concentrations in these regions may indicate reductions in myelin development. While our study did not assess motor coordination or gait analysis in young pigs, future work should seek to assess the effect of early life iron on these measures. Provided there remain differences in both grey and white matter after a 30 day period of dietary iron repletion, future studies should seek to characterize if there is a period of iron repletion that is capable of rendering CONT and ID brains structurally similar.

4.3. Tract-Based Spatial Statistics

Tract-based spatial statistics allows for comparison of diffusion values along predetermined white matter tracts in the brain. Our previous diffusion tensor analysis indicated reductions in whole brain FA values in ID pigs, as well as FA reductions in the caudate, cerebellum, and internal capsule [24]. These previous observations were averaged over all white matter found in a defined brain region and were not specific to white matter tracts. Provided our previous results indicated differences in diffusion values that persisted at PND 61, we used TBSS to visualize white matter tracts where early-life ID pigs exhibited decreased FA values relative to CONT pigs. Assessment of white matter tracts in which CONT pigs exhibited voxels with higher FA values compared with ID pigs indicated differences located exclusively in subcortical brain regions. From our analysis, the regions in which FA values were greater in CONT pigs along white matter tracts appear to be localized to the internal capsule, thalamus, and hypothalamus. Importantly, there were no voxels along white matter tracts in which ID pigs exhibited increased FA values compared with CONT pigs, thereby suggesting that iron deficiency only causes detriments in white matter integrity and does not support white matter maturation. As described above, decreased white matter was observed in the internal capsule of ID pigs compared with CONT pigs. Thus, our VBM findings and the differences in TBSS in the internal capsule may suggest decreased myelin content of this brain region. Moreover, ID and ID anemic infants are known to have delayed motor development [8], and both the internal capsule and thalamus contain motor projections within the brain [50,51]. Previous research in rodents indicates the thalamus is susceptible to dietary iron deficiency, resulting in alterations in monoamine metabolism [4,16,17]. Additionally, increased thalamic axial, radial, and mean diffusivity values were observed in ID pigs at PND 29, suggesting altered myelination in this region [47]. Thus, our findings of altered white matter tracts in these two regions may suggest decreased internal capsule and thalamic myelination, thereby affirming a mechanism through which motor development is delayed in ID infants. It is interesting to note that these differences persist despite a subsequent period of iron repletion in pigs, thus indicating either the period for iron repletion was not long enough or it was applied too late in development to allow for recovery of microstructural changes due to early-life iron deficiency. Future research should seek to quantify myelin content in these brain regions at different time-points during and after iron deficiency to more definitively link iron status and myelination.

4.4. Limitations

While the results of this study are novel, we cannot definitively conclude that iron repletion after a period of early-life iron deficiency is incapable of compensating for developmental differences. Future research should seek to quantify different periods of dietary iron repletion as well as the timing of first providing an iron replete diet. In doing so, researchers will be able to better quantify critical windows during which iron influences particular aspects of brain development. Provided the results of our study, we suggest that early-life iron deficiency through PND 32 in the pig greatly alters myelinating events and may influence morphology of grey matter, but it does not appear to influence overall brain growth.

5. Conclusions

We previously showed that iron deficiency alters whole brain volumes at PND 32 but iron repletion was able to correct for observed differences by PND 61. Here we have shown that despite similar brain volumes, differences in grey matter and white matter, as well as decreased white matter tract integrity, remain at PND 61. Thus, while gross brain morphology appeared unaltered, microstructural detriments in brain development persisted in pigs exposed to early-life iron deficiency followed by a period of iron repletion. Our results also indicate region-specific reductions in brain iron concentrations of ID pigs, regardless of imaging time-point. Notably, characterization of altered brain iron and grey and white matter tissue concentrations were observed through non-invasive techniques, thereby providing clinically relevant methods to assess similar results in human infants. Thus, it is possible that neuroimaging may be used to comprehensively characterize altered brain iron status in infants at risk of iron deficiency, prior to the presence of overt symptoms of iron deficiency or iron deficiency anemia.

Acknowledgments: We would like to thank Brian Berg and Rosaline Waworuntu for their advice in study design. Additionally, we would like to thank Mead Johnson Nutrition for the dietary treatments used in this study. We would like to thank Kristen Karkiewicz and the rest of the Piglet Nutrition and Cognition Laboratory staff for day-to-day pig rearing. Lastly, we would like to thank Brad Sutton and the rest of the Beckman Imaging Center staff for their help in imaging acquisition and data analysis.

Author Contributions: A.T.M., J.E.F., L.C.K., and R.N.D. were involved in study design and implementation. All authors (A.T.M., J.E.F., L.C.K., F.L., Z.-P.L. and R.N.D.) were involved in data acquisition, analysis, and interpretation. All authors read and approved the final version of this manuscript.

References

1. World Health Organization. *Micronutrient Deficiencies—Iron Deficiency Anemia*; World Health Organization: Geneva, Switzerland, 2017.
2. World Health Organization. *Iron Deficiency Anaemia: Assessment, Prevention, and Control: A Guide for Programme Managers*; World Health Organization: Geneva, Switzerland, 2010.
3. McLean, E.; Cogswell, M.; Egli, I.; Wojdyla, D.; de Benoist, B. Worldwide prevalence of anaemia, WHO Vitamin and Mineral Nutrition Information System, 1993–2005. *Public Health Nutr.* **2009**, *12*, 444. [CrossRef] [PubMed]
4. Lozoff, B.; Georgieff, M.K. Iron deficiency and brain development. *Semin. Pediatr. Neurol.* **2006**, *13*, 158–165. [CrossRef] [PubMed]
5. Georgieff, M.K. Iron assessment to protect the developing brain. *Am. J. Clin. Nutr.* **2017**, *106*, 1588S–1593S. [CrossRef] [PubMed]
6. Georgieff, M.K. Nutrition and the developing brain: Nutrient priorities and measurement. *Am. J. Clin. Nutr.* **2007**, *85*, 614–620.
7. Radlowski, E.C.; Johnson, R.W. Perinatal iron deficiency and neurocognitive development. *Front. Hum. Neurosci.* **2013**, *7*, 1–11. [CrossRef] [PubMed]
8. Shafir, T.; Angulo-Barroso, R.; Jing, Y.; Angelilli, M.L.; Jacobson, S.W.; Lozoff, B. Iron deficiency and infant motor development. *Early Hum. Dev.* **2008**, *84*, 479–485. [CrossRef] [PubMed]
9. Congdon, E.L.; Westerlund, A.; Algarin, C.R.; Peirano, P.D.; Gregas, M.; Lozoff, B.; Nelson, C.A. Iron deficiency in infancy is associated with altered neural correlates of recognition memory at 10 years. *J. Pediatr.* **2012**, *160*, 1027–1033. [CrossRef] [PubMed]
10. Lukowski, A.F.; Koss, M.; Burden, M.J.; Jonides, J.; Nelson, C.A.; Kaciroti, N.; Jimenez, E.; Lozoff, B. Iron deficiency in infancy and neurocognitive functioning at 19 years: Evidence of long-term deficits in executive function and recognition memory. *Nutr. Neurosci.* **2010**, *13*, 54–70. [CrossRef] [PubMed]
11. Lozoff, B.; Smith, J.B.; Kaciroti, N.; Clark, K.M.; Guevara, S.; Jimenez, E. Functional significance of early-life iron deficiency: Outcomes at 25 years. *J. Pediatr.* **2013**, *163*, 1260–1266. [CrossRef] [PubMed]
12. Algarín, C.; Peirano, P.; Garrido, M.; Pizarro, F.; Lozoff, B. Iron deficiency anemia in infancy: Long-lasting effects on auditory and visual system functioning. *Pediatr. Res.* **2003**, *53*, 217–223. [CrossRef] [PubMed]
13. Otero, G.A.; Fernández, T.; Pliego-Rivero, F.B.; Mendieta, G.G. Iron therapy substantially restores qEEG maturational lag among iron-deficient anemic infants. *Nutr. Neurosci.* **2017**, 1–10. [CrossRef] [PubMed]
14. Bastian, T.W.; Santarriaga, S.; Nguyen, T.A.; Prohaska, J.R.; Georgieff, M.K.; Anderson, G.W. Fetal and neonatal iron deficiency but not copper deficiency increases vascular complexity in the developing rat brain. *Nutr. Neurosci.* **2015**, *18*, 365–375. [CrossRef] [PubMed]
15. Todorich, B.; Pasquini, J.M.; Garcia, C.I.; Paez, P.M.; Connor, J.R. Oligodendrocytes and myelination: The role of iron. *Glia* **2009**, *57*, 467–478. [CrossRef] [PubMed]
16. Lozoff, B.; Unger, E.; Connor, J.; Felt, B.; Georgieff, M. Early iron deficiency has brain and behavior effects consistent with dopaminergic function. *J. Nutr.* **2011**, *141*, 740–746. [CrossRef] [PubMed]
17. Felt, B.T.; Beard, J.L.; Schallert, T.; Shao, J.; Aldridge, J.W.; Connor, J.R.; Georgieff, M.K.; Lozoff, B. Persistent neurochemical and behavioral abnormalities in adulthood despite early iron supplementation for perinatal iron deficiency anemia in rats. *Behav. Brain Res.* **2006**, *171*, 261–270. [CrossRef] [PubMed]
18. Bastian, T.W.; Von Hohenberg, W.C.; Mickelson, D.J.; Lanier, L.M.; Georgieff, M.K. Iron deficiency impairs developing hippocampal neuron gene expression, energy metabolism, and dendrite complexity. *Dev. Neurosci.* **2016**, *38*, 264–276. [CrossRef] [PubMed]
19. Greminger, A.R.; Lee, D.L.; Shrager, P.; Mayer-Proschel, M. Gestational iron deficiency differentially alters the structure and function of white and gray matter brain regions of developing rats. *J. Nutr.* **2014**, *144*, 1058–1066. [CrossRef] [PubMed]
20. Monk, C.; Georgieff, M.K.; Xu, D.; Hao, X.; Bansal, R.; Gustafsson, H.; Spicer, J.; Peterson, B.S. Maternal prenatal iron status and tissue organization in the neonatal brain. *Pediatr. Res.* **2016**, *79*, 482–488. [CrossRef] [PubMed]
21. Li, X.; Allen, R.P.; Earley, C.J.; Liu, H.; Cruz, T.E.; Edden, R.A.E.; Barker, P.B.; van Zijl, P.C.M. Brain iron deficiency in idiopathic restless legs syndrome measured by quantitative magnetic susceptibility at 7 tesla. *Sleep Med.* **2016**, *22*, 75–82. [CrossRef] [PubMed]

22. Qiu, D.; Chan, G.C.-F.; Chu, J.; Chan, Q.; Ha, S.-Y.; Moseley, M.E.; Khong, P.-L. MR quantitative susceptibility imaging for the evaluation of iron loading in the brains of patients with β-thalassemia. *Am. J. Neuroradiol.* **2014**, *35*, 1085–1090. [CrossRef] [PubMed]
23. Carpenter, K.L.H.; Li, W.; Wei, H.; Wu, B.; Xiao, X.; Liu, C.; Worley, G.; Egger, H.L. Magnetic susceptibility of brain iron is associated with childhood spatial IQ. *Neuroimage* **2016**, *132*, 167–174. [CrossRef] [PubMed]
24. Mudd, A.; Fil, J.; Knight, L.; Dilger, R. Dietary iron repletion following early-life dietary iron deficiency does not correct regional volumetric or diffusion tensor changes in the developing pig brain. *Front. Neurol.* **2017**. [CrossRef]
25. Gan, L.; Yang, B.; Mei, H. The effect of iron dextran on the transcriptome of pig hippocampus. *Genes Genom.* **2017**, *39*, 1–14. [CrossRef]
26. Antonides, A.; Schoonderwoerd, A.C.; Scholz, G.; Berg, B.M.; Nordquist, R.E.; van der Staay, F.J. Pre-weaning dietary iron deficiency impairs spatial learning and memory in the cognitive holeboard task in piglets. *Front. Behav. Neurosci.* **2015**, *9*, 1–16. [CrossRef] [PubMed]
27. National Research Council (USA). *Nutrient Requirements of Swine*, 11th ed.; The National Academies Press: Washington, DC, USA, 2012.
28. Mudd, A.T.; Getty, C.; Sutton, B.; Dilger, R. Perinatal choline deficiency delays brain development and alters metabolite concentrations in the young pig. *Nutr. Neurosci.* **2016**, *19*, 425–433. [CrossRef] [PubMed]
29. Conrad, M.S.; Sutton, B.P.; Dilger, R.N.; Johnson, R. An in vivo three-dimensional magnetic resonance imaging-based averaged brain collection of the neonatal piglet (Sus scrofa). *PLoS ONE* **2014**, *9*, 107650. [CrossRef] [PubMed]
30. Lam, F.; Liang, Z.-P. A subspace approach to high-resolution spectroscopic imaging. *Magn. Reson. Med.* **2014**, *71*, 1349–1357. [CrossRef] [PubMed]
31. Peng, X.; Lam, F.; Li, Y.; Clifford, B.; Liang, Z.-P. Simultaneous QSM and metabolic imaging of the brain using SPICE. *Magn. Reson. Med.* **2018**, *79*, 13–21. [CrossRef] [PubMed]
32. Wang, Y.; Liu, T. Quantitative susceptibility mapping (QSM): Decoding MRI data for a tissue magnetic biomarker. *Magn. Reson. Med.* **2015**, *73*, 82–101. [CrossRef] [PubMed]
33. Zhou, D.; Liu, T.; Spincemaille, P.; Wang, Y. Background field removal by solving the Laplacian boundary value problem. *NMR Biomed.* **2014**, *27*, 312–319. [CrossRef] [PubMed]
34. Smith, S.M.; Jenkinson, M.; Woolrich, M.W.; Beckmann, C.F.; Behrens, T.E.J.; Johansen-Berg, H.; Bannister, P.R.; De Luca, M.; Drobnjak, I.; Flitney, D.E.; et al. Advances in functional and structural MR image analysis and implementation as FSL. *Neuroimage* **2004**, *23*, S208–S219. [CrossRef] [PubMed]
35. Smith, S.M.; Jenkinson, M.; Johansen-Berg, H.; Rueckert, D.; Nichols, T.E.; Mackay, C.E.; Watkins, K.E.; Ciccarelli, O.; Cader, M.Z.; Matthews, P.M.; et al. Tract-based spatial statistics: Voxelwise analysis of multi-subject diffusion data. *Neuroimage* **2006**, *31*, 1487–1505. [CrossRef] [PubMed]
36. Georgieff, M.K. Long-term brain and behavioral consequences of early iron deficiency. *Nutr. Rev.* **2011**, *69*, 43–48. [CrossRef] [PubMed]
37. Haacke, E.M.; Cheng, N.Y.C.; House, M.J.; Liu, Q.; Neelavalli, J.; Ogg, R.J.; Khan, A.; Ayaz, M.; Kirsch, W.; Obenaus, A. Imaging iron stores in the brain using magnetic resonance imaging. *Magn. Reson. Imaging* **2005**, *23*, 1–25. [CrossRef] [PubMed]
38. Bradbury, M.W. Transport of iron in the blood-brain-cerebrospinal fluid system. *J. Neurochem.* **1997**, *69*, 443–454. [CrossRef] [PubMed]
39. Rytych, J.L.; Elmore, M.R.P.; Burton, M.D.; Conrad, M.S.; Donovan, S.M.; Dilger, R.N.; Johnson, R.W. Early life iron deficiency impairs spatial cognition in neonatal piglets. *J. Nutr.* **2012**, *142*, 2050–2056. [CrossRef] [PubMed]
40. Jorgenson, L.A.; Wobken, J.D.; Georgieff, M.K. Perinatal iron deficiency alters apical dendritic growth in hippocampal CA1 pyramidal neurons. *Dev. Neurosci.* **2003**, *25*, 412–420. [CrossRef] [PubMed]
41. Schachtschneider, K.M.; Liu, Y.; Rund, L.A.; Madsen, O.; Johnson, R.W.; Groenen, M.A.M.; Schook, L.B. Impact of neonatal iron deficiency on hippocampal DNA methylation and gene transcription in a porcine biomedical model of cognitive development. *BMC Genom.* **2016**, *17*, 856. [CrossRef] [PubMed]
42. Drobyshevsky, A.; Song, S.; Gamkrelidze, G.; Wyrwicz, A.M.; Derrick, M.; Meng, F.; Li, L.; Ji, X.; Trommer, B.; Beardsley, D.J.; et al. Developmental changes in diffusion anisotropy coincide with immature oligodendrocyte progression and maturation of compound action potential. *J. Neurosci.* **2005**, *25*, 5988–5997. [CrossRef] [PubMed]

43. Hermoye, L.; Saint-Martin, C.; Cosnard, G.; Lee, S.-K.; Kim, J.; Nassogne, M.-C.; Menten, R.; Clapuyt, P.; Donohue, P.K.; Hua, K.; et al. Pediatric diffusion tensor imaging: Normal database and observation of the white matter maturation in early childhood. *Neuroimage* **2006**, *29*, 493–504. [CrossRef] [PubMed]
44. Wu, L.-L.; Zhang, L.; Shao, J.; Qin, Y.-F.; Yang, R.-W.; Zhao, Z.-Y. Effect of perinatal iron deficiency on myelination and associated behaviors in rat pups. *Behav. Brain Res.* **2008**, *188*, 263–270. [CrossRef] [PubMed]
45. Yu, G.S.; Steinkirchner, T.M.; Rao, G.A.; Larkin, E.C. Effect of prenatal iron deficiency on myelination in rat pups. *Am. J. Pathol.* **1986**, *125*, 620–624. [PubMed]
46. Xu, X.; Wang, Q.; Zhang, M. Age, gender, and hemispheric differences in iron deposition in the human brain: An in vivo MRI study. *Neuroimage* **2008**, *40*, 35–42. [CrossRef] [PubMed]
47. Leyshon, B.J.; Radlowski, E.C.; Mudd, A.T.; Steelman, A.J.; Johnson, R.W. Postnatal iron deficiency impairs brain development in piglets. *J. Nutr.* **2016**, *146*, 1420–1427. [CrossRef] [PubMed]
48. Nelissen, E.; De Vry, J.; Antonides, A.; Paes, D.; Schepers, M.; van der Staay, F.J.; Prickaerts, J.; Vanmierlo, T. Early-postnatal iron deficiency impacts plasticity in the dorsal and ventral hippocampus in piglets. *Int. J. Dev. Neurosci.* **2017**, *59*, 47–51. [CrossRef] [PubMed]
49. Conrad, M.S.; Dilger, R.N.; Johnson, R.W. Brain growth of the domestic pig (Sus scrofa) from 2 to 24 weeks of age: A longitudinal MRI study. *Dev. Neurosci.* **2012**, *34*, 291–298. [CrossRef] [PubMed]
50. Rose, J.; Mirmiran, M.; Butler, E.E.; Lin, C.Y.; Barnes, P.D.; Kermoian, R.; Stevenson, D.K. Neonatal microstructural development of the internal capsule on diffusion tensor imaging correlates with severity of gait and motor deficits. *Dev. Med. Child Neurol.* **2007**, *49*, 745–750. [CrossRef] [PubMed]
51. Hartmann-von Monakow, K.; Akert, K.; Künzle, H. Projections of the precentral motor cortex and other cortical areas of the frontal lobe to the subthalamic nucleus in the monkey. *Exp. Brain Res.* **1978**, *33*, 395–403. [CrossRef]

11

Dietary Fructose Intake and Hippocampal Structure and Connectivity during Childhood

Kristi A. Clark [1], Jasmin M. Alves [2,3], Sabrina Jones [2,3], Alexandra G. Yunker [2,3], Shan Luo [2,3,4], Ryan P. Cabeen [5], Brendan Angelo [2,3], Anny H. Xiang [6] and Kathleen A. Page [2,3,*]

1 Department of Neurology, Keck School of Medicine of the University of Southern California, Los Angeles, CA 90033, USA; kristi.clark.999@gmail.com
2 Department of Internal Medicine; Division of Endocrinology, Keck School of Medicine of the University of Southern California, Los Angeles, CA 90033, USA; jalves@usc.edu (J.M.A.); sljones@usc.edu (S.J.); ayunker@usc.edu (A.G.Y.); shanluo@usc.edu (S.L.); angelob@usc.edu (B.A.)
3 Diabetes and Obesity Research Institute of the University of Southern California, Los Angeles, CA 90033, USA
4 Department of Psychology, University of Southern California, Los Angeles, CA 90089, USA
5 Laboratory of Neuro Imaging (LONI), USC Stevens Neuroimaging and Informatics Institute, Keck School of Medicine of USC, Los Angeles, CA 90033, USA; Ryan.Cabeen@loni.usc.edu
6 Department of Research and Evaluation, Kaiser Permanente Southern California, Pasadena, CA 91101, USA; Anny.H.Xiang@kp.org
* Correspondence: kpage@usc.edu

Abstract: In rodent literature, there is evidence that excessive fructose consumption during development has a detrimental impact on hippocampal structure and function. In this study of 103 children ages 7–11 years old, we investigated whether dietary fructose intake was related to alterations in hippocampal volume and connectivity in humans. To examine if these associations were specific to fructose or were related to dietary sugars intake in general, we explored relationships between dietary intake of added sugars and the monosaccharide, glucose, on the same brain measures. We found that increased dietary intake of fructose, measured as a percentage of total calories, was associated with both an increase in the volume of the CA2/3 subfield of the right hippocampus and increased axial, radial, and mean diffusivity in the prefrontal connections of the right cingulum. These findings are consistent with the idea that increased fructose consumption during childhood may be associated with an inflammatory process, and/or decreases or delays in myelination and/or pruning. Increased habitual consumption of glucose or added sugar in general were associated with an increased volume of right CA2/3, but not with any changes in the connectivity of the hippocampus. These findings support animal data suggesting that higher dietary intake of added sugars, particularly fructose, are associated with alterations in hippocampal structure and connectivity during childhood.

Keywords: children; cingulum; development; dietary sugar; fructose; hippocampus

---

1. Introduction

Diets high in added sugars, particularly fructose, have adverse metabolic consequences and are associated with oxidative stress, insulin resistance, and cardiometabolic disorders [1–4]. Beyond its known metabolic health risks, high fructose consumption has been linked to impairments in peripheral and central appetite signaling and may promote feeding behavior [5–10]. Emerging data also indicates that high fructose diets have a profound impact on brain function [11,12], particularly within the hippocampus, a brain region involved in memory, learning, and food intake regulation that is particularly vulnerable to dietary and metabolic insults [13–15]. Experimental studies in animal models have shown that high fructose consumption leads to hippocampal insulin resistance [16,17], neuroinflammation [18,19], and reduced hippocampal neurogenesis [20], and suggests a potential mechanistic basis for fructose induced cognitive deficits [17,18,21].

The findings that hippocampal function is highly sensitive to excess fructose consumption are particularly relevant to the study of obesity and excess weight gain considering the role the hippocampus plays in energy regulation. In rodents, hippocampal lesions [14] or inactivation [15] increase food consumption and body weight. The translation of these findings to humans has been supported by experiments in patients with brain lesions. Patients with lesions to the temporal lobe have been shown to overeat in response to food presentation relative to healthy controls and patients with lesions in other brain regions, even after consuming an energy dense meal [22,23]. Considering these findings together, the hippocampus appears to be highly important in the inhibition of food consumption; therefore, in the case of hippocampal impairment by external insults, such as excessive consumption of fructose, humans and animals may overeat and consequently gain additional weight.

Human hippocampal connectivity has been found to be quite extensive [24], and evidence from animal models suggests that the ability of the hippocampus to inhibit appetitive behaviors may rely on its connections to other brain areas. Prior findings have demonstrated that disconnection lesions (the elimination of all direct and indirect connections) between the ventral hippocampus and the contralateral prefrontal cortex in rodents impairs general behavioral inhibition in a 5-choice reaction time task [25]. More specifically related to obesity, a monosynaptic glutamatergic pathway between the ventral hippocampus and the medial prefrontal cortex has been identified as important in the control of energy regulation. Chemogenic inactivation of this pathway has been shown to increase food consumption, indicating the activation of this pathway may be important in the ability to suppress overeating [26]. The hippocampus is also connected to the lateral septum, and activation of this excitatory pathway inhibits food intake [27]. Other hippocampal-dependent feeding pathways include connections with the amygdala and hypothalamus [18,28]. While diets high in fructose or other added sugars have been found to alter hippocampal physiology [18,20], and metabolic insults, such as obesity, have been shown to decrease hippocampal global brain connectivity [29], the impact of dietary fructose or added sugar intake on the microstructure of pathways that connect the hippocampus to other brain regions has not yet been studied.

Recent studies in rodents have shown that the effects of high fructose diets on hippocampal function are particularly damaging during sensitive periods of neurocognitive development, such as childhood and adolescence [18], but few studies have attempted to translate these findings to humans. To address this gap in knowledge, we used in vivo magnetic resonance imaging (MRI) methods, which provide a non-invasive way to examine the neurodevelopment of the human brain. T1-weighted acquisitions allow quantification of grey matter volume in specific regions of the brain, and diffusion tensor imaging (DTI) is a sensitive imaging method that can characterize the microstructural architecture of white matter tracts that connect distinct brain regions [30]. We used both structural MRI and diffusion MRI to examine the associations between dietary fructose and added sugar intake and hippocampal development in healthy children aged 7 to 11 years. Based on studies in animal models, we hypothesized that higher dietary intake of added sugars, particularly fructose, would be associated with alterations in hippocampal volume and in the microstructure of white matter tracts that connect the hippocampus to other brain regions.

2. Materials and Methods

2.1. Participants

Healthy, typically developing children between the ages of 7–11 years old participated in the BrainChild Study of the impact of intrauterine exposure to metabolic disorders on brain pathways during childhood. Children were born at Kaiser Permanente Southern California (KPSC), a large health care organization that uses an integrated electronic medical record (EMR) system. KPSC member demographics are broadly representative of Southern California residents [31]. Each participating Institutional Review Board approved this study (University of Southern California (USC) #HS-14-00034, KPSC #10282). Participants' parents gave written informed consent. Children provided written informed assent.

The study included two in-person visits. Visit one occurred at the Clinical Research Unit of the USC Diabetes and Obesity Research Institute. Visit two occurred at USC Dana and David Dornsife Neuroimaging Center and included a MRI scan of the brain.

2.2. *Clinical Characteristics and Demographics*

Child's height was measured to the nearest 0.1 cm using a stadiometer and weight to the nearest 0.1 kg using a calibrated digital scale. BMI was calculated using the standard formula, weight (kg) divided by height (m^2). BMI z-scores and BMI percentiles (age and sex-specific standard deviation scores) were determined based on Center for Disease Control (CDC) standards [32]. Participants were given the option of having Tanner stage assessed by physical exam [33,34] and/or by a validated sex-specific assessment questionnaire for children and parents, containing both illustrations and explanatory text [35]. Forty-eight participants opted for both physical exam and questionnaire, and 55 participants opted for self-reported puberty status only. The correlation between Tanner Staging assessed by physical exam and by questionnaire was 0.91.

Socioeconomic status (SES) was assessed using household income at birth, estimated based on census tract of residence and expressed as a continuous variable, and maternal education at birth, which was extracted from birth certificates in the EMR as a categorical variable with the following categories: "high-school or some high-school", "some college", and "college and post-education". Prenatal exposures to maternal gestational diabetes mellitus (GDM) and maternal pre-pregnancy BMI were assessed using the EMR.

2.3. *Dietary Measures*

Diet was assessed using repeated 24-h dietary recalls on non-consecutive days during two in-person visits as part of the BrainChild Study. In a subset of 35 participants, we also obtained 3-day dietary records on one of the two in-person visits, and dietary intake was estimated using a total of four days of dietary assessments for these participants. The mean interval between the two in-person visits was 34 ± 57 days. We used the multi-pass method for dietary recall, in which a trained staff member asked the participant to recall what food and beverages they had consumed over a 24-h time period with the input of both the child and the child's parent. The trained staff member then went through three other "passes" to complete quantity of food/beverages consumed as well as to include missing or forgotten food/beverages. Use of the multi-pass 24-h dietary recall method is a valid method to assess energy intake in children [36]. Once the dietary recalls were collected, the recalls were analyzed using the Nutritional Data System for Research software v.2018 developed by the Nutrition Coordinating Center (NCC), University of Minnesota, Minneapolis, MS [37]. The variables used were percent calories from fructose, percent calories from glucose, and percent calories from added sugar by available carbohydrate. Data from dietary recalls were manually checked for quality. To determine outliers, we performed linear regression analysis, using body weight to predict total energy intake. Residuals were standardized and examined for any values that were >3 or <-3 standard deviations from the mean. Records containing data that exceeded these values were not included in the analysis. Using this method, 267 dietary recalls were included in the analysis, and one dietary recall was excluded.

2.4. Magnetic Resonance Imaging (MRI) Acquisition

After a mock scanner training session, magnetic resonance imaging (MRI) was performed using a Siemens MAGNETOM Prisma^{fit} 3 Tesla MRI scanner (Siemens Medical Systems) with a 20-channel phased array coil. A high-resolution magnetic resonance imaging scan was acquired using a T1-weighted three-dimensional magnetization prepared rapid gradient echo (MP-RAGE) sequence with the parameters: 256 × 256 × 176-matrix size with 1 × 1 × 1-mm^3 resolution; inversion time = 900 ms; repetition time (TR) = 1950 ms; echo time (TE) = 2.26 ms; flip angle = 90°; Total scan duration was 4 min and 14 s. A diffusion weighted image was acquired using a dual spin echo, single shot, pulsed gradient, echo planar imaging sequence in 64 diffusion sensitized gradient directions with the following parameters: TR = 8100 ms; TE = 69 ms; flip angle = 90°; 70 axial slices; 2 mm × 2 mm × 2 mm voxel size; FOV = 256 mm; b value = 1000 s/mm^2; Total scan duration was 9 min and 29 s.

2.5. MRI Data Processing

The T1 MP-RAGE structural image was put into the automated segmentation software, FreeSurfer version 6.0 hippocampal module (http://surfer.nmr.mgh.harvard.edu/, RRID:SCR_001847) to examine total hippocampal grey matter volume and grey matter volume in the hippocampal subfields. The procedure uses Bayesian inference and a probabilistic atlas of the hippocampal formation based on manual delineations of subfields in ultra-high-resolution MRI scans [38]. Manual quality check of automated hippocampal segmentation was performed for each participant following an existing protocol [39]. The segmentation of the hippocampus was visually assessed by an individual trained in hippocampal neuroanatomy and then given a rating of "pass", "pass on condition", and "fail". Images that failed to have defined landmarks due to motion artifacts or segmentation error were excluded. Although twelve subfield volumes are generated by FreeSurfer 6.0, we only included subfields that have been shown to be preferentially affected by high sugar diets, including the CA1, CA2/3, CA4, DG (granule cell layer) and subiculum [40,41]. Previous studies in children have used FreeSurfer to segment the hippocampus and hippocampal subfields [42,43]. The raw volume data were included in the supplemental materials (Table S1).

Tractography models were created from the diffusion-weighted MRI (dMRI) data using FSL [44] and the Quantitative Imaging Toolkit (QIT) [45]. The dMRIs were first skull stripped using FSL BET and then corrected for motion and eddy current artifact using FSL FLIRT. For this, each diffusion scan was affinely registered to the baseline scan using the mutual information metric, and the associated gradient orientations were rotated to account for the registration. Diffusion tensor models were then estimated from the dMRI using QIT, and the following tensor parameters were extracted: fractional anisotropy (FA), mean diffusivity (MD), axial diffusivity (AD), and radial diffusivity (RD). Tensor images were upsampled to 1 mm^3 using model-based interpolation in QIT [46], and a deformation field was computed using DTI-TK [47] to register the data to the IIT brain template [48]. Tractography models of the bundles-of-interest were created using a framework for deterministic streamline integration [49]. For each bundle, seed, inclusion and exclusion masks were manually drawn in the IIT template [50] in reference to a white matter atlas [51]. The template masks were then resampled in each subject's native space image to constrain tractography. Other tractography parameters included a step size of 1.0 mm, a maximum angle of 45 degrees, a minimum FA of 0.15, and 25000 seeds per bundle. Bundle-specific metrics of fractional anisotropy (FA), mean diffusivity (MD), axial diffusivity (AD), and radial diffusivity (RD) were then computed. FA and MD were used as primary metrics of microstructure, with many studies showing that FA increases with age while MD decreases with age [52–55]. AD and RD were used as post-hoc measures in regions that showed a significant effect on MD. The MD measure is a weighted average of AD and RD, which themselves are more biologically specific than MD alone. The bundles of interest included major connections between the hippocampus and the rest of the brain, specifically: the uncinate fasciculus, fornix, and cingulum bundle (separated into prefrontal and temporal lobe sections) (See Figure 1A).

2.6. Statistical Analysis

Hierarchical regression models were implemented in R to estimate the effects of dietary consumption of fructose on the volume of the hippocampus and its connectivity with the rest of the brain. The dependent variables for the volume of the hippocampus included the following regions of interest (ROIs): (i) Whole hippocampus, (ii) CA1, (iii) CA2/3, (iv) CA4, (v) DG/GC/ML, (vi) subiculum. Left and right values were tested separately for a total of 12 tests, which led to a per-test p-value of 0.004 to reach an overall alpha of $p < 0.05$ using Bonferroni correction. The dependent variables for the connectivity between the hippocampus and the rest of the brain included the following tracts: (i) uncinate, (ii) fornix, (iii) cingulum–prefrontal section, and (iv) cingulum–temporal section. Left and right values were tested separately and MD and FA were tested separately for a total of 16 tests, which led to a per-test p-value of 0.003 to reach an overall alpha of $p < 0.05$ using Bonferroni correction. Planned post-hocs included: testing the associations of dietary added sugar and glucose intake on brain metrics that showed evidence of being affected by fructose, and testing the effects of axial and radial diffusivity for any tests that showed significant effects in FA or MD. Associations of sugar consumption with total intracranial volume were also computed as a negative control.

Model 1 was the unadjusted model for percent calories from fructose. Model 2 included age and sex (and intracranial volume for analyses of the volume of the hippocampus). Model 3 included the child's BMI z-score. Model 4 included two categorical variables aimed at measuring socioeconomic status: the highest education level attained by the mother and the family income level. Model 5 included maternal measures that impact prenatal environment, i.e., gestational diabetes (binary) and pre-pregnancy BMI. As variables were added, an F-test was used to determine whether the newly added variables showed a significant improvement in R^2. Semi-partial r values were calculated as an indication of effect size, where $r < 0.1$ is a small effect size, $0.1 < r < 0.3$ is a medium effect size, and $r > 0.3$ is a large effect size.

Effects of Tanner stage and potential interactions with sex were tested as Models 2A and 2B respectively. If either or both were found to explain significantly more variance than Model 2, then models 3–5 included a covariate for Tanner stage and/or an interaction between the dietary measure and sex.

3. Results

3.1. Participant Characteristics

A total of 103 children participated in this study. Child demographic and clinical characteristics are reported in Table 1. The mean ± SD age of the children was 8.55 ± 1.03 years old, 91% of the children were pre-pubertal (Tanner Stage <2), and 62% were girls. Children's BMI ranged from 13.62 to 34.01 kg/m^2; BMI percentiles ranged from 5.28 to 99.58; BMI z-scores ranged from −1.78 to 2.64. According to CDC standards, 61 (59%) children were healthy-weight, 16 (15%) children were overweight, and 26 (25%) children were obese. Overall, the participants consumed an average (±SD) of 1763 ± 359 kcal per day; 4.57 ± 2.19% of their total calories came from fructose, 4.32 ± 1.81% of their total calories came from glucose, and 13.91 ± 6.89% of total calories from added sugar. Total energy and added sugar intake in our cohort are in line with the general population of the children in the United States [56]. Familial demographics, including maternal education, family income, and mother's self-reported race/ethnicity, are shown in Table 2. Maternal pre-pregnancy BMI ranged from 18.97 to 50.38 kg/m^2, and 58% of mothers had GDM during pregnancy.

Table 1. Child demographic and clinical characteristics

	Mean (SD) or N (%) [1]	Range
Age, years	8.55 (1.03)	7.33–11.34
BMI, kg/m^2	19.00 (4.12)	13.62–34.01
BMI percentile	69.96 (27.33)	5.28–99.58
BMI z-score	0.77 (1.08)	−1.78–2.64
BMI category	Healthy-weight: 61 (59%) Overweight: 16 (16%) Obese: 26 (25%)	
Sex	Boys: 41 (40%) Girls: 62 (60%)	
Tanner Stage of Pubertal Development	Tanner stage 1: 94 (91%) Tanner stage 2: 5 (5%) Tanner stage 3: 3 (3%) Tanner stage 4: 1 (1%)	
Energy Intake (kcal)	1763 (359)	825–2708
Percent Calories from Added Sugar (%)	13.91 (6.89)	2.65–39.90
Percent Calories from Glucose (%)	4.32 (1.81)	1.21–8.40
Percent Calories from Fructose (%)	4.57 (2.19)	0.93–11.44

[1] Percentages were rounded to the nearest percent, therefore sum of variables do not equal 100%; BMI: body mass index.

Table 2. Familial demographics.

	Mean (SD) or N (%) [1]
Maternal education [2]	LN: 21 (20%) SC: 29 (28%) CN: 51 (50%)
Mother's race/ethnicity	Hispanic: 59 (57%) Black: 11 (11%) Non-Hispanic White: 20 (19%) Other: 13 (13%)
Family income [2]	0–$30 K: 10 (10%) $30 K–50 K: 29 (29%) $50 K–70 K: 33 (33%) $70 K–90 K: 14 (14%) ≥$90 K: 15 (15%)

[1] Percentages were rounded to the nearest percent, therefore sum of variables do not equal 100%; [2] Missing maternal education and family income data from 2 participants.

3.2. Influence of Diet on Hippocampal Volumes

A total of 101 participants were included in the hippocampal volume analyses, after excluding the two participants who were missing data for the mother's education level. The amount of fructose children consumed as a percentage of calories in their diet was significantly associated with an increase in the volume of the right CA2/3 hippocampal subfield (ß = 3.34, sr = 0.25, $p < 0.01$; Model 1)) (Table 3; Figure 1B). Results remained significant after adjusting for ICV, age, and sex (ß = 2.56, sr = 0.19, $p < 0.02$; Model 2), further adjusting for child BMI z-score (ß = 2.80, sr = 0.21, $p < 0.01$; Model 3), and additionally adjusting for SES (ß = 2.70, sr = 0.19, $p < 0.02$; Model 4), as well as in fully adjusted models (ß = 3.33, sr = 0.24, $p < 0.003$; Model 5). These findings suggest that dietary fructose has an effect on hippocampal CA 2/3 volume that is independent of child's age, sex, BMI Z-score, SES, or prenatal exposures. Of note, Model 2, which included covariates for intracranial volume, age, and sex, explained significantly more variance than the unadjusted Model 1, which only contained a covariate for percentage of calories from fructose ($F(3,96) = 16.78$, $p < 0.001$). This result is unsurprising because the volume of the hippocampus and its subfields are highly dependent upon total brain volume. Model 5, which included all covariates, explained significantly more variance than Model 4, which included all covariates except maternal GDM status and maternal pre-pregnancy BMI (F(2,90) = 6.56, $p < 0.002$). All other hippocampal subfield volumes were non-significant. None of the models tested showed significant interactions of sex with dietary intake, nor did they show significant effects of Tanner stage. Additionally, neither fructose (ß = 6893, $p < 0.30$, $R^2 = 0.0008$), glucose (ß = 7583, $p < 0.30$, $R^2 = 0.0008$), nor added sugar consumption (ß = −277, $p < 0.89$, $R^2 = -0.0097$) were significantly associated with intracranial volume.

Table 3. Associations between dietary fructose intake and the volume of right CA2/3.

Predictor Variables	Model 1 ß (sr)	Model 2 ß (sr)	Model 3 ß (sr)	Model 4 ß (sr)	Model 5 ß (sr)
Percent Calories from Fructose	3.34 (0.25) **	2.56 (0.19) *	2.80 (0.21) *	2.70 (0.19) *	3.33 (0.24) **
Age, years		−1.06 (−0.04)	−1.14 (−0.04)	−1.27 (−0.04)	−1.71 (−0.06)
Sex (1, male; 0, female)		5.17 (0.07)	5.44 (0.08)	6.18 (0.08)	2.52 (0.03)
Intracranial Volume (mm^3)		1.31×10^{-4} (0.49) ***	1.30×10^{-4} (0.48) ***	1.34×10^{-4} (0.47) ***	1.24×10^{-4} (0.43) ***
BMI z-score			3.13 (0.11)	3.05 (0.11)	5.80 (0.20) *
Family income (1: <$30 K; 5: >$90 K)				−1.67 (−0.01)	−1.90 (−0.07)
Mom's education (CN)					
LN				3.24 (0.04)	2.56 (0.03)
SC				2.01 (0.03)	1.81 (0.03)
Maternal GDM (1, yes; 0, no)					4.29 (0.07)
Maternal pre-pregnancy BMI, kg/m^2					−1.31 (−0.28) ***
R^2	0.064	0.365	0.378	0.380	0.459
ΔR^2		0.301	0.013	0.002	0.079
ΔF		16.78 ***	2.13	0.11	6.56 **

Model 1 is percent calories from fructose only; Model 2 includes age, sex and intracranial volume; Model 3 includes BMI z-score; Model 4 includes family income and mom's education; Model 5 includes prenatal exposures to maternal GDM and maternal pre-pregnancy BMI. Successive models include all covariates from earlier models. BMI: body mass index; LN: <high school; SC: some college; CN: college and post-graduate; GDM: gestational diabetes mellitus; sr = semi-partial r; * $p < 0.05$; ** $p < 0.01$; *** $p < 0.001$.

In planned post-hoc analyses, we explored whether the associations between dietary fructose intake and hippocampal CA 2/3 volume were specific to fructose, or if alternatively the associations were also observed between dietary added sugar and/or glucose intake and CA 2/3 volume. We found that associations between percent of calories from added sugar and volume of the right CA2/3 were also significant ($R^2 = 0.448$, F(10,90) = 7.29, $p < 0.001$). Likewise, planned post-hoc analyses on the effects of percent of calories from glucose on the volume of the right CA2/3 were also significant ($R^2 = 0.471$, F(10,90) = 8.00, $p < 0.001$). These findings indicated that effects of dietary fructose, added sugar, and glucose intake on right CA2/3 volume were all similar suggesting that increases in the volume of right CA2/3 were non-specific with regards to whether the increased sugar intake was from glucose, fructose, or added sugars. In fact, the effect sizes for glucose intake (sr = 0.27), fructose intake (sr = 0.25), and added sugar intake (sr = 0.23) were nearly identical, indicating each of these types of sugar explained a similar amount of variance. The percent calories from fructose and percent calories from glucose were highly correlated (r = 0.87, $p < 0.001$), and there were moderate correlations between percent calories from fructose and percent calories from added sugar (r = 0.31, $p < 0.001$) and between percent calories from glucose and percent calories from added sugar (r = 0.48, $p < 0.001$). Given that dietary intake of fructose, glucose, and added sugar were correlated, we did not include them in the same model to test independent effects. It is important to note that added sugars are classified as sugars that are added to foods or beverages when they are processed or prepared, whereas naturally occurring sugars, such as those in fruit or milk, are not classified as added sugars [57].

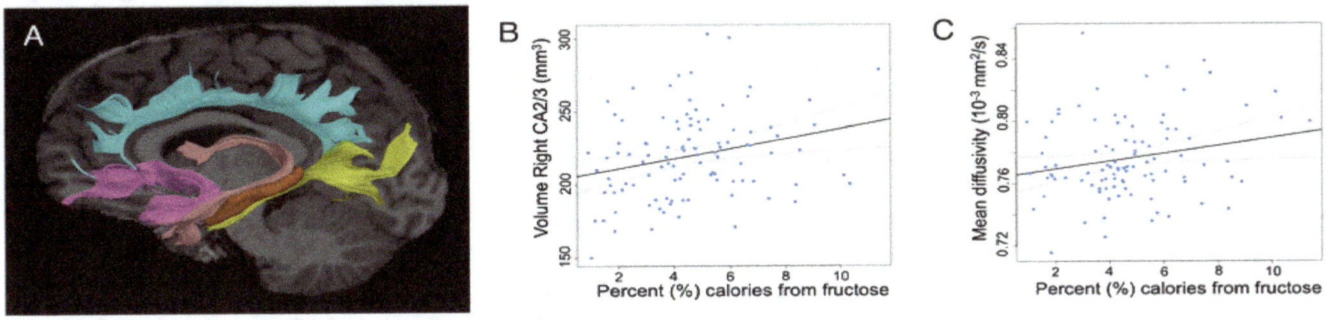

Figure 1. Associations with fructose consumption. (**A**) Using regions of interest for the hippocampus (orange) and its major connections (fornix: pink, uncinate: purple, and the cingulum, which was segmented into the temporal part: yellow and the prefrontal part: turquoise), we identified associations between fructose consumption and the volume of the right CA2/3 subfield of the hippocampus (**B**) and the mean diffusivity of the right cingulum, prefrontal connections (**C**). (**B**,**C**) Graphs show the unadjusted model with no covariates. Solid line indicates the best fit linear trend, with dotted lines showing the confidence interval. Notably, these graphs show the results from Model 1 (Tables 1 and 2, respectively).

3.3. *Influence of Diet on Hippocampal Connectivity*

A total of 98 participants were included in the diffusion imaging analyses, after excluding the 6 participants who were missing data for either the mother's education level ($n = 2$) or who failed quality control for the diffusion imaging data ($n = 4$). The amount of fructose children consumed as a percentage of calories was significantly associated with an increase in the mean diffusivity (MD) of the right cingulum, prefrontal connections (ß = 2.51×10^{-6}, sr = 0.21, $p < 0.04$; Model 1) (Table 4; Figure 1C). Results remained significant after adjusting for age and sex (ß = 2.66×10^{-6}, sr = 0.22, $p < 0.02$; Model 2), further adjusting for child BMI z-score (ß = 2.79×10^{-6}, sr = 0.23, $p < 0.02$; Model 3), and additionally adjusting for SES (ß = 3.51×10^{-6}, sr = 0.28, $p < 0.003$; Model 4), as well as in fully adjusted models (ß = 3.64×10^{-6}, sr = 0.29, $p < 0.002$; Model 5). The outcome of the hierarchical modeling indicated that Model 4 explained significantly more variance than Models 1–3, but Model 5 did not explain more variance than Model 4. Therefore, Model 4 was used for the planned post-hoc analyses. The MD for all other tracts and the FA for all the tracts were non-significant. None of the models tested showed significant interactions of sex with dietary intake, nor did they show significant effects of Tanner stage.

Planned post-hoc analyses on the effects of percent of calories from added sugar on the MD of the right cingulum, prefrontal connections resulted in a significant model overall ($R^2 = 0.167$, $F(7,90) = 2.58$, $p < 0.02$). Although the overall model was significant, the covariate of interest (i.e., percent calories from added sugar) was not significantly associated with MD of the right cingulum, prefrontal connections (ß = -2.56×10^{-7}, sr = -0.07, $p < 0.50$), indicating that the overall model for added sugar associations with MD of the right cingulum, prefrontal connections was driven by significant associations with decreased age and increased family income. Planned post-hoc analyses on the effects of percent of calories from glucose on the MD of the right cingulum, prefrontal connections also resulted in a significant model overall ($R^2 = 0.184$, $F(7,90) = 2.89$, $p < 0.009$). However, similar to findings with added sugar, there was not a significant association of percent calories from glucose on the MD of the right cingulum, prefrontal connections (ß = 2.25×10^{-6}, sr = 0.15, $p < 0.13$). Likewise, similar to added sugar, the overall model for glucose associations with MD of the right cingulum, prefrontal connections was driven by significant associations with decreased age and increased family income. These result are different from the effects we observed in the volume of the right CA2/3 because MD was only associated with fructose intake and not added sugar or glucose intake.

Table 4. Effects of fructose consumption on the mean diffusivity (MD) of right cingulum, prefrontal connections.

Predictor Variables	Model 1 ß (sr)	Model 2 ß (sr)	Model 3 ß (sr)	Model 4 ß (sr)	Model 5 ß (sr)
Percent Calories from Fructose	2.51×10^{-6} (0.21) *	2.66×10^{-6} (0.22) *	2.79×10^{-6} (0.23) *	3.51×10^{-6} (0.28) **	3.64×10^{-6} (0.29) **
Age, years		-7.52×10^{-6} (−0.28) **	-7.50×10^{-6} (−0.28) **	-6.78×10^{-6} (−0.25) **	-6.95×10^{-6} (−0.26) **
Sex (1, male; 0, female)		-9.79×10^{-6} (−0.19)	-9.82×10^{-6} (−0.19)	-8.65×10^{-6} (−0.17)	-8.37×10^{-6} (−0.16)
BMI z-score			1.67×10^{-6} (0.07)	1.68×10^{-6} (0.07)	2.40×10^{-6} (0.10)
Family income (1: <$30 K; 5: >$90 K)				6.71×10^{-6} (0.29) **	6.56×10^{-6} (0.28) **
Mom's education (CN)					
LN				3.64×10^{-6} (0.05)	5.09×10^{-6} (0.07)
SC				4.69×10^{-6} (0.08)	5.67×10^{-6} (0.09)
Maternal GDM (1, yes; 0, no)					-3.99×10^{-6} (−0.08)
Maternal pre-pregnancy BMI, kg/m^2					-3.51×10^{-7} (−0.09)
R^2	0.044	0.152	0.157	0.243	0.257
ΔR^2		0.108	0.005	0.086	0.014
ΔF		6.87 **	0.57	3.42 *	0.83

Model 1 includes percent calories from fructose only; Model 2 includes age and sex; Model 3 includes BMI z-score; Model 4 includes family income and mom's education; Model 5 includes maternal GDM and maternal pre-pregnancy BMI. Successive models include all covariates from earlier models. BMI: body mass index; LN: <high school; SC: some college; CN: college and post-graduate; GDM: gestational diabetes mellitus; sr = semi-partial r; * $p < 0.05$; ** $p < 0.01$.

3.4. *Post-hocs for Diffusion Imaging Measures*

Because MD is defined as the average diffusivity, it is not as biologically specific as axial diffusivity (AD) or radial diffusivity (RD). Therefore, we ran post-hoc analyses using Model 4 only to determine whether the observed association of increased fructose intake on MD of the right cingulum, prefrontal connections, was driven by axial diffusivity (AD), radial diffusivity (RD), or both. The AD for the right cingulum, prefrontal connections was significantly associated with increased percentage of calories from fructose (ß = 4.62×10^{-6}, sr = 0.27, $p < 0.005$; Model 4). The RD for the right cingulum, prefrontal connections was significantly associated with increased percentage of calories from fructose (ß = 2.89×10^{-6}, sr = 0.23, $p < 0.01$; Model 4). This pattern was quite similar to the pattern observed with MD. Comparing the effect sizes of sr = 0.27 for AD and sr = 0.23 for RD, we conclude that the effects were similar, but slightly larger for AD.

4. Discussion

In this study, we examined the influence of dietary sugar intake on hippocampal neuroanatomy, both gray matter and white matter, in children. We found that increased volume in the right hippocampal CA2/3 subfield was associated with increased consumption of the monosaccharides, fructose or glucose, and/or added sugars in general, while increased MD in the right cingulate-prefrontal cortex connections were only associated with increased dietary intake of fructose. We found associations on the right but not the left hemisphere, which is broadly consistent with prior work showing lateralities on the impact of environmental insults in the hippocampus [58,59]. These associations between dietary sugar intake and hippocampal volume and fructose intake and cingulate-prefrontal cortex connections remained significant after adjusting for child's intracranial volume, age, sex, BMI, SES, and prenatal exposures suggesting an effect of dietary fructose, added sugar, and glucose intake on hippocampal volume and an effect of dietary fructose on cingulate-prefrontal cortex white matter connectivity that is independent of a number of potential confounding factors.

The observed association between dietary sugar intake and increased hippocampal volume during childhood may be driven by a few factors. A larger hippocampal CA2/3 volume during childhood could be due to a delay in synaptic pruning, a process that typically occurs during early adolescence. During adolescence, the hippocampus reaches peak volume, and begins to undergo synaptic pruning, eliminating unused connections [60,61], and prior studies have shown that the CA3 hippocampal subfield gradually begins to decrease in volume during mid childhood [61,62]. Work by Vuong et al. found that synaptic pruning is delayed in juvenile rats exposed in utero to obese mothers with GDM [63]. In their findings, inflammation and recruitment of microglial cells occurred during post-natal development in the hippocampus, along with a reduction in synaptic pruning, and the animals presented with altered hippocampal morphology. These findings suggest that prenatal environmental insults can result in hippocampal inflammation, reductions in synaptic pruning and altered hippocampal development [63]. Interestingly, Hershey et al., found that children with Type 1 diabetes had increased hippocampal volume, despite the commonly reported decreased volume in adults with Type 1 and Type 2 diabetes [64]. There is substantial research that a diet high in added sugar contributes to a pro-inflammatory environment [13,19,65]. Therefore, increased volume in the CA2/3 hippocampal subfield may be due to inflammation and/or a delay in synaptic pruning. Future studies that examine inflammation specifically, such as T2 scans for gliosis, could potentially address this possibility [66].

Notably, we found that the CA2/3 hippocampal subfield was preferentially impacted by dietary sugar intake. Coincidentally, the CA3 subfield is among the last subfields to undergo postnatal maturation, paralleling DG development [67,68]. Additionally, substantial work in animals has shown that the CA3 subfield is altered by a host of prenatal and early life environmental insults, such as prenatal exposure to GDM [69,70] or postnatal exposure to chronic stress [71–73]. Therefore, our findings are in line with prior research in animals indicating a preferential sensitivity of the CA3 subfield. It is worth noting, due to the predetermined boundaries delineated by FreeSurfer, we were unable to decipher the boundary between the CA2 and CA3 subfield. Future studies that incorporate manual tracing should be considered to confirm if excessive added sugar intake preferentially impacts the CA3 subfield of the hippocampus.

Many studies have observed that MD decreases while FA increases over the course of development [52–55]. We found that increased dietary fructose intake was associated with increased mean diffusivity (MD) in the white matter cingulum tract that connects the right hippocampus and the right prefrontal cortex. MD has been shown to increase in many different white matter diseases that lead to demyelination, dysmyelination, and/or wallerian degeneration [74–76]. For example, increases in MD have been observed prior to the appearance of lesions on a gadolinium-enhanced scan in multiple sclerosis, which is a complex disease that involves not only demyelination and wallerian degeneration, but also edema and inflammation, indicating that changes in the MD may be sensitive to pre-lesion changes in the blood brain barrier [77]. Patients with chronic epilepsy and hippocampal sclerosis show increased MD values in the hippocampus [78,79]. Together, these results are consistent with the idea that the increased MD values associated with fructose could reflect an inflammatory process, possibly associated with a loss of myelin, or delayed axonal pruning.

Because mean diffusivity is a weighted average of axial (AD) and radial diffusivity (RD), we conducted post-hoc analyses on these measures to obtain more biological specificity about what might be underlying the observed associations with MD. In general, AD is thought to reflect intracellular water mobility and is influenced by the integrity and arrangement of axonal membranes and cytoskeletal proteins, while RD is thought to reflect more of the extracellular water mobility and is primarily influenced by myelin [80]. Previous studies have shown that over the course of normal neurodevelopment, both RD and AD decrease with age [81–85]. Decreases in RD are typically attributed to myelination, while the decreases in AD are thought to correspond more to axonal pruning [86]. In our study, we found that both AD and RD were increased in the cingulum tract in children with increased dietary fructose intake, consistent with the idea that increases in fructose intake could be associated with a decrease or delay in the myelination process and the normal pruning process. Future studies could use multi-compartment diffusion imaging models, such as Neurite Orientation Dispersion and Density Imaging (NODDI), to further investigate this tract to determine whether these changes in diffusivity are more related to cellular density and/or orientation dispersion, thus adding more biological specificity [87].

Self-reported dietary assessments have known limitations, including under-reporting of dietary intake. Given that eating behavior can vary from day to day, the collection of multiple 24-hr recalls on non-consecutive days is recommended to improve the accuracy of habitual dietary intake estimates [88]. Some studies have recommended obtaining at least three 24-hr dietary recalls on non-consecutive days to provide better accuracy of energy intake [36]. Dietary assessments in our study were obtained from repeated 24-hr recalls obtained during in-person visits on non-consecutive days. We obtained two days of dietary assessments on the majority of participants, and four days of dietary assessments on a subset of 35 participants. We implemented techniques to improve the accuracy of our dietary data collection method, including the Multiple Pass 24-h recall method, which was previously shown to significantly reduce levels of under-reporting [89]. We also used a consensus recall method, in which the child and parent were interviewed together, which has been suggested to improve the accuracy of dietary assessments compared to interviews with the child or parent alone [90]. Estimates of total energy intake in our cohort are similar to national averages for children in this age range [91], while the average percent calories from added sugar in our cohort was 2.5% lower than the average of 16.4% reported in the 2009 to 2012 National Health and Nutrition Examination Survey for children age 6–11 [92]. Thus, while total energy intake estimates in our cohort are in line with those of national averages of children in the U.S., it is possible that our cohort under-reported intake of foods and beverages that contain added sugars. It is also possible that the children in our cohort consumed, on average, slightly lower amounts of added sugars than average children in the U.S. population.

In summary, our findings suggest that increases in dietary fructose are associated with alterations in hippocampal structure and connectivity in children. These findings should be interpreted cautiously given the limitations of self-reported dietary intake assessments, and it is important to note that our observations are correlational and do not confer causality. Future studies that include experimental designs that manipulate dietary intake of fructose and/or added sugars are necessary to determine the effects of fructose and added sugar on hippocampal structure and connectivity during childhood. Moreover, the potential cognitive consequences of the observed associations between dietary fructose and alterations in hippocampal structure and connectivity remains an important consideration. Our findings support the need for future studies that include cognitive testing in addition to neuroimaging to examine whether increased dietary fructose intake in childhood is associated with altered hippocampal structure and hippocampal function in childhood.

Supplementary Materials: ,
Figure S1: Raw data plots of added sugar consumption and the mean diffusivity of the right cingulum, prefrontal connections, Figure S2: Raw data plots of added sugar consumption and the volume of the right CA2/3 subfield of the hippocampus, Figure S3: Raw data plots of glucose consumption and the mean diffusivity of the right cingulum, prefrontal connections, Figure S4: Raw data plots of glucose consumption and the volume of the right CA2/3 subfield of the hippocampus, Table S1: Table of hippocampal and total brain volumes.

Author Contributions: K.A.C., K.A.P., J.M.A., S.J. were responsible for conceptualization of the study; K.A.C., J.M.A., R.P.C., B.A. contributed to methodology and formal analysis; J.M.A., A.G.Y., B.A., S.L. were responsible for management and coordination of the study execution; K.A.P. and A.H.X. were responsible for supervision of the research activities; K.A.C., K.A.P., S.J., J.M.A. wrote the original draft; K.A.C., K.A.P., S.J., J.M.A., S.L., A.G.Y., R.C., A.H.X. provided critical review, commentary and revisions to the manuscript; K.A.P., A.H.X., S.L., J.M.A. provided funding for this study. Prior Presentation. Some of the data from the BrainChild Cohort were used to address a separate research question related to prenatal exposure to maternal obesity and hippocampal volume in children, which was accepted for publication in *Brain and Behavior* on December 8, 2019. All authors have read and agreed to the published version of the manuscript.

Acknowledgments: The authors would like to thank the families who participate in the BrainChild Study. The authors would also like to thank Ana Romero for managing the BrainChild study, Mayra Martinez and Janet Mora-Marquez for recruiting volunteers, Alexis Defendis for helping with study execution, and the staff at Dana and David Dornsife Cognitive Neuroimaging Center at USC and at the USC Diabetes and Obesity Research Institute for their assistance with these studies.

References

1. Bray, G.A.; Nielsen, S.J.; Popkin, B.M. Consumption of high-fructose corn syrup in beverages may play a role in the epidemic of obesity. *Am. J. Clin. Nutr.* **2004**, *79*, 537–543. [CrossRef]
2. Basciano, H.; Federico, L.; Adeli, K. Fructose, insulin resistance, and metabolic dyslipidemia. *Nutr. Metab.* **2005**, *2*, 5. [CrossRef]
3. Tappy, L.; Le, K.A. Metabolic Effects of Fructose and the Worldwide Increase in Obesity. *Physiol. Rev.* **2010**, *90*, 23–46. [CrossRef]
4. Johnson, R.J.; Segal, M.S.; Sautin, Y.; Nakagawa, T.; Feig, D.I.; Kang, D.-H.; Gersch, M.S.; Benner, S.; Sánchez-Lozada, L.G. Potential role of sugar (fructose) in the epidemic of hypertension, obesity and the metabolic syndrome, diabetes, kidney disease, and cardiovascular disease. *Am. J. Clin. Nutr.* **2007**, *86*, 899–906.
5. Lindqvist, A.; Baelemans, A.; Erlanson-Albertsson, C. Effects of sucrose, glucose and fructose on peripheral and central appetite signals. *Regul. Pept.* **2008**, *150*, 26–32. [CrossRef]
6. Page, K.A.; Chan, O.; Arora, J.; Belfort-DeAguiar, R.; Dzuira, J.; Roehmholdt, B.; Cline, G.W.; Naik, S.; Sinha, R.; Constable, R.T.; et al. Effects of Fructose vs Glucose on Regional Cerebral Blood Flow in Brain Regions Involved with Appetite and Reward Pathways. *JAMA* **2013**, *309*, 63. [CrossRef]
7. Luo, S.; Monterosso, J.R.; Sarpelleh, K.; Page, K.A. Differential effects of fructose versus glucose on brain and appetitive responses to food cues and decisions for food rewards. *Proc. Natl. Acad. Sci. USA* **2015**, *112*, 6509–6514. [CrossRef]
8. Teff, K.L.; Elliott, S.S.; Tschöp, M.; Kieffer, T.J.; Rader, D.; Heiman, M.; Townsend, R.R.; Keim, N.L.; D'Alessio, D.; Havel, P.J. Dietary Fructose Reduces Circulating Insulin and Leptin, Attenuates Postprandial Suppression of Ghrelin, and Increases Triglycerides in Women. *J. Clin. Endocrinol. Metab.* **2004**, *89*, 2963–2972. [CrossRef]
9. Cha, S.H.; Wolfgang, M.; Tokutake, Y.; Chohnan, S.; Lane, M.D. Differential effects of central fructose and glucose on hypothalamic malonyl—CoA and food intake. *Proc. Natl. Acad. Sci. USA* **2008**, *105*, 16871–16875. [CrossRef]
10. Erlanson-Albertsson, C.; Lindqvist, A. Fructose affects enzymes involved in the synthesis and degradation of hypothalamic endocannabinoids. *Regul. Pept.* **2010**, *161*, 87–91. [CrossRef]
11. Lowette, K.; Roosen, L.; Tack, J.; Vanden Berghe, P. Effects of high-fructose diets on central appetite signaling and cognitive function. *Front. Nutr.* **2015** 2, 5. [CrossRef]

12. Lakhan, S.E.; Kirchgessner, A. The emerging role of dietary fructose in obesity and cognitive decline. *Nutr. J.* **2013**, *12*, 114. [CrossRef]
13. Hsu, T.M.; Kanoski, S.E. Blood-brain barrier disruption: Mechanistic links between Western diet consumption and dementia. *Front. Aging Neurosci.* **2014**, *6*, 88. [CrossRef]
14. Davidson, T.L.; Chan, K.; Jarrard, L.E.; Kanoski, S.E.; Clegg, D.J.; Benoit, S.C. Contributions of the Hippocampus and Medial Prefrontal Cortex to Energy and Body Weight Regulation. *Hippocampus* **2009**, *19*, 235–252. [CrossRef]
15. Hannapel, R.C.; Henderson, Y.H.; Nalloor, R.; Vazdarjanova, A.; Parent, M.B. Ventral hippocampal neurons inhibit postprandial energy intake. *Hippocampus* **2017**, *27*, 274–284. [CrossRef]
16. Agrawal, R.; Gomez-Pinilla, F. "Metabolic syndrome" in the brain: Deficiency in omega-3 fatty acid exacerbates dysfunctions in insulin receptor signalling and cognition. *J. Physiol.* **2012**, *590*, 2485–2499. [CrossRef]
17. Wu, H.-W.; Ren, L.-F.; Zhou, X.; Han, D.-W. A high-fructose diet induces hippocampal insulin resistance and exacerbates memory deficits in male Sprague-Dawley rats. *Nutr. Neurosci.* **2015**, *18*, 323–328. [CrossRef]
18. Hsu, T.M.; Konanur, V.R.; Taing, L.; Usui, R.; Kayser, B.D.; Goran, M.I.; Kanoski, S.E. Effects of sucrose and high fructose corn syrup consumption on spatial memory function and hippocampal neuroinflammation in adolescent rats. *Hippocampus* **2015**, *25*, 227–239. [CrossRef]
19. Djordjevic, A.; Bursać, B.; Veličković, N.; Vasiljević, A.; Matić, G. The impact of different fructose loads on insulin sensitivity, inflammation, and PSA-NCAM-mediated plasticity in the hippocampus of fructose-fed male rats. *Nutr. Neurosci.* **2015**, *18*, 66–75. [CrossRef]
20. Van der Borght, K.; Köhnke, R.; Göransson, N.; Deierborg, T.; Brundin, P.; Erlanson-Albertsson, C.; Lindqvist, A. Reduced neurogenesis in the rat hippocampus following high fructose consumption. *Regul. Pept.* **2011**, *167*, 26–30. [CrossRef]
21. Ross, A.P.; Bartness, T.J.; Mielke, J.G.; Parent, M.B. A high fructose diet impairs spatial memory in male rats. *Neurobiol. Learn. Mem.* **2009**, *92*, 410–416. [CrossRef]
22. Hebben, N.; Corkin, S.; Eichenbaum, H.; Shedlack, K. Diminished ability to interpret and report internal states after bilateral medial temporal resection: Case, H.M. *Behav. Neurosci.* **1985**, *99*, 1031–1039. [CrossRef]
23. Rozin, P.; Dow, S.; Moscovitch, M.; Rajaram, S. What Causes Humans to Begin and End a Meal? A Role for Memory for What Has Been Eaten, as Evidenced by a Study of Multiple Meal Eating in Amnesic Patients. *Psychol. Sci.* **1998**, *9*, 392–396. [CrossRef]
24. Maller, J.J.; Welton, T.; Middione, M.; Callaghan, F.M.; Rosenfeld, J.V.; Grieve, S.M. Revealing the Hippocampal Connectome through Super-Resolution 1150-Direction Diffusion MRI. *Sci. Rep.* **2019**, *9*, 2418. [CrossRef] [PubMed]
25. Chudasama, Y.; Doobay, V.M.; Liu, Y. Hippocampal-Prefrontal Cortical Circuit Mediates Inhibitory Response Control in the Rat. *J. Neurosci.* **2012**, *32*, 10915–10924. [CrossRef] [PubMed]
26. Hsu, T.M.; Noble, E.E.; Liu, C.M.; Cortella, A.M.; Konanur, V.R.; Suarez, A.N.; Reiner, D.J.; Hahn, J.D.; Hayes, M.R.; Kanoski, S.E. A hippocampus to prefrontal cortex neural pathway inhibits food motivation through glucagon-like peptide-1 signaling. *Mol. Psychiatry* **2018**, *23*, 1555–1565. [CrossRef] [PubMed]
27. Sweeney, P.; Yang, Y. An excitatory ventral hippocampus to lateral septum circuit that suppresses feeding. *Nat. Commun.* **2015**, *6*, 10188. [CrossRef] [PubMed]
28. Russo, C.; Russo, A.; Pellitteri, R.; Stanzani, S. Hippocampal Ghrelin-positive neurons directly project to arcuate hypothalamic and medial amygdaloid nuclei. Could they modulate food-intake? *Neurosci. Lett.* **2017**, *653*, 126–131. [CrossRef] [PubMed]
29. Geha, P.; Cecchi, G.; Constable, R.T.; Abdallah, C.; Small, D.M. Reorganization of brain connectivity in obesity. *Hum. Brain Mapp.* **2017**, *38*, 1403–1420. [CrossRef]
30. Alexander, A.L.; Lee, J.E.; Lazar, M.; Field, A.S. Diffusion Tensor Imaging of the Brain. *Neurotherapeutics* **2007**, *4*, 316–329. [CrossRef]
31. Koebnick, C.; Langer-Gould, A.M.; Gould, M.K.; Chao, C.R.; Iyer, R.L.; Smith, N.; Chen, W.; Jacobsen, S.J. Sociodemographic Characteristics of Members of a Large, Integrated Health Care System: Comparison with US Census Bureau Data. *Perm. J.* **2012**, *16*, 37–41. [CrossRef] [PubMed]

32. Defining Childhood Obesity|Overweight & Obesity|CDC. Available online: https://www.cdc.gov/obesity/childhood/defining.html (accessed on 1 November 2019).
33. Marshall, W.A.; Tanner, J.M. Variations in pattern of pubertal changes in girls. *Arch. Dis. Child.* **1969**, *44*, 291–303. [CrossRef] [PubMed]
34. Marshall, W.A.; Tanner, J.M. Variations in the pattern of pubertal changes in boys. *Arch. Dis. Child.* **1970**, *45*, 13–23. [CrossRef] [PubMed]
35. Rasmussen, A.R.; Wohlfahrt-Veje, C.; Tefre de Renzy-Martin, K.; Hagen, C.P.; Tinggaard, J.; Mouritsen, A.; Mieritz, M.G.; Main, K.M. Validity of self-assessment of pubertal maturation. *Pediatrics* **2015**, *135*, 86–93. [CrossRef]
36. Johnson, R.K.; Driscoll, P.; Goran, M.I. Comparison of Multiple-Pass 24-Hour Recall Estimates of Energy Intake with Total Energy Expenditure Determined by the Doubly Labeled Water Method in Young Children. *J. Am. Diet. Assoc.* **1996**, *96*, 1140–1144. [CrossRef]
37. Schakel, S.F.; Buzzard, I.M.; Gebhardt, S.E. Procedures for Estimating Nutrient Values for Food Composition Databases. *J. Food Compos. Anal.* **1997**, *10*, 102–114. [CrossRef]
38. Iglesias, J.E.; Augustinack, J.C.; Nguyen, K.; Player, C.M.; Player, A.; Wright, M.; Roy, N.; Frosch, M.P.; McKee, A.C.; Wald, L.L.; et al. A computational atlas of the hippocampal formation using ex vivo, ultra-high resolution MRI: Application to adaptive segmentation of in vivo MRI. *NeuroImage* **2015**, *115*, 117–137. [CrossRef]
39. Backhausen, L.L.; Herting, M.M.; Buse, J.; Roessner, V.; Smolka, M.N.; Vetter, N.C. Quality Control of Structural MRI Images Applied Using FreeSurfer—A Hands-On Workflow to Rate Motion Artifacts. *Front. Neurosci.* **2016**, *10*, 558. [CrossRef]
40. Calvo-Ochoa, E.; Hernández-Ortega, K.; Ferrera, P.; Morimoto, S.; Arias, C. Short-term high-fat-and-fructose feeding produces insulin signaling alterations accompanied by neurite and synaptic reduction and astroglial activation in the rat hippocampus. *J. Cereb. Blood Flow Metab.* **2014**, *34*, 1001–1008. [CrossRef]
41. Molteni, R.; Barnard, R.J.; Ying, Z.; Roberts, C.K.; Gómez-Pinilla, F. A high-fat, refined sugar diet reduces hippocampal brain-derived neurotrophic factor, neuronal plasticity, and learning. *Neuroscience* **2002**, *112*, 803–814. [CrossRef]
42. Al-Amin, M.; Zinchenko, A.; Geyer, T. Hippocampal subfield volume changes in subtypes of attention deficit hyperactivity disorder. *Brain Res.* **2018**, *1685*, 1–8. [CrossRef] [PubMed]
43. Tamnes, C.K.; Walhovd, K.B.; Engvig, A.; Grydeland, H.; Krogsrud, S.K.; Østby, Y.; Holland, D.; Dale, A.M.; Fjell, A.M. Regional Hippocampal Volumes and Development Predict Learning and Memory. *Dev. Neurosci.* **2014**, *36*, 161–174. [CrossRef] [PubMed]
44. Jenkinson, M.; Beckmann, C.F.; Behrens, T.E.J.; Woolrich, M.W.; Smith, S.M. FSL. *Neuroimage* **2012**, *62*, 782–790. [CrossRef] [PubMed]
45. Cabeen, R.P.; Laidlaw, D.H.; Toga, A.W. Quantitative Imaging Toolkit: Software for Interactive 3D Visualization, Processing, and Analysis of Neuroimaging Datasets. In Proceedings of the Annual Meeting of the International Society for Magnetic Resonance in Medicine (ISMRM), Paris, France, 2018.
46. Arsigny, V.; Fillard, P.; Pennec, X.; Ayache, N. Log-Euclidean metrics for fast and simple calculus on diffusion tensors. *Magn. Reson. Med.* **2006**, *56*, 411–421. [CrossRef] [PubMed]
47. Zhang, H.; Yushkevich, P.A.; Alexander, D.C.; Gee, J.C. Deformable registration of diffusion tensor MR images with explicit orientation optimization. *Med. Image Anal.* **2006**, *10*, 764–785. [CrossRef] [PubMed]
48. Zhang, S.; Peng, H.; Dawe, R.J.; Arfanakis, K. Enhanced ICBM Diffusion Tensor Template of the Human Brain. *Neuroimage* **2011**, *54*, 974–984. [CrossRef]
49. Cabeen, R.P.; Bastin, M.E.; Laidlaw, D.H. Kernel Regression Estimation of Fiber Orientation Mixtures in Diffusion MRI. *Neuroimage* **2016**, *127*, 158–172. [CrossRef]
50. Wakana, S.; Caprihan, A.; Panzenboeck, M.M.; Fallon, J.H.; Perry, M.; Gollub, R.L.; Hua, K.; Zhang, J.; Jiang, H.; Dubey, P.; et al. Reproducibility of quantitative tractography methods applied to cerebral white matter. *Neuroimage* **2007**, *36*, 630–644. [CrossRef]
51. Catani, M.; Thiebaut de Schotten, M. A diffusion tensor imaging tractography atlas for virtual in vivo dissections. *Cortex* **2008**, *44*, 1105–1132. [CrossRef]
52. Neil, J.; Miller, J.; Mukherjee, P.; Hüppi, P.S. Diffusion tensor imaging of normal and injured developing human brain—A technical review. *NMR Biomed.* **2002**, *15*, 543–552. [CrossRef]

53. Snook, L.; Paulson, L.-A.; Roy, D.; Phillips, L.; Beaulieu, C. Diffusion tensor imaging of neurodevelopment in children and young adults. *NeuroImage* **2005**, *26*, 1164–1173. [CrossRef] [PubMed]
54. Mukherjee, P.; McKinstry, R.C. Diffusion tensor imaging and tractography of human brain development. *Neuroimaging Clin. N. Am.* **2006**, *16*, 19–43. [CrossRef] [PubMed]
55. Bonekamp, D.; Nagae, L.M.; Degaonkar, M.; Matson, M.; Abdalla, W.M.; Barker, P.B.; Mori, S.; Horská, A. Diffusion tensor imaging in children and adolescents: Reproducibility, hemispheric, and age-related differences. *Neuroimage* **2007**, *34*, 733–742. [CrossRef] [PubMed]
56. Drewnowski, A.; Rehm, C.D. Energy intakes of US children and adults by food purchase location and by specific food source. *Nutr. J.* **2013**, *12*, 59. [CrossRef] [PubMed]
57. CDC Know Your Limit for Added Sugars. Available online: https://www.cdc.gov/nutrition/data-statistics/know-your-limit-for-added-sugars.html (accessed on 19 December 2019).
58. Zach, P.; Mrzílková, J.; Stuchlík, A.; Valeš, K. Delayed Effects of Elevated Corticosterone Level on Volume of Hippocampal Formation in Laboratory Rat. *Physiol. Res.* **2010**, *59*, 12.
59. Teicher, M.H.; Anderson, C.M.; Polcari, A. Childhood maltreatment is associated with reduced volume in the hippocampal subfields CA3, dentate gyrus, and subiculum. *Proc. Natl. Acad. Sci. USA* **2012**, *109*, E563–E572. [CrossRef]
60. Andersson, J.L.; Skare, S.; Ashburner, J. How to correct susceptibility distortions in spin-echo echo-planar images: Application to diffusion tensor imaging. *Neuroimage* **2003**, *20*, 870–888. [CrossRef]
61. Tamnes, C.K.; Bos, M.G.N.; van de Kamp, F.C.; Peters, S.; Crone, E.A. Longitudinal development of hippocampal subregions from childhood to adulthood. *Dev. Cogn. Neurosci.* **2018**, *30*, 212–222. [CrossRef]
62. Canada, K.L.; Ngo, C.T.; Newcombe, N.S.; Geng, F.; Riggins, T. It's All in the Details: Relations Between Young Children's Developing Pattern Separation Abilities and Hippocampal Subfield Volumes. *Cereb. Cortex* **2019**, *29*, 3427–3433. [CrossRef]
63. Vuong, B.; Odero, G.; Rozbacher, S.; Stevenson, M.; Kereliuk, S.M.; Pereira, T.J.; Dolinsky, V.W.; Kauppinen, T.M. Exposure to gestational diabetes mellitus induces neuroinflammation, derangement of hippocampal neurons, and cognitive changes in rat offspring. *J. Neuroinflamm.* **2017**, *14*, 80. [CrossRef]
64. Hershey, T.; Perantie, D.C.; Wu, J.; Weaver, P.M.; Black, K.J.; White, N.H. Hippocampal Volumes in Youth with Type 1 Diabetes. *Diabetes* **2010**, *59*, 236–241. [CrossRef]
65. Beilharz, J.E.; Maniam, J.; Morris, M.J. Short-term exposure to a diet high in fat and sugar, or liquid sugar, selectively impairs hippocampal-dependent memory, with differential impacts on inflammation. *Behav. Brain Res.* **2016**, *306*, 1–7. [CrossRef] [PubMed]
66. Lee, J.K.; Ekstrom, A.D.; Ghetti, S. Volume of hippocampal subfields and episodic memory in childhood and adolescence. *NeuroImage* **2014**, *94*, 162–171. [CrossRef] [PubMed]
67. Jabès, A.; Lavenex, P.B.; Amaral, D.G.; Lavenex, P. Postnatal Development of the Hippocampal Formation: A Stereological Study in Macaque Monkeys. *J. Comp. Neurol.* **2011**, *519*, 1051–1070. [CrossRef] [PubMed]
68. Lu, D.; He, L.; Xiang, W.; Ai, W.-M.; Cao, Y.; Wang, X.S.; Pan, A.; Luo, X.-G.; Li, Z.; Yan, X.-X. Somal and Dendritic Development of Human CA3 Pyramidal Neurons from Midgestation to Middle Childhood: A Quantitative Golgi Study. *Anat. Rec.* **2013**, *296 Pt 8*, 123–132. [CrossRef] [PubMed]
69. Golalipour, M.J.; Kafshgiri, S.K.; Ghafari, S. Gestational diabetes induced neuronal loss in CA1 and CA3 subfields of rat hippocampus in early postnatal life. *Folia Morphol.* **2012**, *71*, 71–77. [PubMed]
70. Lotfi, N.; Hami, J.; Hosseini, M.; Haghir, D.; Haghir, H. Diabetes during pregnancy enhanced neuronal death in the hippocampus of rat offspring. *Int. J. Dev. Neurosci.* **2016**, *51*, 28–35. [CrossRef]
71. Schoenfeld, T.J.; McCausland, H.C.; Morris, H.D.; Padmanaban, V.; Cameron, H.A. Stress and Loss of Adult Neurogenesis Differentially Reduce Hippocampal Volume. *Biol. Psychiatry* **2017**, *82*, 914–923. [CrossRef]
72. Kumar, R.S.; Narayanan, S.N.; Kumar, N.; Nayak, S. Exposure to Enriched Environment Restores Altered Passive Avoidance Learning and Ameliorates Hippocampal Injury in Male Albino Wistar Rats Subjected to Chronic Restraint Stress. *Int. J. Appl. Basic Med. Res.* **2018**, *8*, 231–236.
73. Baran, S.E.; Campbell, A.M.; Kleen, J.K.; Foltz, C.H.; Wright, R.L.; Diamond, D.M.; Conrad, C.D. Combination of high fat diet and chronic stress retracts hippocampal dendrites. *Neuroreport* **2005**, *16*, 39–43. [CrossRef]
74. Guo, A.C.; Jewells, V.L.; Provenzale, J.M. Analysis of normal-appearing white matter in multiple sclerosis: Comparison of diffusion tensor MR imaging and magnetization transfer imaging. *AJNR Am. J. Neuroradiol.* **2001**, *22*, 1893–1900. [PubMed]

75. Pierpaoli, C.; Barnett, A.; Pajevic, S.; Chen, R.; Penix, L.R.; Virta, A.; Basser, P. Water diffusion changes in Wallerian degeneration and their dependence on white matter architecture. *Neuroimage* **2001**, *13*, 1174–1185. [CrossRef] [PubMed]
76. Horsfield, M.A.; Jones, D.K. Applications of diffusion-weighted and diffusion tensor MRI to white matter diseases—A review. *NMR Biomed.* **2002**, *15*, 570–577. [CrossRef] [PubMed]
77. Werring, D.J.; Brassat, D.; Droogan, A.G.; Clark, C.A.; Symms, M.R.; Barker, G.J.; MacManus, D.G.; Thompson, A.J.; Miller, D.H. The pathogenesis of lesions and normal-appearing white matter changes in multiple sclerosis: A serial diffusion MRI study. *Brain* **2000**, *123*, 1667–1676. [CrossRef] [PubMed]
78. Wieshmann, U.C.; lark, C.A.C.; Symms, M.R.; Barker, G.J.; Birnie, K.D.; Shorvon, S.D. Water diffusion in the human hippocampus in epilepsy. *Magn. Reson. Imaging* **1999**, *17*, 29–36. [CrossRef]
79. Yoo, S.Y.; Chang, K.-H.; Song, I.C.; Han, M.H.; Kwon, B.J.; Lee, S.H.; Yu, I.K.; Chun, C.-K. Apparent diffusion coefficient value of the hippocampus in patients with hippocampal sclerosis and in healthy volunteers. *AJNR Am. J. Neuroradiol.* **2002**, *23*, 809–812.
80. Schwartz, E.D.; Cooper, E.T.; Fan, Y.; Jawad, A.F.; Chin, C.-L.; Nissanov, J.; Hackney, D.B. MRI diffusion coefficients in spinal cord correlate with axon morphometry. *Neuroreport* **2005**, *16*, 73–76. [CrossRef]
81. Zhang, Y.; Zhang, J.; Oishi, K.; Faria, A.V.; Jiang, H.; Li, X.; Akhter, K.; Rosa-Neto, P.; Pike, G.B.; Evans, A.; et al. Atlas-guided tract reconstruction for automated and comprehensive examination of the white matter anatomy. *Neuroimage* **2010**, *52*, 1289–1301. [CrossRef]
82. Lebel, C.; Walker, L.; Leemans, A.; Phillips, L.; Beaulieu, C. Microstructural maturation of the human brain from childhood to adulthood. *NeuroImage* **2008**, *40*, 1044–1055. [CrossRef]
83. Bava, S.; Thayer, R.; Jacobus, J.; Ward, M.; Jernigan, T.L.; Tapert, S.F. Longitudinal characterization of white matter maturation during adolescence. *Brain Res.* **2010**, *1327*, 38–46. [CrossRef]
84. Suzuki, Y.; Matsuzawa, H.; Kwee, I.L.; Nakada, T. Absolute eigenvalue diffusion tensor analysis for human brain maturation. *NMR Biomed.* **2003**, *16*, 257–260. [CrossRef]
85. Kumar, R.; Nguyen, H.D.; Macey, P.M.; Woo, M.A.; Harper, R.M. Regional brain axial and radial diffusivity changes during development. *J. Neurosci. Res.* **2012**, *90*, 346–355. [CrossRef]
86. Bockhorst, K.H.; Narayana, P.A.; Liu, R.; Ahobila-Vijjula, P.; Ramu, J.; Kamel, M.; Wosik, J.; Bockhorst, T.; Hahn, K.; Hasan, K.M.; et al. Early postnatal development of rat brain: In vivo diffusion tensor imaging. *J. Neurosci. Res.* **2008**, *86*, 1520–1528. [CrossRef]
87. Zhang, H.; Schneider, T.; Wheeler-Kingshott, C.A.; Alexander, D.C. NODDI: Practical in vivo neurite orientation dispersion and density imaging of the human brain. *NeuroImage* **2012**, *61*, 1000–1016. [CrossRef]
88. Tucker, K.L. Assessment of usual dietary intake in population studies of gene—Diet interaction. *Nutr. Metab. Cardiovasc. Dis.* **2007**, *17*, 74–81. [CrossRef]
89. Moshfegh, A.J.; Rhodes, D.G.; Baer, D.J.; Murayi, T.; Clemens, J.C.; Rumpler, W.V.; Paul, D.R.; Sebastian, R.S.; Kuczynski, K.J.; Ingwersen, L.A.; et al. The US Department of Agriculture Automated Multiple-Pass Method reduces bias in the collection of energy intakes. *Am. J. Clin. Nutr.* **2008**, *88*, 324–332. [CrossRef]
90. Foster, E.; Bradley, J. Methodological considerations and future insights for 24-hour dietary recall assessment in children. *Nutr. Res.* **2018**, *51*, 1–11. [CrossRef]
91. Herrick, K.A.; Rossen, L.; Parsons, R.; Dodd, K. Estimating usual dietary intake from National Health and Nutrition Examination Survey data using the National Cancer Institute method. *Natl. Cent. Health Stat.* **2018**, *178*, 1–63.
92. Vos, M.B.; Kaar, J.L.; Welsh, J.A.; Van Horn, L.V.; Feig, D.I.; Anderson, C.A.M.; Patel, M.J.; Munos, J.C.; Krebs, N.F.; Xanthakos, S.A.; et al. Added Sugars and Cardiovascular Disease Risk in Children. *Circulation* **2017**, *135*, e1017–e1034. [CrossRef]

12

Evaluating the Memory Enhancing Effects of *Angelica gigas* in Mouse Models of Mild Cognitive Impairments

Minsang Kim [1], Minah Song [2], Hee-Jin Oh [2], Jin Hui [3], Woori Bae [2], Jihwan Shin [2], Sang-Dock Ji [4], Young Ho Koh [5,6], Joo Won Suh [3], Hyunwoo Park [7,*] and Sungho Maeng [2,*]

1 Graduate School of Interdisciplinary Program of Biomodulation Collage of Natural Science, Myongji University, Yongin 17058, Korea; kms0177@naver.com

2 Graduate School of East-West Medical Science, Kyung Hee University, Yongin 17104, Korea; bungu20@naver.com (M.S.); julia110892@naver.com (H.-J.O.); wrbae0328@naver.com (W.B.); junikk0@naver.com (J.S.)

3 Center for Nutraceutical and Pharmaceutical Materials, Myongji University, Yongin 17058, Korea; kimhwi83@gmail.com (J.H.); jwsuh@mju.ac.kr (J.W.S.)

4 Department of Agricultural Biology, National Academy of Agricultural Science, Rural Development Administration, Wanju-gun, Jeollabuk-do 55365, Korea; sdji11@korea.kr

5 ILSONG Institute of Life Science, Hallym University, Anyang 14066, Korea; kohyh@hallym.ac.kr

6 Department of Bio-Medical Gerontology, Hallym University Graduate School, Chuncheon 24252, Korea

7 Health Park Co., Ltd., #2502, Gangnam-dae-Ro 305, Sucho-gu, Seoul 06628, Korea

* Correspondence: hwpark75@gmail.com (H.P.); jethrot@khu.ac.kr (S.M.)

Abstract: (1) Background: By 2050, it is estimated that 130 million people will be diagnosed with dementia, and currently approved medicines only slow the progression. So preventive intervention is important to treat dementia. Mild cognitive impairment is a condition characterized by some deterioration in cognitive function and increased risk of progressing to dementia. Therefore, the treatment of mild cognitive impairment (MCI) is a possible way to prevent dementia. *Angelica gigas* reduces neuroinflammation, improves circulation, and inhibits cholinesterase, which can be effective in the prevention of Alzheimer's disease and vascular dementia and the progression of mild cognitive impairment. (2) Methods: *Angelica gigas* (AG) extract 1 mg/kg was administered to mildly cognitive impaired mice, models based on mild traumatic brain injury and chronic mild stress. Then, spatial, working, and object recognition and fear memory were measured. (3) Result: *Angelica gigas* improved spatial learning, working memory, and suppressed fear memory in the mild traumatic brain injury model. It also improved spatial learning and suppressed cued fear memory in the chronic mild stress model animals. (4) Conclusions: *Angelica gigas* can improve cognitive symptoms in mild cognitive impairment model mice.

Keywords: *Angelica gigas*; mild cognitive impairment; traumatic brain injury; chronic mild stress

1. Introduction

Mild cognitive impairment (MCI) refers to a condition in which one's cognitive function is lower than that of normal peers but not considered dementia [1,2]. However, patients with MCI have an approximately 50% chance of developing Alzheimer's disease within five years [3]. Dementia is not curable. Therefore, it is important to prevent MCI from progressing into dementia. However, there is no established treatment that prevents the progression of MCI to dementia [4].

Animal models are needed to study MCI and develop therapeutics. An appropriate MCI model may have symptoms aggravating with age, but with only subtle memory impairment [5]. Animal models that meet these criteria include middle-aged rodents and transgenic mice that overexpress A β at an early stage before the dementia onset [4]. Spontaneously hypertensive rats (SHRs) appear to be appropriate as MCI models for vascular dementia, since hypertensive astrogliosis, cytoskeleton breakdown, hippocampal atrophy, and cholinergic deficit prematurely appear prematurely in this animal [6–8]. In contrast, drug-induced memory impairment models (such as those using scopolamine, NMDA blockers, and benzodiazepines) are not appropriate because they do not represent the various aspects of MCI [5].

Traumatic brain injury (TBI) is one of the most common brain injuries that causes a progressive decline of memory and cognition [9]. Unlike severe TBI, moderate to minimal TBI tends to be overlooked. However, even mild TBI can cause gradual amnesia, altered executive function, concentration disorders, depression, apathy, and anxiety [8,10,11]. In particular, repetitive head injuries, such as those caused by collision sports or motor vehicle accidents, are known to cause dementia [12]. Animal models of TBI show a decrease in cognitive function that correlates to the extent of injury, the number of impacts, and progressively worsens [13–15]. Therefore, the TBI model is a useful MCI research tool because it is simple, progressive, reproducible, and the severity of cognitive decline is relative to the number of impacts [16].

Chronic mild stress (CMS) is a behavioral model of depression that is caused by sequential exposure to variable mild stressors. CMS is characterized by anhedonia that may be reversed by chronic treatment with antidepressants [17]. However, most depression models show cognitive decline. Also, in the CMS animal model, mild cognitive deficit is accompanied, and antidepressants improve cognitive function in this model [18]. These memory deficits were related to the increased phosphorylation of Tau and APP processing, and the application of stress to wild type mice was suggested as an animal model of sporadic AD (Alzheimer's disease) [19].

Currently, there are many methods on trial to prevent the progression of MCI to dementia. In particular, nonpharmacological methods, such as cognitive leisure activities, education and exercise, and pharmacological methods, such as vitamin E, donepezil, and intranasal insulin, have been tried [20–23]. However, more research is needed to prove their efficacy.

Angelica gigas (AG) has been used in traditional medicine to improve circulation, physical weakness, headache, dizziness, joint pain, abdominal pain, constipation, irregular menstruation, and bruises, etc. [24]. Known bioactive components of AG include decursin, decursinol angelate, and nodakenin [24]. It has been shown to improve liver function in rats treated with long-term ethanol. AG also lowered LDL cholesterol and inhibited nicotine sensitization in rats [25,26]. Finally, AG attenuated acetylcholinesterase activity and was neuroprotective against beta-amyloid peptide-induced memory impairment [27]. According to these findings, the AG extract was tested in TBI and CMS models to evaluate whether it would improve memory impairment in MCI.

2. Results

2.1. AG Improved TBI- and CMS-Induced Spatial Learning Deficit

The effect of AG on spatial learning and memory was measured using the Morris water maze (Figure 1). During the five-day training, TBI impaired spatial learning. Supplementation of AG improved the TBI-induced deficit in spatial learning (Figure 1A). CMS impaired spatial learning (control vs. CMS), which improved following AG supplementation (CMS vs. CMS + AG) (Figure 1B). The sucrose preference of the CMS mice gradually decreased over six weeks. This declining preference meant that the mice developed an anhedonia-like tendency. AG did not affect this anhedonia-like behavior (Figure S1).

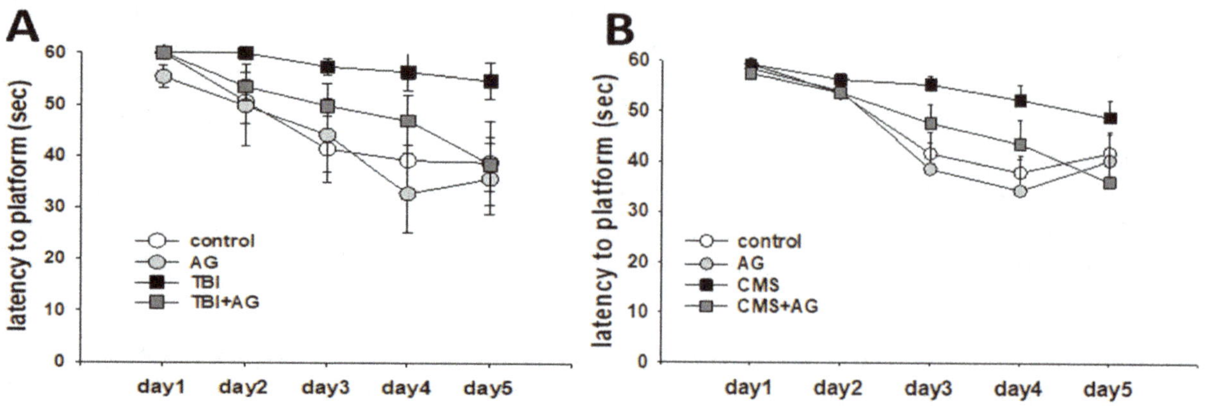

Figure 1. Spatial learning by *Angelica gigas* (AG) in traumatic brain injury (TBI) and chronic mild stress (CMS) mice as measured by the latency to the platform in the Morris water maze (MWM). (**A**) TBI model. There were repetitive training (within) effects [F(4,104) = 13.9, $p < 0.001$] and treatment group (between) effects [F(3,26) = 2.27, $p = 0.044$], but with non-significant within–between interaction differences [F(12,104) = 1.1, $p = 0.36$]. The post-hoc pairwise comparison showed a difference between control vs. TBI ($p = 0.033$), TBI vs. TBI + AG ($p = 0.041$). (**B**) CMS model. There were repetitive training effects [F(4,196) = 31.3, $p < 0.001$], treatment group effects [F(3,49) = 3.1, $p = 0.034$], and within–between interactions [F(12,196) = 2.2, $p = 0.012$]. Post-hoc pairwise comparison revealed a difference between the control and CMS groups ($p = 0.019$), AG vs. CMS ($p = 0.01$), CMS vs. CMS + AG ($p = 0.042$). All data were normally distributed and are represented as means ± S.E.M. Control: vehicle (DW) treated; AG: *Angelica gigas* 1 mg/kg; TBI: vehicle treated + traumatic brain injury; TBI + AG: *Angelica gigas* 1 mg/kg + traumatic brain injury; CMS: vehicle treated + chronic mild stress; CMS + AG: *Angelica gigas* 1 mg/kg + chronic mild stress. Repeated measure ANOVA, Tukey's HSD post-hoc test.

2.2. AG Improved Short-Term Working Memory

The effect of AG on short-term working memory was measured using the Y-maze test (Figure 2). TBI did not have a significant effect on the alternation behaviors. However, AG increased the alternation behavior in both TBI and normal mice (Figure 2A). Similarly, CMS did not affect the alternation behavior in CMS mice. In contrast, AG treatment increased the alternation behavior (Figure 2B)

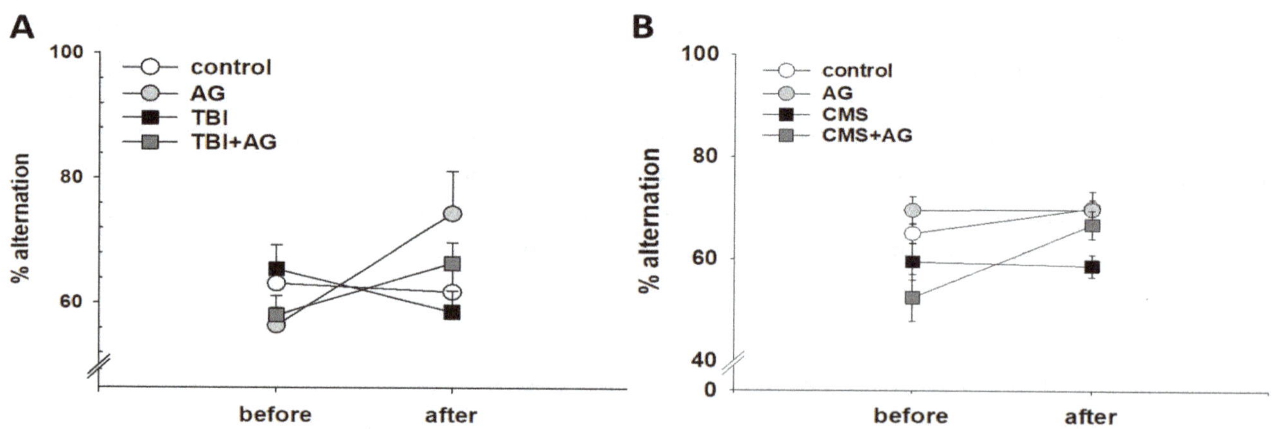

Figure 2. Short-term working memory by AG in TBI and CMS mice, measured by the percent alternation in the Y-maze. (**A**) TBI model. There were before–after (within) effects [F(1,28) = 3.57, $p = 0.012$], treatment group (between) effects [F(3,28) = 3.23, $p = 0.081$], and within–between interactions [F(3,28) = 3.28, $p = 0.036$]. There were no before–after changes in the control ($p = 0.6$) and TBI ($p = 0.38$), but improvements in the AG ($p = 0.008$) and TBI + AG ($p = 0.047$). (**B**) CMS model. There were before–after effects [F(1,36) = 6.2, $p = 0.018$] and treatment group effects [F(3,36) = 11.8, $p < 0.001$], but no significant within–between interaction differences [F(3,36) = 1.5, $p = 0.24$]. There was no before–after

change in the control group (p = 031), AG (p = 0.97) or CMS (p = 0.33) groups. However, there was an increase of % alternation in the CMS + AG group (p = 0.006). All data were normally distributed and are represented as means ± S.E.M. Control: vehicle (DW) treated; AG: *Angelica gigas* 1 mg/kg; TBI: vehicle treated + traumatic brain injury; TBI+AG: *Angelica gigas* 1 mg/kg + traumatic brain injury; CMS: vehicle treated + chronic mild stress; CMS+AG: *Angelica gigas* 1 mg/kg + chronic mild stress. Repeated measures ANOVA, Tukey's HSD post-hoc test.

2.3. AG Had No Effect on Object Recognition Memory

The effect of AG on recognition memory was measured in the novel object test (Figure 3). AG had no effect on normal mice. However, the recognition memory in TBI model mice declined with AG treatment. The absence of a before–after change in the AG treated TBI group meant that AG prevented the adverse effect of TBI (Figure 3A). There was no significant effect of CMS and AG treatment on the recognition memory (Figure 3B)

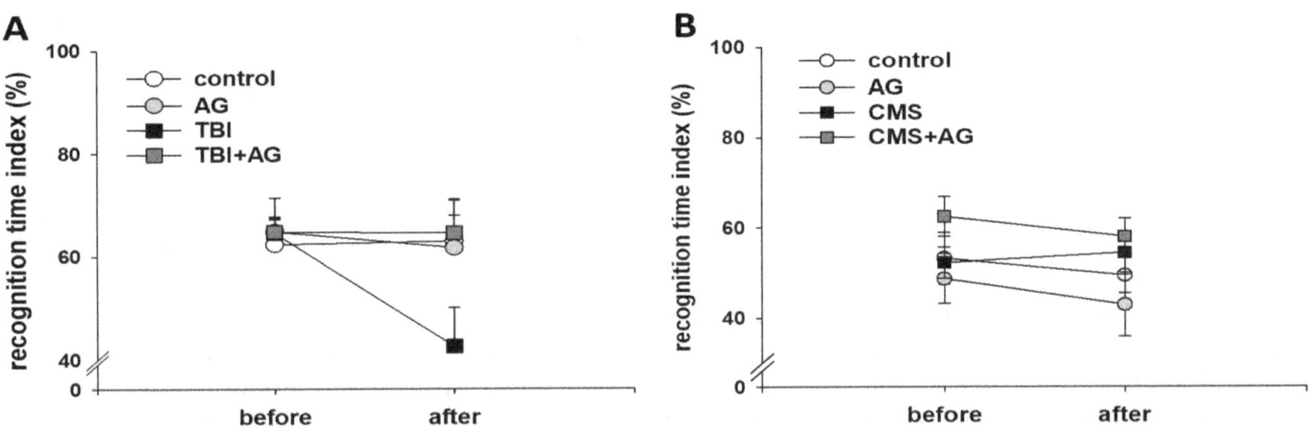

Figure 3. Object recognition memory by AG in the TBI and CMS mice as measured by the recognition time index in the novel object test. (**A**) TBI model. There were before–after (within) effects [F(1,28) = 8.3, p = 0.008], treatment group (between) effects [F(3,28) = 0.67, p = 0.58], and within–between interaction effects [F(3,28) = 3.6, p = 0.026]. There was no before–after change in the control (p = 0.93), AG (p = 0.59) and TBI + AG (p = 0.97) groups, but there were decreases in the TBI (p = 0.001) group. (**B**) CMS model. There were no before-after effects [F(1,36) = 0.32, p = 0.57], treatment group effects [F(3,36) = 1.2, p = 0.31], or within–between interactions [F(3,36) = 0.12, p = 0.95]. All data were normally distributed and are represented as means ± S.E.M. Control: vehicle (DW) treated; AG: *Angelica gigas* 1 mg/kg; TBI: vehicle treated + traumatic brain injury; TBI + AG: *Angelica gigas* 1 mg/kg + traumatic brain injury; CMS: vehicle treated + chronic mild stress; CMS+AG: *Angelica gigas* 1 mg/kg + chronic mild stress. Repeated measures ANOVA, Tukey's HSD post-hoc test.

2.4. The Effect of AG on Fear Memory

The effect of AG on fear memory was measured using the fear conditioning paradigm (Figure 4). The acquisition of fear memory in the TBI mouse model was not statistically higher than that of the control animals. AG treatment lowered the acquisition of fear memory in the TBI model mice (Figure 4A). There was no significant effect of TBI and AG on the consolidated contextual and cued fear memory (Figure 4B,C). The acquisition of fear memory in the CMS mice was lower than that of controls. There was no difference in the fear acquisition after AG treatment in CMS mice (Figure 4D). Compared to the normal mice, the CMS, AG, and CMS + AG mouse groups had lower levels of consolidated contextual fear memory. However, there were no differences among the CMS, AG, and CMS + AG groups (Figure 4E). Compared to normal mice, the AG and CMS + AG groups had lower levels of consolidated cued fear memory. In addition, AG reduced the consolidated cued fear memory in the CMS group of mice (Figure 4F).

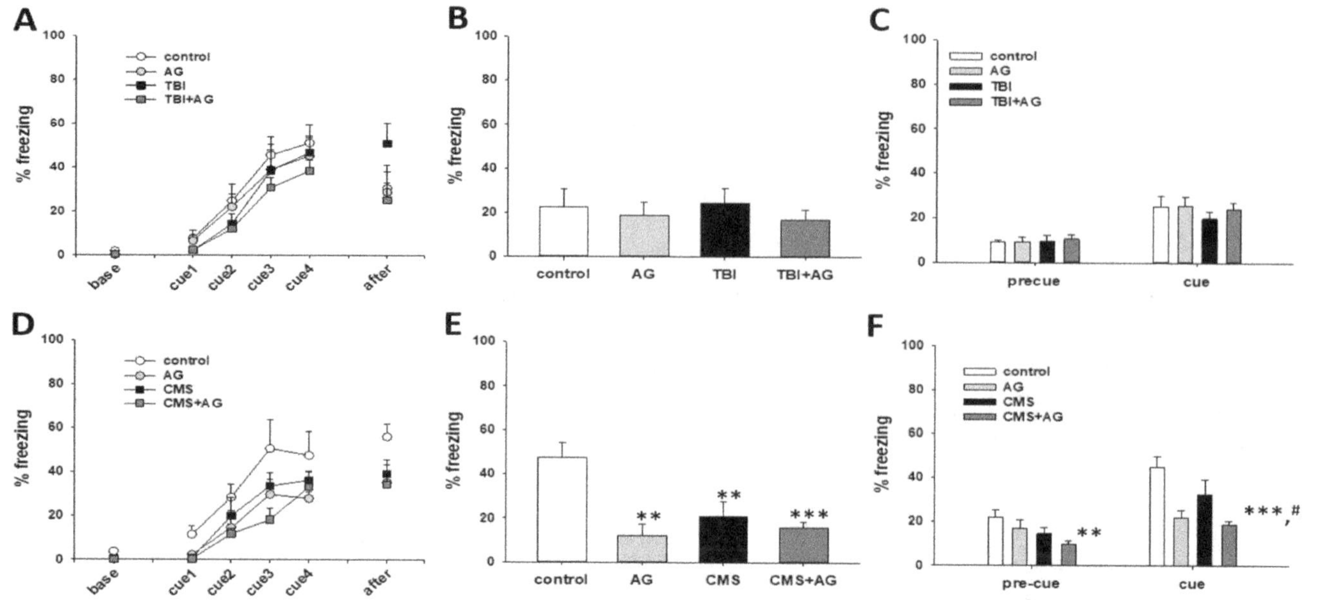

Figure 4. Fear memory by AG in TBI and CMS mice, as measured by the freezing time in the fear conditioning test. (**A**) Fear acquisition in the TBI model. There were time (within) effects [$F(5,140) = 45.7$, $p < 0.001$], treatment group (between) effects [$F(3,28) = 3.25$, $p = 0.03$], but no within–between interaction differences [$F(15,140) = 1.1$, $p = 0.36$]. There were no differences between the treatment groups at base, cue1, cue2, cue3, or cue4. However, the differences between the TBI and TBI + AG groups were significant ($p = 0.039$). In addition, the differences between the TBI and control groups ($p = 0.16$), and TBI vs. AG ($p = 0.13$) groups were not significant. (**B**) Consolidated contextual fear memory in TBI model. There were no group differences in the freezing response to the context [$F(3,28) = 0.36$, $p = 0.78$). (**C**) Consolidated cued fear in the TBI model. There were procedure (within) effects [$F(1, 28) = 61.6$, $p < 0.001$], no treatment group (between) effects [$F(3,28) = 0.29$, $p = 0.83$], or within–between interactions [$F(3,28) = 0.64$, $p = 0.59$]. There was a significant increase in the freezing comparing cue vs. precue in the control ($p < 0.001$), AG ($p < 0.001$), TBI ($p = 0.005$), and TBI + AG groups ($p < 0.001$). (**D**) Fear acquisition in the CMS model. There were time (within) effects [$F(5,95) = 27.8$, $p < 0.001$], treatment group (between) effects [$F(3,19) = 4.9$, $p = 0.011$], but no within–between interaction effects [$F(15,95) = 0.47$, $p = 0.95$]. Fear acquisition in AG ($p = 0.021$), CMS ($p = 0.035$), and CMS + AG ($p = 0.001$) were lower than controls throughout the fear acquisition procedure. There were no statistical differences among the AG, CMS, and CMS + AG groups. (**E**) Consolidated contextual fear memory in the CMS model. There were group differences in the freezing response to the context [$F(3,19) = 9.8$, $p < 0.001$). The contextual fear in AG ($p = 0.002$), CMS ($p = 0.008$), and CMS + AG ($p < 0.001$) was lower than those of the controls. (**F**) Consolidated cued fear in the CMS model. There were procedure (within) effects [$F(1,19) = 54.7$, $p < 0.001$], treatment group (between) effects [$F(3,19) = 9.3$, $p = 0.001$], and within–between interaction differences [$F(3,19) = 4.8$, $p = 0.012$]. There was a significant increase in freezing between cue and precue in the control ($p < 0.001$), CMS ($p < 0.001$), and CMS + AG ($p = 0.002$) groups, but not in the AG group ($p = 0.31$). At pre-cue, the control vs. CMS + AG ($p = 0.001$) groups were statistically different. At cue, the control vs. AG, ($p = 0.004$); control vs. CMS + AG, ($p < 0.001$); CMS vs. CMS + AG, ($p = 0.017$) were all statistically different. All data were normally distributed and are represented as means ± S.E.M. Control: vehicle (DW) treated; AG: *Angelica gigas* 1 mg/kg; TBI: vehicle treated + traumatic brain injury; TBI + AG: *Angelica gigas* 1 mg/kg + traumatic brain injury; CMS: vehicle treated + chronic mild stress; CMS + AG: *Angelica gigas* 1 mg/kg + chronic mild stress. ** $p < 0.01$, *** $p < 0.001$ vs. control. $^{\#}$ $p < 0.05$ vs. CMS. ANOVA and repeated measures ANOVA, Tukey's HSD post-hoc test.

3. Discussion

We investigated whether AG extract could prevent the progression of cognitive decline or improve memory in MCI models. We found that AG improved spatial learning and working memory but suppressed fear memory in the TBI model. In the CMS model, AG improved spatial learning and suppressed the cued fear memory.

MCI is a condition that increases a patient's risk of developing dementia. Therefore, it is important that MCI is diagnosed early in order to prevent or limit dementia development [4]. Methods to improve sleep disorders, depression, one's social network, and physical exercise are considered for the treatment of MCI [28–30]. Pharmacological interventions, such as cholinesterase inhibitors, nonsteroidal anti-inflammatory drugs, estrogen replacement therapy, Gingko biloba, and vitamin E, have not shown to prevent MCI progression to dementia [4].

The roots of AG have been used in traditional medicine to improve blood flow and anemia. They have also been used for their analgesic properties [31]. AG improves spatial memory, avoidance memory, and working memory in dementia models [27]. Among the components of AG, decursinol showed the highest inhibitory activity toward acetylcholinesterase [32]. Therefore, AG is expected to improve cognitive impairment in animal models.

In order to develop a valid MCI animal model, there must be subtle memory impairment [5]. The presence of depression-like symptoms may also be an important factor in the MCI model. Dementia and depression are known to have many associations. For instance, 60% of MCI cases that progress to AD are accompanied by depression [33].

The defect in a TBI model varies depending on the hitting area and velocity [14]. In contrast with severe TBI, mild TBI has minimal histological changes but apparent cognitive and emotional problems [8]. This association suggests that mild TBI can be used as an MCI model [34]. Such spatial memory deficit occurred in our TBI model mice, but other reflexes (such as the paw withdrawal reflex, righting reflex, and corneal reflex) were maintained (data not shown). Also, TBI is commonly known to cause disturbances in working memory. TBI in the parietotemporal regions has been shown to cause working memory deficits in mice [35]. However, working memory was normal in the mild TBI model made by repeated frontal impact; therefore, working memory is not always compromised in TBI [36]. Our measurements of working memory did not differ in the TBI model. Another common problem in TBI is the inability to recognize the source of information, such as facial recognition [37]. Face recognition memory corresponds to animal object recognition memory. There was a deficit in animal object recognition memory in the TBI models [38]. The TBI mice in this study also had decreased object recognition memory. These model mice also showed heightened fear memory; however, the results are controversial. One group found that there was no difference between normal animals and a mild repeated frontal TBI model with regard to conditioned fear after a severe CCI impact to the left parietal cortex [36]. However, a single impact above the skull increased anxiety and contextual fear in rats [39]. In mice, hippocampal-dependent fear memory decreased, but cued-dependent fear memory was not affected by TBI [40]. In our results, there was an enhanced acquisition of contextual fear in the TBI mice. However, after 24 h, the consolidated level of contextual and cued memory was not different with control animals.

Stress has a variety of effects on cognitive function [41]. CMS is a depression model also characterized by a decrease in cognitive function associated with neuroimmune, neuroendocrine, and neurogenesis functions [4]. In this experiment, the CMS animals displayed anhedonia-like behaviors in the sucrose preference test and deficits in spatial memory. In other studies using CMS models, working memory was reduced in rats but was maintained in mice [42,43]. Our study similarly found that there was no working memory deficit in CMS mice. Reduction in object recognition memory in mice and increased contextual fear in rats were reported previously [42,44]. In the present study, CMS did not affect object recognition memory, but fear acquisition and contextual consolidation were reduced. These findings were inconsistent; however, rats that were exposed to social instability stress (daily 1-h isolation, change of cage partners) showed deficits in contextual and cued memory [45,46]. Taken together, in the TBI mice, spatial learning and object recognition memory were degraded. However, spatial memory, working memory, and fear memory were intact. In the CMS model, spatial memory was degraded, but working and object recognition memory were not affected, and cued fear memory was reduced.

AG has known antibacterial, immune-stimulating, antiplatelet aggregation, neuroprotective, anti-inflammatory, and antioxidant properties [31]. We found that AG did not improve spatial memory in normal mice. However, it did improve memory in TBI and CMS animals. In addition, AG treatment led to improved working memory in normal mice of the TBI cohort. AG did not increase the recognition memory of the normal mice. However, recognition memory was only abnormal in the TBI mice at baseline. In the TBI and AG co-administration group, recognition memory was maintained. This result suggests that AG can prevent TBI-induced deficit. In the CMS cohort, however, the object memory of the CMS group was not affected. Therefore, AG also did not improve object memory in either the normal or the CMS mice. With regard to fear memory, the contextual and cued consolidated fear memory of normal and CMS mice were reduced in the CMS cohort. However, consolidated fear levels were not affected in the TBI cohort. Among AG's known effects, its cholinesterase inhibition, improved blood flow, and anti-inflammatory properties may prevent cognitive decline and improve memory in these mouse models [31,32].

In conclusion, AG prevented the deterioration of spatial learning and object recognition memory in a mouse TBI model. AG also prevented the deterioration of spatial learning in the CMS model mice and improved working memory in normal mice. As TBI is a cognitive impairment gradually progresses, and chronic stress can cause AD-like pathologies, these findings suggest that AG may also prevent progressive cognitive decline in MCI animal models, which may be worth further research.

4. Materials and Methods

4.1. Preparation of AG Extract

The dried AG root was purchased from the Junbu, Bonghwa, and Jecheon area and authenticated by professor Hui Jin. A voucher specimen was deposited in the Myongji Bioefficiency Research Center, Myongji University. AG was immersed in 70% ethanol and boiled for 4 h at 90 °C, 2 times. Then, filtered extracts were concentrated up to 25 Brix at 60 °C by depressurized evaporation, and then stored at 4 °C before using. The crude extract yield was 42.1% (*w*/*w*). The extract was dissolved in distilled water for administration into animals. HPLC was used to examine whether extracts contained nodakenin and decursin (Figure S2).

4.2. Animals and Experimental Groups

Seven-week-old male C57Bl/6 mice were purchased from Central Laboratory animals Inc. (Seoul, Korea) ($n = 32$ for cohort 1, $n = 40$ for cohort 2). The mice were housed under constant temperature and humidity with 12-h cycles of light/darkness. They had *ad libitum* access to rodent chow and water. After a week of habituation, the mice were randomly assigned into experimental groups. The mice in the TBI cohort were assigned to the following assignments: (1) control ($n = 6$): DW p.o. + no TBI; (2) AG ($n = 6$): *Angelica gigas* 1 mg/kg p.o + no TBI; (3) TBI ($n = 8$): DW p.o. + TBI; (4) TBI + AG ($n = 12$): *Angelica gigas* 1 mg/kg p.o. + TBI. The mice in the CMS cohort were assigned to the following assignments: (1) control ($n = 10$): DW p.o. + no CMS; (2) AG ($n = 10$): *Angelica gigas* 1 mg/kg p.o + no CMS; 3) CMS ($n = 10$): DW p.o. + CMS; 4) CMS + AG ($n = 10$): *Angelica gigas* 1 mg/kg p.o. + CMS. The outline of the experimental procedures is schematically represented in Figure 5. Animal studies were conducted in accordance with the Guide for the Care and Use of Laboratory Animals by the NIH. The protocols were approved by the Institutional Animal Care and Use Committee of Kyung Hee University (KHUASP(GC)-17-024).

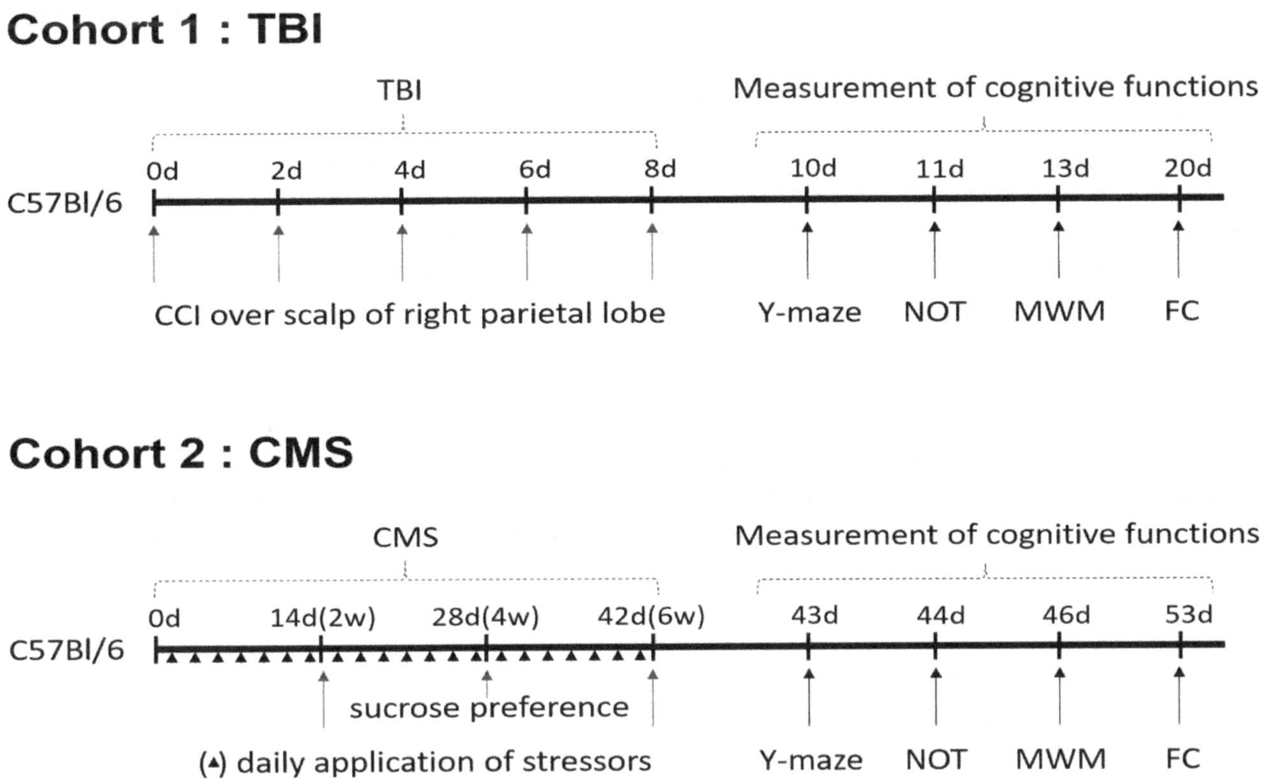

Figure 5. Experimental outline of mild cognitive impairment mice models induced by TBI (Cohort 1) and CMS (Cohort 2). TBI: Traumatic brain injury, CCI: Controlled cortical impact, Y-maze: Y shaped maze test, NOT: Novel object test, MWM: Morris water maze, FC: Fear conditioning, CMS: Chronic mild stress.

4.3. Creating Animal Models

4.3.1. TBI Model

A Cortical Contusion Injury device, which was purchased from Custom Design and Fabrication, Inc., (model eCCI-6.3), was used to simulate TBI. The mice were anesthetized with 3% isoflurane during the procedure. In order to induce TBI, a 3 mm rod impacted the scalp over the right hippocampal region at the velocity of 4 m/second and depth of 0.5 mm. This was repeated five times, with two days between each impact. Animals in the control and AG groups also underwent isoflurane anesthesia, but no impact.

4.3.2. CMS Model

The stress procedure lasted for six weeks. The mice were randomly subjected to two types of stressors each day. The potential stressors included 2 h of immobilization, strobe light exposure, white noise exposure, cat urine exposure, and overnight food deprivation, water deprivation, or light exposure. During the weekend, the mice were exposed to wet bedding or a tilted cage for 24 h. The control mice were left undisturbed in their home cage.

4.4. Behavioral Tests

4.4.1. Sucrose Preference

Anhedonia-like changes in the CMS mice were monitored using the sucrose preference test, which was performed at the 2nd, 4th, and 6th week. Consumption of water and sucrose by a single caged mouse was measured from 6 p.m. to 9 a.m. The preference index was calculated as follows: [sucrose consumption/(DW consumption + sucrose consumption)].

4.4.2. Morris Water Maze

The water tank (200 cm diameter) was filled 0.5 cm above the platform with tap water and made opaque by white paint. For 5 days, the mice were trained to locate the submerged platform within 60 s according to the symbols placed around the walls. If the mouse was unable to escape within 60 s, it was guided to the platform. Each day of training included 4 sessions, each of which started in a different quadrant.

4.4.3. Y-Maze

The maze consisted of three corridors that were joined at the center at equal angles. After placing a mouse in the maze, the movements were recorded for five minutes. An alternation was defined as a sequential visit to each arm without the repetition of either of the two previous arms. The percent alternation was calculated as the number of correct alternations per total arm visits minus 2.

4.4.4. Novel Object Test

In a plexiglas box (50 × 50 × 40 cm), two cylinder-shaped tin cans were introduced in two corners, 30 cm apart from each other. The mice were allowed to explore each object for 5 min. On the next day, the object of the right corner was replaced with a box-shaped novel object. The time that the mice spent exploring each object was recorded during the 5-min period. The animals were considered to be exploring an object when they were facing or sniffing the object. The recognition index was calculated by the ratio of time spent exploring the novel object over the total time spent exploring both objects.

4.4.5. Fear Conditioning

The fear conditioning test consisted of acquisition, contextual consolidation, and cued consolidation phases. For the acquisition, the mice were placed in the Passive/Active avoidance system chamber from Scitech Korea (model No. PAAS) and left undisturbed for two minutes. The subsequent sessions comprised a conditioned stimulus (2000 Hz tone, 30 s) that co-terminated with an unconditioned stimulus (electric foot shock, 0.45 mA, 2 s), and intertrial intervals (30 s) were repeated four times. The mice were left in the chamber for an additional two minutes. Freezing was measured during the first two minutes and last two minutes of the 4 intertrial intervals. On the following day, the animals were placed in the chamber for five minutes. Freezing was measured as a contextual fear memory. On the third day, the mice were placed in a novel chamber for three minutes, followed by three minutes of exposure to a 2000 Hz tone. Freezing was measured before and during the tone exposure.

4.5. Statistical Analysis

Analysis of variance (ANOVA) and repeated measures ANOVA, following Tukey's HSD post-hoc test, were performed using SPSS 23 (IBM). p-Values < 0.05 were considered significantly different. The normality of distribution of variables was tested by the Shapiro-Wilk test.

Author Contributions: Conceptualization, S.-D.J. and Y.H.K.; methodology, J.S.; formal analysis and investigation, M.K., M.S. and H.-J.O.; investigation, W.B.; data curation, J.H.; writing—original draft preparation, S.M.; writing—review and editing, H.P.; supervision, J.W.S. All authors have read and agreed to the published version of the manuscript.

References

1. Ebly, E.M.; Hogan, D.B.; Parhad, I.M. Cognitive impairment in the nondemented elderly. Results from the Canadian Study of Health and Aging. *Arch. Neurol.* **1995**, *52*, 612–619. [CrossRef] [PubMed]

2. Graham, J.E.; Rockwood, K.; Beattie, B.L.; Eastwood, R.; Gauthier, S.; Tuokko, H.; McDowell, I. Prevalence and severity of cognitive impairment with and without dementia in an elderly population. *Lancet* **1997**, *349*, 1793–1796. [CrossRef]
3. Tuokko, H.; Frerichs, R.; Graham, J.; Rockwood, K.; Kristjansson, B.; Fisk, J.; Bergman, H.; Kozma, A.; McDowell, I. Five-year follow-up of cognitive impairment with no dementia. *Arch. Neurol.* **2003**, *60*, 577–582. [CrossRef] [PubMed]
4. Chertkow, H.; Massoud, F.; Nasreddine, Z.; Belleville, S.; Joanette, Y.; Bocti, C.; Drolet, V.; Kirk, J.; Freedman, M.; Bergman, H. Diagnosis and treatment of dementia: 3. Mild cognitive impairment and cognitive impairment without dementia. *CMAJ Can. Med. Assoc. J. J. De L'association Med. Can.* **2008**, *178*, 1273–1285. [CrossRef]
5. Pepeu, G. Mild cognitive impairment: Animal models. *Dialogues Clin. Neurosci.* **2004**, *6*, 369–377.
6. Hernandez, C.M.; Hoifodt, H.; Terry, A.V., Jr. Spontaneously hypertensive rats: Further evaluation of age-related memory performance and cholinergic marker expression. *J. Psychiatry Neurosci. JPN* **2003**, *28*, 197–209.
7. Terry, A.V., Jr.; Hernandez, C.M.; Buccafusco, J.J.; Gattu, M. Deficits in spatial learning and nicotinic-acetylcholine receptors in older, spontaneously hypertensive rats. *Neuroscience* **2000**, *101*, 357–368. [CrossRef]
8. Kibby, M.Y.; Long, C.J. Minor head injury: Attempts at clarifying the confusion. *Brain Inj.* **1996**, *10*, 159–186. [CrossRef]
9. Stern, R.A.; Riley, D.O.; Daneshvar, D.H.; Nowinski, C.J.; Cantu, R.C.; McKee, A.C. Long-term consequences of repetitive brain trauma: Chronic traumatic encephalopathy. *PM R J. Inj. Funct. Rehabil.* **2011**, *3*, S460–S467. [CrossRef]
10. Arciniegas, D.; Adler, L.; Topkoff, J.; Cawthra, E.; Filley, C.M.; Reite, M. Attention and memory dysfunction after traumatic brain injury: Cholinergic mechanisms, sensory gating, and a hypothesis for further investigation. *Brain Inj.* **1999**, *13*, 1–13. [CrossRef]
11. Levin, H.S.; Mattis, S.; Ruff, R.M.; Eisenberg, H.M.; Marshall, L.F.; Tabaddor, K.; High, W.M., Jr.; Frankowski, R.F. Neurobehavioral outcome following minor head injury: A three-center study. *J. Neurosurg.* **1987**, *66*, 234–243. [CrossRef]
12. Guskiewicz, K.M.; Marshall, S.W.; Bailes, J.; McCrea, M.; Cantu, R.C.; Randolph, C.; Jordan, B.D. Association between recurrent concussion and late-life cognitive impairment in retired professional football players. *Neurosurgery* **2005**, *57*, 719–726. [CrossRef] [PubMed]
13. Langlois, J.A.; Rutland-Brown, W.; Wald, M.M. The epidemiology and impact of traumatic brain injury: A brief overview. *J. Head Trauma Rehabil.* **2006**, *21*, 375–378. [CrossRef] [PubMed]
14. Xiong, Y.; Mahmood, A.; Chopp, M. Animal models of traumatic brain injury. *Nat. Rev. Neurosci.* **2013**, *14*, 128–142. [CrossRef]
15. Mouzon, B.C.; Bachmeier, C.; Ferro, A.; Ojo, J.O.; Crynen, G.; Acker, C.M.; Davies, P.; Mullan, M.; Stewart, W.; Crawford, F. Chronic neuropathological and neurobehavioral changes in a repetitive mild traumatic brain injury model. *Ann. Neurol.* **2014**, *75*, 241–254. [CrossRef] [PubMed]
16. Creeley, C.E.; Wozniak, D.F.; Bayly, P.V.; Olney, J.W.; Lewis, L.M. Multiple episodes of mild traumatic brain injury result in impaired cognitive performance in mice. *Acad. Emerg. Med.* **2004**, *11*, 809–819. [CrossRef]
17. Willner, P. Validity, reliability and utility of the chronic mild stress model of depression: A 10-year review and evaluation. *Psychopharmacology* **1997**, *134*, 319–329. [CrossRef]
18. Song, L.; Che, W.; Min-Wei, W.; Murakami, Y.; Matsumoto, K. Impairment of the spatial learning and memory induced by learned helplessness and chronic mild stress. *Pharmacol. Biochem. Behav.* **2006**, *83*, 186–193. [CrossRef]
19. Cuadrado-Tejedor, M.; Ricobaraza, A.; Del Rio, J.; Frechilla, D.; Franco, R.; Perez-Mediavilla, A.; Garcia-Osta, A. Chronic mild stress in mice promotes cognitive impairment and CDK5-dependent tau hyperphosphorylation. *Behav. Brain Res.* **2011**, *220*, 338–343. [CrossRef]
20. Sattler, C.; Toro, P.; Schonknecht, P.; Schroder, J. Cognitive activity, education and socioeconomic status as preventive factors for mild cognitive impairment and Alzheimer's disease. *Psychiatry Res.* **2012**, *196*, 90–95. [CrossRef]
21. Geda, Y.E.; Roberts, R.O.; Knopman, D.S.; Christianson, T.J.; Pankratz, V.S.; Ivnik, R.J.; Boeve, B.F.; Tangalos, E.G.; Petersen, R.C.; Rocca, W.A. Physical exercise, aging, and mild cognitive impairment: A population-based study. *Arch. Neurol.* **2010**, *67*, 80–86. [CrossRef] [PubMed]

22. Craft, S.; Baker, L.D.; Montine, T.J.; Minoshima, S.; Watson, G.S.; Claxton, A.; Arbuckle, M.; Callaghan, M.; Tsai, E.; Plymate, S.R.; et al. Intranasal insulin therapy for Alzheimer disease and amnestic mild cognitive impairment: A pilot clinical trial. *Arch. Neurol.* **2012**, *69*, 29–38. [CrossRef] [PubMed]
23. Petersen, R.C.; Thomas, R.G.; Grundman, M.; Bennett, D.; Doody, R.; Ferris, S.; Galasko, D.; Jin, S.; Kaye, J.; Levey, A.; et al. Alzheimer's Disease Cooperative Study Group. Vitamin E and donepezil for the treatment of mild cognitive impairment. *N. Engl. J. Med.* **2005**, *352*, 2379–2388. [CrossRef] [PubMed]
24. Sarker, S.D.; Nahar, L. Natural medicine: The genus Angelica. *Curr. Med. Chem.* **2004**, *11*, 1479–1500. [CrossRef]
25. Cha, Y.S.; Choi, D.S.; Oh, S.H. Effects of *Angelica gigas* Nakai diet on lipid metabolism, alcohol metabolism and liver function of rats administered with chronic ethanol. *Appl. Biol. Chem.* **1999**, *42*, 29–33.
26. Zhao, R.J.; Koo, B.S.; Kim, G.W.; Jang, E.Y.; Lee, J.R.; Kim, M.R.; Kim, S.C.; Kwon, Y.K.; Kim, K.J.; Huh, T.L.; et al. The essential oil from *Angelica gigas* NAKAI suppresses nicotine sensitization. *Biol. Pharm. Bull.* **2005**, *28*, 2323–2326. [CrossRef]
27. Yan, J.J.; Kim, D.H.; Moon, Y.S.; Jung, J.S.; Ahn, E.M.; Baek, N.I.; Song, D.K. Protection against beta-amyloid peptide-induced memory impairment with long-term administration of extract of *Angelica gigas* or decursinol in mice. *Prog. Neuro-Psychopharmacol. Biol. Psychiatry* **2004**, *28*, 25–30. [CrossRef]
28. Reischies, F.M.; Neu, P. Comorbidity of mild cognitive disorder and depression–a neuropsychological analysis. *Eur. Arch. Psychiatry Clin. Neurosci.* **2000**, *250*, 186–193. [CrossRef]
29. Fratiglioni, L.; Wang, H.X.; Ericsson, K.; Maytan, M.; Winblad, B. Influence of social network on occurrence of dementia: A community-based longitudinal study. *Lancet* **2000**, *355*, 1315–1319. [CrossRef]
30. Laurin, D.; Verreault, R.; Lindsay, J.; MacPherson, K.; Rockwood, K. Physical activity and risk of cognitive impairment and dementia in elderly persons. *Arch. Neurol.* **2001**, *58*, 498–504. [CrossRef]
31. Sowndhararajan, K.; Kim, S. Neuroprotective and Cognitive Enhancement Potentials of *Angelica gigas* Nakai Root: A Review. *Sci. Pharm.* **2017**, *85*, 21. [CrossRef] [PubMed]
32. Kang, S.Y.; Lee, K.Y.; Sung, S.H.; Park, M.J.; Kim, Y.C. Coumarins isolated from *Angelica gigas* inhibit acetylcholinesterase: Structure-activity relationships. *J. Nat. Prod.* **2001**, *64*, 683–685. [CrossRef] [PubMed]
33. Visser, P.J.; Verhey, F.R.; Ponds, R.W.; Kester, A.; Jolles, J. Distinction between preclinical Alzheimer's disease and depression. *J. Am. Geriatr. Soc.* **2000**, *48*, 479–484. [CrossRef] [PubMed]
34. Milman, A.; Rosenberg, A.; Weizman, R.; Pick, C.G. Mild traumatic brain injury induces persistent cognitive deficits and behavioral disturbances in mice. *J. Neurotrauma* **2005**, *22*, 1003–1010. [CrossRef]
35. Eakin, K.; Baratz-Goldstein, R.; Pick, C.G.; Zindel, O.; Balaban, C.D.; Hoffer, M.E.; Lockwood, M.; Miller, J.; Hoffer, B.J. Efficacy of N-acetyl cysteine in traumatic brain injury. *PLoS ONE* **2014**, *9*, e90617. [CrossRef]
36. Cheng, J.S.; Craft, R.; Yu, G.Q.; Ho, K.; Wang, X.; Mohan, G.; Mangnitsky, S.; Ponnusamy, R.; Mucke, L. Tau reduction diminishes spatial learning and memory deficits after mild repetitive traumatic brain injury in mice. *PLoS ONE* **2014**, *9*, e115765. [CrossRef]
37. Dywan, J.; Segalowitz, S.J.; Henderson, D.; Jacoby, L. Memory for source after traumatic brain injury. *Brain Cogn.* **1993**, *21*, 20–43. [CrossRef]
38. Gauthier, I.; Tarr, M.J.; Anderson, A.W.; Skudlarski, P.; Gore, J.C. Activation of the middle fusiform 'face area' increases with expertise in recognizing novel objects. *Nat. Neurosci.* **1999**, *2*, 568–573. [CrossRef]
39. Meyer, D.L.; Davies, D.R.; Barr, J.L.; Manzerra, P.; Forster, G.L. Mild traumatic brain injury in the rat alters neuronal number in the limbic system and increases conditioned fear and anxiety-like behaviors. *Exp. Neurol.* **2012**, *235*, 574–587. [CrossRef]
40. Lifshitz, J.; Witgen, B.M.; Grady, M.S. Acute cognitive impairment after lateral fluid percussion brain injury recovers by 1 month: Evaluation by conditioned fear response. *Behav. Brain Res.* **2007**, *177*, 347–357. [CrossRef]
41. McEwen, B.S.; Sapolsky, R.M. Stress and cognitive function. *Curr. Opin. Neurobiol.* **1995**, *5*, 205–216. [CrossRef]
42. Henningsen, K.; Andreasen, J.T.; Bouzinova, E.V.; Jayatissa, M.N.; Jensen, M.S.; Redrobe, J.P.; Wiborg, O. Cognitive deficits in the rat chronic mild stress model for depression: Relation to anhedonic-like responses. *Behav. Brain Res.* **2009**, *198*, 136–141. [CrossRef] [PubMed]
43. Pothion, S.; Bizot, J.C.; Trovero, F.; Belzung, C. Strain differences in sucrose preference and in the consequences of unpredictable chronic mild stress. *Behav. Brain Res.* **2004**, *155*, 135–146. [CrossRef] [PubMed]

44. Haridas, S.; Kumar, M.; Manda, K. Melatonin ameliorates chronic mild stress induced behavioral dysfunctions in mice. *Physiol. Behav.* **2013**, *119*, 201–207. [CrossRef]
45. Wright, R.L.; Conrad, C.D. Chronic stress leaves novelty-seeking behavior intact while impairing spatial recognition memory in the Y-maze. *Stress* **2005**, *8*, 151–154. [CrossRef]
46. Morrissey, M.D.; Mathews, I.Z.; McCormick, C.M. Enduring deficits in contextual and auditory fear conditioning after adolescent, not adult, social instability stress in male rats. *Neurobiol. Learn. Mem.* **2011**, *95*, 46–56. [CrossRef]

13

The Food-Specific Serum IgG Reactivity in Major Depressive Disorder Patients, Irritable Bowel Syndrome Patients and Healthy Controls

Hanna Karakula-Juchnowicz [1,2,*], Mirosława Gałęcka [3], Joanna Rog [1,*], Anna Bartnicka [3], Zuzanna Łukaszewicz [3], Pawel Krukow [2], Justyna Morylowska-Topolska [2], Karolina Skonieczna-Zydecka [4], Tomasz Krajka [5], Kamil Jonak [1,6] and Dariusz Juchnowicz [7]

1 1st Department of Psychiatry, Psychotherapy and Early Intervention Medical University of Lublin, Gluska Street 1, 20-439 Lublin, Poland; jonak.kamil@gmail.com

2 Department of Clinical Neuropsychiatry Medical University of Lublin, Gluska Street 1, 20-439 Lublin, Poland; pawelkrukow@umlub.pl (P.K.); justynamorylowska@op.pl (J.M.-T.)

3 Institute of Microecology, Sielska Street 10, 60-129 Poznan, Poland; drgalecka@instytut-mikroekologii.pl (M.G.); anna.bartnicka@instytut-mikroekologii.pl (A.B.); dietetyk@instytut-mikroekologii.pl (Z.L.)

4 Department of Biochemistry and Human Nutrition, Pomeranian Medical University in Szczecin, Broniewskiego Street 24, 71-460 Szczecin, Poland, karzyd@pum.edu.pl

5 Faculty of Mechanical Engineering, Department of Mathematics, Lublin University of Technology, Nadbystrzycka Street 36, 20-618 Lublin, Poland; t.krajka@pollub.pl

6 Department of Biomedical Engineering, Lublin University of Technology, Nadbystrzycka Street 38D, 20-618 Lublin, Poland

7 Department of Psychiatric Nursing Medical University of Lublin, Szkolna Street 18, 20-124 Lublin, Poland; juchnowiczdariusz@wp.pl

* Correspondence: karakula.hanna@gmail.com (H.K.-J.); rog.joann@gmail.com (J.R.)

Abstract: There is an increasing amount of evidence which links the pathogenesis of irritable bowel syndrome (IBS) with food IgG hyperreactivity. Some authors have suggested that food IgG hyperreactivity could be also involved in the pathophysiology of major depressive disorder (MDD). The aim of this study was to compare levels of serum IgG against 39 selected food antigens between three groups of participants: patients with MDD (MDD group), patients with IBS (IBS group) and healthy controls (HC group). The study included 65 participants (22 in the MDD group, 22 in the IBS group and 21 in the HC group). Serum IgG levels were examined using enzyme-linked immunosorbent assay (ELISA). Medical records, clinical data and laboratory results were collected for the analysis. IgG food hyperreactivity (interpreted as an average of levels of IgG antibodies above 7.5 μg/mL) was detected in 28 (43%) participants, including 14 (64%) from the MDD group, ten (46%) from the IBS group and four (19%) from the HC group. We found differences between extreme IgG levels in MDD versus HC groups and in IBS versus HC groups. Patients with MDD had significantly higher serum levels of total IgG antibodies and IgG against celery, garlic and gluten compared with healthy controls. The MDD group also had higher serum IgG levels against gluten compared with the IBS group. Our results suggest dissimilarity in immune responses against food proteins between the examined groups, with the highest immunoreactivity in the MDD group. Further studies are needed to repeat and confirm these results in bigger cohorts and also examine clinical utility of IgG-based elimination diet in patients with MDD and IBS.

Keywords: major depressive disorder; irritable bowel syndrome; immunoglobulin G antibody; food antigen; low-grade inflammation; gut-brain axis; food hypersensitivity; food allergy; intestinal permeability

1. Introduction

Depression is an etiologically and clinically heterogeneous psychiatric disorder [1] which affects more than 300 million people worldwide [2]. Its development is connected with both genetic determinants and environmental factors [3,4]. In 1991, Smith formulated the macrophage theory of depression which suggested that mechanisms involved in the pathogenesis of the disease are macrophage activation and excessive secretion of pro-inflammatory cytokines. Pro-inflammatory cytokines, due to their ability to penetrate the blood–brain barrier (BBB), may influence the metabolism and secretion of neurotransmitters which, consequently, leads to dysregulation of Central Nervous System (CNS) homeostasis [5]. There is a vast body of evidence in support of this theory: (1) the imbalance of pro-inflammatory and anti-inflammatory mediators is observed before the onset of the illness [6]; (2) significantly higher levels of pro-inflammatory cytokines are observed in the acute phase of depression [7]; (3) higher levels of inflammation markers are linked to a higher risk of recurrence of the next depressive episode [8]; (4) higher concentrations of markers of inflammation are connected with progression of the illness [9]; (5) a wide range of anti-inflammatory agents have been successfully tested in patients suffering from major depressive disorder (MDD) [10].

Factors related to systemic inflammation include i.a. excessive stress, environmental pollution, stimulants (cigarettes, alcohol), excessive body weight, poor diet [11] and leaky gut syndrome [12,13]. An increasing number of studies show a probable relationship between systemic inflammation and gut permeability in such conditions as: coeliac disease [14], autoimmune hepatitis [15], Parkinson's disease [16], autism spectrum disorders [17,18]. In 2017, Karakula-Juchnowicz et al. suggested that IgG food hypersensitivity could lead to systemic inflammation and be a trigger factor for the development of MDD. Proteins that occur in food and protein-derived compounds may modulate the immune response of the body. Increased gut permeability may lead to translocation of food-borne components into blood circulation, resulting in an abnormal immune response and increased levels of circulating pro-inflammatory cytokines, and thus, the development or maintenance of MDD. Elimination of trigger foods may inhibit the pathological response of the immune system and restore the pro/anti-inflammatory balance of the body [19] (see Figure 1 for an overview).

There is growing evidence that one of the most visible manifestations of gut permeability is irritable bowel syndrome (IBS) which affects 10–13% people around the world [20]. What is more, it is documented that individuals with IBS present low-grade intestinal inflammatory process [21], which is not always connected with a history of a gastrointestinal infection [22]. Irritable bowel syndrome, the most common group of gastrointestinal symptoms characterized by diarrhoea, constipation and bloating, can affect quality of life in those patients [23]. Abdominal pain or discomfort associated with IBS is relieved by defecation. Subtypes of IBS are distinguished based on the manifested symptoms: IBS with constipation (IBS-C), IBS with diarrhoea (IBS-D), mixed IBS (IBS-M), unsubtyped IBS [24].

The etiology of IBS has not been fully elucidated. However, some determinants known as gut-permeability-inducers (e.g., microbiota alternation and diet), have been suggested to play a role in pathophysiology of IBS [25]. Due to the characteristics of IBS (no organic changes), the treatment is based on changes of lifestyle, dietary interventions, counselling, psychological therapies, and dealing with symptoms [26]. Pharmacological therapies that target IBS symptoms include: antispasmodic medication with laxative or anti-diarrhoeal therapies; antibiotics, probiotics, bulking agents, stool softeners or stimulant laxatives [27,28]. Elimination diets are key to reducing IBS symptoms like bloating, gas and pain. The most recommended one is a low FODMAP diet (eliminating fermentable oligosaccharides, disaccharides, monosaccharides and polyols) [29,30] which is followed by a gluten-free diet according to non-celiac gluten sensitivity (NCGS) [31,32], a lactose-free diet [33] or a diet based on measurements of individual levels of IgG antibodies to food antigens in patients [34]. The efficacy of a low FODMAP diet is around 75% in patients with visceral hypersensitivity [35], but on the other hand, a low FODMAP diet might alter gut microbiota. FODMAPs belong to foods that have prebiotic functions, therefore their restriction may lead to reduction in beneficial bacteria in faeces (*Bifidobacteria*) [36].

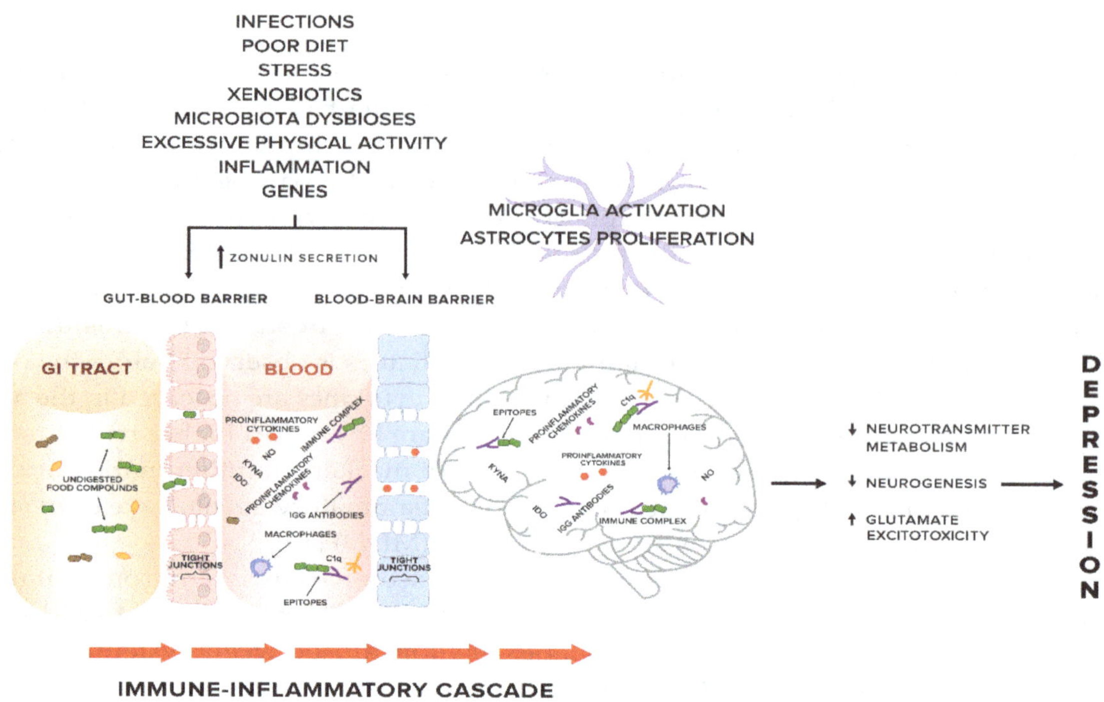

Figure 1. The gut-immune-inflammatory-brain model for Major Depressive Disorder associated with food IgG hyperreactivity. According to the hypothesis proposed in our previous work [19], we present a possible mechanism underlying the MDD development, suggesting that the interplay between genetic and environmental factors may lead to disruption of tight junctions, the loss of their integrity and both gut and BBB permeability. Undigested food compounds, which would normally break down in the gut, translocate into the blood circulation, and trough epitopes combine with food IgG antibodies to form immune complexes. This, in turn, provokes an abnormal response and triggers immune-inflammatory cascade. Uncontrolled release of the proinflammatory mediators may contribute to low-grade systemic inflammation and low-grade neuroinflammation, which, via pathological processes in CNS, i.e., changes in neurotransmitter metabolism, neurogenesis, glutamate excitotoxicity, may in consequence induce and then maintain and prolong depression. Abbreviations: GI tract, gastrointestinal tract; KYNA, kynurenic acid; NO, nitrogen oxide; IDO, indoleamine 2,3-dioxygenase; C1q, complement component 1q.

An elimination diet based on specific IgG antibodies against food has been shown to improve symptoms in patients with IBS [27,37,38]. In 2006, Monsbakken suggested that food hyperreactivity can affect up to 70% of IBS patients [39] and the number of studies confirming this finding is still growing [40,41].

Given that there is:

(1) increasing evidence linking IBS and food IgG hyperreactivity, and
(2) a suggested relationship between food IgG reactivity and MDD.

We decided to compare IgG reactions to food proteins in the serum of patients with IBS, MDD and healthy controls.

2. Material and Methods

2.1. Participants

Sixty five subjects aged 18–60 years participated in the study, including: 22 outpatients with a *DSM-5* diagnosis of major depressive disorder (MDD) [42], 22 outpatients who met Rome III Criteria [24] for the diagnosis of irritable bowel syndrome (IBS) and 21 healthy controls (HC) with no current or past history of IBS or psychiatric disorders. The mean age and sex ratio were matched across the three groups.

Exclusion criteria were as follows: (1) Body Mass Index (BMI) below 18.5 kg/m^2 or above 30 kg/m^2 (due to the possibility of either excessive or insufficient exposure to antigens, abnormal gut permeability [43–45] and changes in the gut microbiota among underweight and overweight subjects [45–47]); (2) prior or current medical history of organic brain dysfunctions; (3) a lifetime IBS diagnosis in the MDD group; (4) a lifetime MDD diagnosis in the IBS group (5) meeting criteria for substance abuse/dependence or mental retardation; (6) current use of anti-inflammatory or anti-allergic medications or antibiotics; (7) any inflammatory, oncological or systemic immune disease, diabetes mellitus, infectious diseases; (8) following any types of specific diets; (9) pregnancy or lactation.

The study was conducted in accordance with the Declaration of Helsinki, and the protocol was approved by the Ethics Committee of Medical University of Lublin (the project identification code: KE-0254/127/2016). After description of the study, a written informed consent was obtained from every subject.

2.2. *Concentration of Specific IgG Antibodies*

The fasting sera were examined for the concentration of specific IgG against 39 selected foods using enzyme-linked immunosorbent assay (ELISA), according to the manufacturer's recommendations (ImuPro test; R-Biopharm, Darmstadt, Germany), which was described previously [48]. Standardized calibration curve for IgG was performed according to 1st WHO IRP 67/86 for human IgG. Quantitative measurements are shown in μg/mL. All values above 7.5 μg/mL were considered as a positive reaction to a certain food. The full list of food antigens tested includes: vegetables (broccoli, carrot, cucumber, sweet pepper, red cabbage, tomato, celery, soya beans); fruits (pineapple, watermelon, cherry); spices (horseradish, garlic, mustard seed); meat (pork, beef, chicken); eggs (chicken egg); cereals with gluten (gluten, barley, oat, wheat, spelt, rye); seeds and nuts (poppy seed, almond, hazelnut, peanut, pistachio, linseed, sunflower seed); fish & seafood (crayfish); milk products (cow's: milk, sour-milk products, rennet cheese, goat's: milk and cheese, sheep's: milk and cheese); sugar products (honey) and yeast (bakery yeast).

2.3. *Statistical Analysis*

Earlier studies demonstrated the skewed distributions of data on IgG antibodies concentrations [49]. In view of the possibility of weakness of results obtained from classical statistical analysis and changes the reliability of analysis after a log-transformation we decided to use the ex-Gaussian statistics which is more advanced and could detect an important dissimilarity in groups with extreme results of IgG plasma levels.

The ex-Gaussian modelling of raw biological data was conducted to illustrate the specificity of quantitative results in a way that best reflects the distribution of the parameters studied. The ex-Gaussian statistics were used to compare the unprocessed results we obtained for the groups, without the need to remove the selected results or to convert the results artificially in order to adjust them to Gaussian distribution, but to take into account their exponential specificity.

The use of the ex-Gaussian statistics makes it possible to estimate three independent parameters: mu (μ) representing the mean of the normal component, reflecting the average IgG results in each group, sigma (σ) corresponding to the symmetrical standard deviation of the normal component, showing the variability of raw results, and tau (τ), containing the exponential part of the distribution, displaying the extremes in IgG results. Comparisons of mu and tau between three studied groups will show factual differences in two separated aspects of IgG outcomes: averaged, most frequently occurring results, and the comparison of tau will indicate which group has the highest number of individuals with clinically high IgG titers.

The modelling of ex-Gaussian parameters was performed with the MATLAB toolbox "DISTRIB". Data pre-processing allowing correct export of the results to the MATLAB software was proceeded with an individually customized Excel macro. All further operations were conducted according to Lacouture and Cousineau [50] recommendations for applying ex-Gaussian modelling to experimental data. Figure 2 confirms that the data obtained for all IgG results in all three groups match closely to the specificity of the ex-Gaussian distribution.

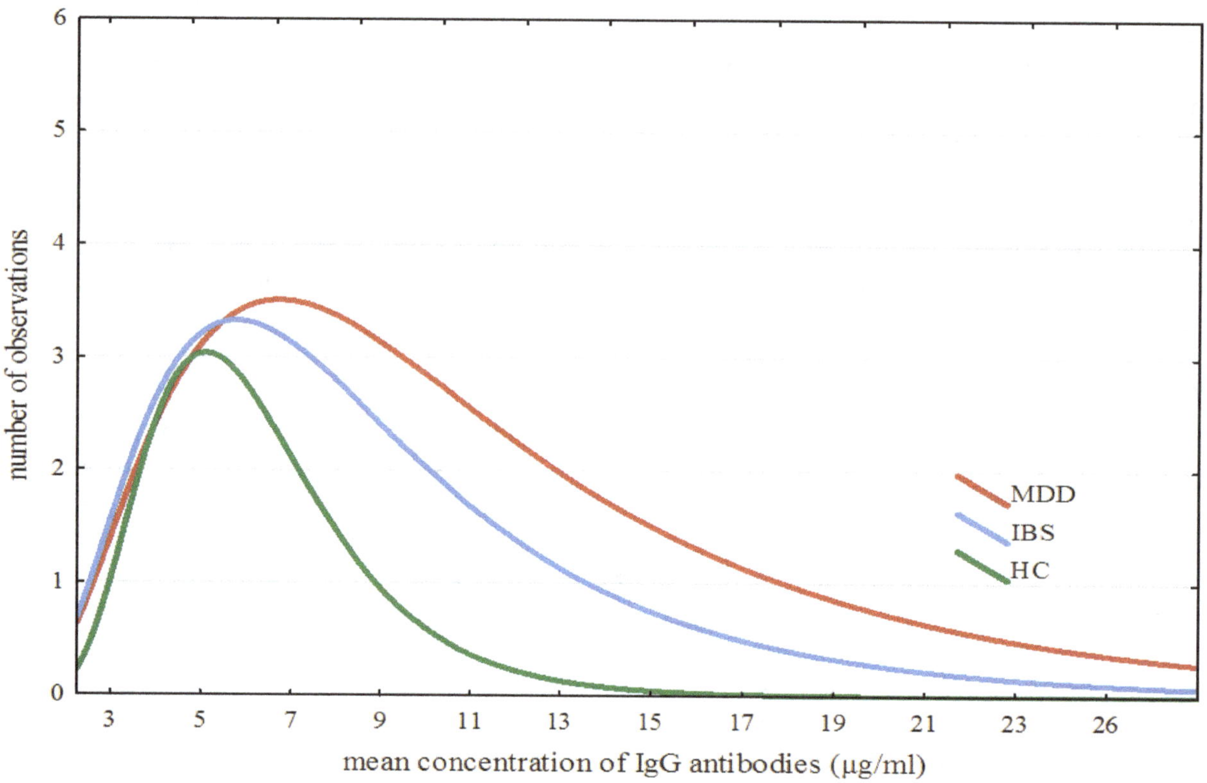

Figure 2. Specific traits of distribution of averaged results across all groups.

Due to the skewed distribution of IgG data, the comparison of obtained ex-Gaussian parameters (μ, σ and τ) for three groups was conducted with the omnibus Kruskal–Wallis rank-based nonparametric H test for comparison of more than two groups. In the case of results confirming the significant between-group difference, *post-hoc* analysis was performed with the median test, an extension of Kruskal–Wallis test enabling the comparison of all groups in pairs. This solution has been chosen instead of Mann–Whitney statistics as a *post-hoc* test, because the ranks that the pair-wise Mann–Whitney test use are not the ranks used by the Kruskal–Wallis test. Relinquishing of the Mann-Whitney test as a *post-hoc* analysis method will also reduce the risk of type I error occurrence [51].

The further statistical exploration was focused on establishing the between-group differences regarding the individual IgG results. This step of the statistical analysis was dependent on the result of the comparison concerning the ex-Gaussian parameters. When the comparison showed a significant difference between two groups, the Mann–Whitney test was used. When the difference concerned three groups, the Kruskal–Wallis test was applied, similarly as with the ex-Gaussian parameters.

All statistical analyses were performed using STATISTICA 12 (TIBCO Software Inc., CA, USA) for Windows and MATLAB software (version: R2017a, Mathworks Inc., Natick, MA, USA).

3. Results

3.1. Characteristics of the Examined Groups

General characteristics of the participants are shown in Table 1. There were no differences in age or alcohol intake between the examined groups. The MDD group had higher BMI and lower levels of physical activity compared with the IBS group. The median of coffee intake (cups/day) was higher in MDD (two cups of coffee a day) compared with IBS and HC group (0 cup of coffee a day). Interestingly, both MDD and the IBS group had more severe gastric complaints (measured during the week prior to the examination by the scale which subjectively assessed frequency and severity of symptoms; the sum of complaints ranged from 0 to 10) compared with the HC group.

Duration of illness ranged from 0.5 to 22 years across the MDD group and from 3 to 36 years across the IBS group. Three (13.63%) of the MDD patients experienced their first episode of depression, 18 (86.37%) patients had a recurrent episode of depression (the number of episodes ranging from two to 11 episodes). Eleven (50%) from MDD patients received selective serotonin reuptake inhibitors (SSRIs), four (18.18%) patients were taking Venlafaxine, five (22.73%) patients were treated with Trazodone and two (9.09%) with Mianserine. Six (31.82%) from the IBS patients had IBS with constipation, four (18.18%) IBS with diarrhoea, five (22.73%) mixed IBS and three (13.64%) unspecific IBS.

Twenty-nine (44.62%) of the patients reported using a diet in the past. Five (7.70%) patients had tried a diet with caloric restriction, including two (9.09%), two (9.09%) and one (4.76%) participants from MDD, IBS and HC group, respectively. Among sixteen (24.62%) patients who had been following an elimination diet, there had been six (27.27%) patients from the MDD group, six (27.27%) from the IBS group and four (19.05%) from HC group (see Supplementary Materials Table S1). At the moment of the examination, none of the patients were on a diet, which was one of the exclusion criteria.

Table 1. Characteristic of studied groups.

	MDD (n = 22)	IBS (n = 22)	HC (n = 21)	Analysis	*Post-hoc* Analysis
Age	31.5 (14.5)	38.5 (15.3)	34 (25)	H = 1.36, p = 0.506	–
Gender (% male)	50	45.4	57.1	χ^2 = 1.17, p = 0.554	–
BMI	28.6 (3.2)	22.8 (5.5)	25.8 (5.9)	H = 9.59, p = 0.005	MDD > IBS
Physical activity *	1 (0)	2 (0.3)	2 (1.5)	H = 7.77, p = 0.021	MDD < IBS
Number of cigarettes per day	0 (2.25)	0 (0)	0 (0)	H = 2.45, p = 0.294	–
Number of cups of coffee per day	2 (2)	0 (0)	0 (2)	H = 22.32, p <0.001	MDD > IBS MDD > HC
Intake of alcohol	4 (7.5)	4 (1)	3.5 (3.3)	H = 2.11, p = 0.348	–
Gastric complaints *	6.5 (6)	5 (5.5)	1 (3)	H = 16.25, p <0.001	MDD > HC IBS > HC
Duration of illness	5 (8)	3 (11.5)	–	Z = 0.94, p = 0.35	–

Values are shown as median (interquartile range); MDD—major depressive disorder; IBS—irritable bowel syndrome; HC—healthy controls; BMI—body mass index; H—H-value; p—p-value; χ^2—χ^2-value; Z—Z-value; * based on 10-point scale.

3.2. Seroreactivity to Food Antigens in the Examined Groups

IgG food hyperreactivity (interpreted as an average of levels of IgG antibodies above 7.5 μg/mL) was detected in 28 (43%) participants: 14 (64%) from the MDD group, ten (46%) from the IBS group and four (19%) from the HC group.

Due to substantially skewed data with increased exponential part of distribution, we decided to examine the differences in the ex-Gaussian parameters (which include differences of the normal component— σ and the extremes— τ) of total IgG serum levels between the three groups.

Figure 2 shows specific traits of distribution of averaged results across all three groups. Detailed analysis of ex-Gaussian distribution of total IgG values suggests a dissimilarity in immune responses between participants from the examined groups. The outliers of IgG levels are shaped from approximately 19–28, from approximately 14–20 and from approximately 9–13 in the MDD, IBS and HC groups, respectively.

As shown in Table 2, there were no significant differences in μ and σ parameters between the three groups. However, statistically significant differences were found in τ parameter between the examined groups. The *post-hoc* analysis revealed differences between MDD and HC groups and between IBS and HC groups.

Table 2. Differences in IgG normal part of data distribution (μ), symmetrical standard deviation (σ) and exponential part of IgG levels dispersion (τ).

ex-Gaussian Parameters	MDD *M*	IBS *M*	HC *M*	H (2, 65)	*p*	*Post-hoc* Analysis
μ	1.640	1.820	2.027	1.178	0.554	–
σ	0.001	0.175	0.463	0.883	0.642	–
τ	8.088	5.692	2.616	19.389	0.0001	MDD > HC IBS > HC

Post-hoc analysis: MDD-HC: major depressive disorder–healthy controls, $p < 0.00001$; IBS–HC: irritable bowel syndrome–healthy controls, $p = 0.018$; *M*—median; H—Kruskal-Wallis non-parametric ANOVA; *p*—*p*-value.

The comparison of serum IgG levels against various food proteins between the examined groups analysed by Kruskal–Wallis non-parametric ANOVA and the results after *post-hoc* test are shown in Table 3. We present only statistically significant results. A comparison of IgG antibodies against all analysed food proteins was summarized in Supplementary Materials (see Tables S2 and S3).

Table 3. Differences in serum IgG levels against tested food proteins.

IgG	G	M	IQR	Min	Max	Kruskal–Wallis H Test for 3 Groups		Post-hoc Analysis	
						H	p	Groups	p
Total IgG	MDD IBS HC	403.9 308.6 219.3	365.1 282.1 70.2	109.68 108.07 130.20	1075.11 1041.08 657.15	7.90	0.019	MDD > HC	0.004
Broccoli	MDD IBS HC	5.29 4.73 3.56	3.16 2.72 1.04	1.52 1.79 1.62	21.85 10.43 6.40	6.20	0.045	MDD > HC	0.039
Celery	MDD IBS HC	6.15 4.53 2.87	6.80 4.74 2.14	1.58 1.52 1.14	28.20 12.43 7.32	8.03	0.017 *	MDD > HC	0.019
Horseradish	MDD IBS HC	4.08 4.02 2.77	3.66 2.68 0.89	1.42 1.51 1.08	48.10 11.43 6.79	6.98	0.030	MDD > HC	0.024
Garlic	MDD IBS HC	6.33 2.92 2.49	7.02 4.98 1.19	1.01 0.75 0.95	75.64 15.83 10.77	7.88	0.017 *	MDD > HC	0.015
Gluten	MDD IBS HC	16.44 8.87 11.74	16.10 10.43 7.40	5.26 2.26 3.94	112.61 117.87 43.01	10.37	0.005 *	MDD > HC MDD > IBS	0.025 0.010
Wheat	MDD IBS HC	15.26 9.31 8.60	16.38 8.05 5.53	4.56 2.28 3.28	99.42 122.13 47.22	6.79	0.033	MDD > HC	0.043
Rye	MDD IBS HC	11.41 7.38 5.59	8.42 8.14 4.94	3.73 2.10 2.08	108.92 28.52 38.05	7.23	0.026	MDD > HC	0.032
Sunflower seed	MDD IBS HC	6.22 3.06 3.13	5.84 2.94 2.45	1.43 0.91 0.74	46.15 68.05 61.62	7.07	0.029	MDD > IBS	0.038
Milk products	MDD IBS HC	27.57 20.00 6.86	39.82 42.78 5.46	1.62 1.24 0.96	110.57 119.30 86.24	7.59	0.025	MDD > HC	0.019

* Differences statistically significant also after *post-hoc* analysis; G—group; *M*—median; IQR—interquartile range; H—H-value; *p*—*p*-value. MDD—major depressive disorder; IBS—irritable bowel syndrome; HC—healthy controls.

There was a difference in total serum IgG levels between MDD and HC groups. Patients suffering from MDD had significantly higher serum levels of total examined IgG antibodies. An analysis of individual IgG levels revealed that patients with MDD had significantly higher IgG levels against broccoli, celery, horseradish, garlic, gluten, wheat, rye and milk products compared with HC group. The MDD group also had statistically higher serum IgG levels against gluten and sunflower seed compared with IBS patients. After *post-hoc* analysis, statistical significance was achieved only by results in differences of serum concentrations of IgG against celery, garlic and gluten between MDD and HC groups and against gluten between MDD and the IBS groups.

We find no correlations between gender, age, BMI, number of cigarettes and cups of coffee per day, intake of alcohol, physical activity, duration of illness and serum total IgG levels across the examined groups. Similarly, correlations between gastric complaints and serum IgG levels were not found in IBS and HC groups. However, there was a positive correlation between total IgG level and gastric complaints in the MDD group ($p < 0.05$; $R = 0.66$).

We performed another statistical analysis on the group of IBS patients divided into two subgroups, i.e., with diarrhoea (IBS-D) and non-diarrhoea (IBS-ND). We did not find any differences either in the total IgG levels ($p > 0.05$) or in the levels of specific IgG antibodies ($p > 0.05$) between the IBS-D and IBS-ND patients. Focusing on differences between IBS subtypes seems to be a promising avenue for future research on bigger groups of patients suffering from IBS. As for our study, due to unequal numbers of patients in 4 groups resulting from the division of the IBS group, multiple-group analysis could not be conducted.

4. Discussion

There are numerous studies which confirm IgG hyperreactivity to food antigens in patients with IBS [27,38,52–59].

Due to this substantial amount of evidence and an unclear association between MDD and IgG hyperreactivity, we decided to compare levels of IgG antibodies against food between IBS, MDD patients and healthy controls.

The results of our study indicate differences between the examined groups in the proportion of people whose total IgG values exceeded the cut off level (>7.5 μg/mL). Unusually, most cases of hyperreactivity were found in MDD (64%) group and the least number in HC (19%) group. As revealed by the *post-hoc* comparisons of the paired groups, total IgG in the examined groups showed differences between MDD patients and healthy controls, no such dissimilarity was found between the IBS group and HC group. It was the application of ex-Gaussian modelling (due to substantially skewed data with increased exponential part of distribution) that revealed differences in tau (τ) (which displays the extremes in IgG results) between MDD and HC groups and also between the IBS and HC groups.

Further analysis demonstrated the presence of many distinctions in individual levels of IgG depending on the type of illness. There were differences in levels of IgG against celery, garlic and gluten between MDD and HC groups and levels of IgG against gluten between the IBS and MDD groups.

Our results indicate a dissimilarity in the immune response to food antigens among the three studied groups, surprisingly, with the highest immunoreactivity in patients suffering from MDD compared with healthy controls. A possible mechanism of the phenomenon remains obscure.

On the one hand, a possible cause of the hyperreactivity among patients with MDD may be disruption of gut-microbiome-brain axis, which is related to low-grade inflammation occurring peripherally and in the CNS [19]. It is suggested that altered gut microbiota could be responsible for increased gut permeability.

Evidence from model studies confirms that intragastric administration of *Clostridium butyricum* contributes to improvements in mucosa and BBB integrity and inhibition of neuroinflammation processes [60]. What is more, one recent study on patients with mood disorders revealed that the disruption of gut barrier integrity could be a result of gut dysbiosis. Based on the analysis of fecal microbiota, researchers demonstrated that patients with MDD and anxiety were characterized by over-representation of genes involved in LPS biosynthesis and deleterious metabolism of mood neurotransmitter pathways. The patients with mood disorders had also higher levels of plasma LPS, zonulin and fatty-acid binding protein 2 (FABP2) which reflected gut permeability [61]. However, it is still poorly understood whether intestinal barrier dysfunction is a cause or a consequence of MDD or it exists merely in some group of patients regardless of the disease.

On the other hand, there is some evidence that due to gut-brain signaling, inflammation of CNS could lead to secondary disruptions of the digestive tract. More and more studies show that neuroinflammation is a cause of chronic mucosal damage in the gut and hyperreactivity of enteric glial cells. The intestinal barrier disruptions manifest themselves by long-term neurobehavioral changes [62,63]. Post-mortem studies demonstrated that neuroinflammation was involved in pathophysiology of depression [64,65].

A scenario proposed by Karakula-Juchnowicz et al. that links the inflammatory theory of depression with IgG food hypersensitivity and leaky gut syndrome assumes that loss of integrity of the tight-junction barrier could be caused by food antigens [19]. Overproduction of zonulin triggered, for example, by gliadin through activation of the epidermal growth factor receptor and protease-activated receptor causes loosening of the tight junction barrier and an increase in permeability of the gut wall. Afterwards, intestinal permeability allows food-derived compounds cross into bloodstream and activate the immune response which is involved in overproduction of proinflammatory cytokines, their transport across BBB and, consequently, the presence of clinical manifestation of depression [19]. There is a substantial body of evidence that there is a link between food-derived antigens and other psychiatric disorders with the suggested role of inflammation in their pathogenesis [66]. Okusaga et al. revealed a possible relationship between non-celiac gluten sensitivity dependent on IgG antibodies and inflammatory pathways. In the mentioned study, schizophrenic patients with elevated anti-gliadin IgG had increased serum kynurenine levels and kynurenine to tryptophan ratio compared with patients without increased anti-gliadin IgG. Tryptophan to kynurenine conversion is linked with inflammation and raised cortisol levels [67]. Another study found that anti-casein IgG antibodies are linked with type I bipolar disorder, psychotic symptoms and mania severity [68].

So far, the number of studies exploring seroreactivity to food antigens in patients with MDD has been insufficient. Only one observation has been made and its results remain inconclusive. The paper in question reports no differences in mean IgG concentrations between MDD patients and healthy persons. The researchers observed lower levels of IgG against dietary proteins in patients with MDD who had high exposure to milk proteins compared with the control group with high exposure. Surprisingly, the authors found lower levels of tumour necrosis factor-alpha (TNF-alpha) and higher levels of cortisol in sera of the patients relative to the control subjects [69]. TNF-alpha and interleukin 6 (IL-6) are considered to be well-known inflammatory factors involved in pathophysiology of depression, as supported by a meta-analysis done by Köhler et al. in 2017 [70]. Also, the results of the studies on anti-inflammatory effects of cortisol [71] have not been confirmed in MDD patients where excess cortisol secretion was associated with higher levels of proinflammatory cytokines [72]. These findings confirmed the notion that glucocorticoid resistance, cortisol hypersecretion and increased inflammation are indeed coexistent and related biological abnormalities [73]. An interesting observation made by Rudzki et al. [69] is the link between TNF-alpha concentration and total food IgG level, indicating a potential relationship between IgG reactivity to dietary proteins and low-grade inflammation. Some explanation for the discrepant results obtained by Rudzki et al. [69] may be provided by findings from the study by Lamers at al. [74] pointing to a differential role of HPA-axis function, inflammation and metabolic syndrome in melancholic versus atypical depression. The proportion of 50% of patients with melancholic depression versus 11.76% of patients with atypical depression in the study by Rudzki et al. [69] could have had a substantial influence on a lack of differences in IgG levels between the patients and the healthy controls. A relatively small size of the group of patients and statistical analysis conducted by means of classical methods may also have affected the validity of the observations.

Our results regarding differences between IBS and HC are partly consistent with findings from other studies and indicated that serum IgG antibody levels of some common foods are abnormally elevated in IBS patients [75,76]. We did not find differences in total IgG levels between IBS and HC groups until we applied ex-Gaussian modelling which allowed us find differences in the extreme results (τ) of IgG levels between these two groups. Based on elevated IgG above the cut-off point we detected dissimilarity between IBS (46%) and HC (19%). However, we did not find differences in individual levels of IgG.

This lack of consistency with findings from other studies could be a consequence of a relatively small size of the group. On the other hand, this may be explained by attempts of IBS patients to cut down on foods aggravating their symptoms such as bloating or constipation. Taking into account that gastrointestinal complaints are the core of IBS [77], patients suffering from this disorder might intuitively cut down on the food products that, in their opinion, worsen the symptoms [39,78], yet without calling this practice "following a diet". From a clinical perspective, such behaviour is not tantamount to an elimination diet, which was an exclusion criterion from our study. However, it might lead to decreased exposure to a specific food antigen, possibly affecting IgG levels. For this reason, further research aimed at finding differences in food IgG levels between the groups studied should determine food intake and eating frequency in order to evaluate exposure to the food products studied. It is worth mentioning that an elimination diet is a method used to reduce IgG antibodies in the case of high concentrations of IgG against food proteins [78]. On the other hand, results of studies concentrated on the relationship between food-IgG exposure and dietary habits are contradictory [69,79], so research aimed at assessing differences in IgG antibodies against food, especially food with high FODMAP concentration levels (e.g., garlic, gluten, broccoli), between healthy controls and IBS patients should strictly determine the time between the discontinuation of the diet and IgG examination.

A positive response to a diet based on IgG antibodies against food has been reported in several different diseases, such as migraine [49,80], obesity [81], Crohn disease [82]. A common thread of all above cases is inflammation. Recent data provide evidence that inflammatory processes are considered to be an important factor for the development of both depression and IBS [12,83,84]. To our knowledge, there are no randomized control trials supporting potential utility of an elimination diet in patients with MDD, however, it has been shown that an elimination diet based on specific IgG antibodies against food may alleviate symptoms in patients suffering from IBS [27,37–39].

In a double blind, randomized, controlled, parallel study, Atkinson et al. [27] showed significant reduction in severity of symptoms in patients with IBS due to an elimination diet based on a IgG test compared to a sham diet (not based on increased quantities of IgG-antibodies). The quality of life also improved after following an IgG-based diet. The authors calculated that three patients out of four should be treated with this approach. After reintroduction of the respective foods the researchers observed the reverse response in the patients. Those findings are consistent with a study by Drisko et al. [38]. They also show a significant improvement of symptoms in patients with IBS. The researchers demonstrated increased titres of specific IgG antibodies for selected food in this group of patients. After 6 months on a diet without products with increased IgG concentration, patients with IBS demonstrated improvement in stool frequency, pain relief and the quality of life.

In turn, Zuo et al. [52] analysed patients with IBS and FD (functional dyspepsia) in comparison to the control group in terms of specific IgG, IgE antibody and total IgE antibody titres. They demonstrated that IBS patients had significantly higher titres of IgG antibody to crab, egg, shrimp, soybean and wheat than controls. FD patients had significantly higher titres of IgG antibody to egg and soybean than controls. Interestingly, there was no correlation in percent of patients with positive specific IgE antibodies in the three groups. There were no significant differences between IBS patients, FD patients and controls in the serum total IgE antibody levels. Guo et al. [57] evaluated the benefit of an IgG-based diet in patients with IBS with diarrhoea form (IBS-D) of the disease. The phase of 12-week elimination of food products with increased IgG resulted in improvement in IBS-D participants compared with the baseline. The researchers showed amelioration in abdominal pain (bloating level and frequency), diarrhoea frequency, abdominal distension, stool shape, general feelings of distress and total symptom score.

An interesting study was conducted by Aydinlar et al. [56]. In this double-blind, randomized, controlled, cross-over clinical trial individuals suffering from both migraine and IBS could take advantage of IgG-based elimination diet. An individual diet approach may effectively alleviate conditions such as migraine attack, maximum attack duration, mean attack duration, maximum attack severity and number of attacks with acute medication, as well as abdominal symptoms: pain-bloating severity, pain-bloating within the last 10 days, and also improvement in quality of life. Nonetheless, the small sample (21 patients) and funding bias of the examination should be pointed out as a weakness of the study.

Despite many results confirming the clinical manifestation of elevated levels of IgG antibodies against food antigens, the diagnosis based on their elimination is controversial. Numerous allergy societies question the usefulness of IgG antibodies tests as a diagnostic method for assessing adverse reactions to food intake [85–88], nevertheless, some recommend using IgG antibodies tests for research purposes [88]. It is known that IgG4 is an antibody involved in the desensitization of type I allergies (IgE-dependent) [89]. There is some new evidence that patients with IBS my present increased IgG4 titres [76], but this still needs clarification. It is worth mentioning that not all subclasses of IgG are involved in desensitization. Furthermore, they are able to form an immune complex with bounded food antigens. Such complexes are destroyed by pathogenic cells which leads to the release of proinflammatory cytokines. Aljada et al. showed that food intake is able to induce significant inflammatory changes, which has been characterized by a decrease in IkappaBalpha and an increase in NF-kappaB binding, plasma C-reactive protein (CRP), and the expression of IKKalpha, IKKbeta as well as p47 (phox) subunit [90]. This state induces a low-grade inflammation condition which may be aggravating for the body. It is documented that individuals with IBS may present low-grade inflammatory process in the gut mucosa which is not always connected with a history of a gastrointestinal infection [22]. Therefore, testing IgG against food could be one of the novel diagnostic approach to identify triggers leading to inflammation in these conditions, and administration of diet based on concentration of specific IgG may exert a beneficial effect in patients with IBS and depression.

5. Conclusions

Multiple lines of evidence increasingly point towards a role of environmental factors and disrupted gut–brain axis function both in many neuropsychiatric disorders, including depression, and in gastrointestinal disorders, including IBS [19,91–93]. The wide range of factors involved in the disturbances are considered, including changes in the mucosal immune system, the microbiota dysbioses and amounts of short chain fatty acids dependent on microbiota, exposure to xenobiotics, gut permeability, food IgG antibodies [91–95].

Our findings suggest more common food-specific serum IgG hyperreactivity among patients with IBS and MDD compared with HC, which may be one of the mechanisms leading to the development of immune activation and low-grade inflammation observed in these disorders.

Interestingly, the highest reactivity was observed in the group of MDD patients, the fact that may be of great importance for both theoretical considerations on MDD etiopathogenesis and therapeutic implications for this disorder. There is no causal relationship which could confirm clinical utility of an elimination diet in patients with MDD, however, some evidence suggests reduction of symptoms in patients with IBS who followed an IgG-based elimination diet.

To the best of our knowledge, this is the first paper published worldwide to compare IgG reactivity to food antigens in patients with these two disorders and we are of the opinion that further studies are needed to repeat and confirm these results in bigger cohorts and to examine clinical utility and duration of IgG-based elimination diet in patients with MDD and with IBS.

Author Contributions: H.K-J., M.G. and D.J. conceived and designed the experiments; H.K-J., M.G., D.J., A.B. and Z.L. performed the experiments; P.K., J.R., K.J., J.M-T. K.S-Z., and T.K. analyzed the data; M.G., K.J. contributed reagents and analysis tools. Writing of the manuscript was done by H.K-J, J.R., A.B., D.J. and Z.L. with final content reviewed by H.K-J. All authors have given approval of the final manuscript.

Acknowledgments: The authors would like to thank Ewa Wisniewska-Ligeza for excellent language and technical assistance. This study was supported by a research grant from the Medical University of Lublin (DS 192/18).

References

1. Klein, D.N.; Hajcak, G. Heterogeneity of Depression: Clinical Considerations and Psychophysiological Measures. *Psychol. Inq.* **2015**, *26*, 247–252. [CrossRef]
2. World Health Organization. Depression. Available online: http://www.who.int/mediacentre/factsheets/fs369/en/ (accessed on 5 December 2017).
3. Uher, R. Gene-environment interactions in common mental disorders: An update and strategy for a genome-wide search. *Soc. Psychiatry Psychiatr. Epidemiol.* **2014**, *49*, 3–14. [CrossRef] [PubMed]
4. Dunn, E.C.; Brown, R.C.; Dai, Y.; Rosand, J.; Nugent, N.R.; Amstadter, A.B.; Smoller, J.W. Genetic determinants of depression: Recent findings and future directions. *Harv. Rev. Psychiatry* **2015**, *23*, 1. [CrossRef] [PubMed]
5. Smith, R.S. The macrophage theory of depression. *Med. Hypotheses* **1991**, *35*, 298–306. [CrossRef]
6. Dantzer, R. Role of the Kynurenine metabolism pathway in inflammation-induced depression: Preclinical approaches. In *Inflammation-Associated Depression: Evidence, Mechanisms and Implications*; Springer: Berlin, Germany, 2016; pp. 117–138.
7. Dahl, J.; Ormstad, H.; Aass, H.; Sandvik, L.; Malt, U.; Andreassen, O. Recovery from major depressive disorder episode after non-pharmacological treatment is associated with normalized cytokine levels. *Acta Psychiatr. Scand.* **2016**, *134*, 40–47. [CrossRef] [PubMed]
8. Lopresti, A.L.; Maker, G.L.; Hood, S.D.; Drummond, P.D. A review of peripheral biomarkers in major depression: The potential of inflammatory and oxidative stress biomarkers. *Prog. Neuro-Psychopharmacol. Biol. Psychiatry* **2014**, *48*, 102–111. [CrossRef] [PubMed]
9. Young, J.J.; Bruno, D.; Pomara, N. A review of the relationship between proinflammatory cytokines and major depressive disorder. *J. Affect. Disord.* **2014**, *169*, 15–20. [CrossRef] [PubMed]
10. Köhler, O.; Benros, M.E.; Nordentoft, M.; Farkouh, M.E.; Iyengar, R.L.; Mors, O.; Krogh, J. Effect of anti-inflammatory treatment on depression, depressive symptoms, and adverse effects: A systematic review and meta-analysis of randomized clinical trials. *JAMA Psychiatry* **2014**, *71*, 1381–1391. [CrossRef] [PubMed]
11. Ruiz-Núñez, B.; Pruimboom, L.; Dijck-Brouwer, D.J.; Muskiet, F.A. Lifestyle and nutritional imbalances associated with Western diseases: Causes and consequences of chronic systemic low-grade inflammation in an evolutionary context. *J. Nutr. Biochem.* **2013**, *24*, 1183–1201. [CrossRef] [PubMed]
12. Maes, M.; Kubera, M.; Leunis, J.-C. The gut-brain barrier in major depression: Intestinal mucosal dysfunction with an increased translocation of LPS from gram negative enterobacteria (leaky gut) plays a role in the inflammatory pathophysiology of depression. *Neuroendocrinol. Lett.* **2008**, *29*, 117–124. [CrossRef]
13. Thevaranjan, N.; Puchta, A.; Schulz, C.; Naidoo, A.; Szamosi, J.; Verschoor, C.P.; Loukov, D.; Schenck, L.P.; Jury, J.; Foley, K.P. Age-Associated Microbial Dysbiosis Promotes Intestinal Permeability, Systemic Inflammation, and Macrophage Dysfunction. *Cell Host Microbe* **2017**, *21*, 455–466.e454. [CrossRef] [PubMed]
14. Fasano, A. Zonulin and its regulation of intestinal barrier function: The biological door to inflammation, autoimmunity, and cancer. *Physiol. Rev.* **2011**, *91*, 151–175. [CrossRef] [PubMed]
15. Lin, R.; Zhou, L.; Zhang, J.; Wang, B. Abnormal intestinal permeability and microbiota in patients with autoimmune hepatitis. *Int. J. Clin. Exp. Pathol.* **2015**, *8*, 5153. [PubMed]
16. Clairembault, T.; Leclair-Visonneau, L.; Coron, E.; Bourreille, A.; Le Dily, S.; Vavasseur, F.; Heymann, M.-F.; Neunlist, M.; Derkinderen, P. Structural alterations of the intestinal epithelial barrier in Parkinson's disease. *Acta Neuropathol. Commun.* **2015**, *3*, 12. [CrossRef] [PubMed]
17. Szachta, P.; Bartnicka, A.; Galecka, M.; Skonieczna-Zydecka, K. Microbiota disorders and food hypersensitivity in autism spectrum disorders; what do we know? *J. Exp. Integr. Med.* **2015**, *5*, 117–120. [CrossRef]

18. Esnafoglu, E.; Cırrık, S.; Ayyıldız, S.N.; Erdil, A.; Ertürk, E.Y.; Daglı, A.; Noyan, T. Increased serum zonulin levels as an intestinal permeability marker in autistic subjects. *J. Pediatr.* **2017**, *188*, 240–244. [CrossRef] [PubMed]
19. Karakuła-Juchnowicz, H.; Szachta, P.; Opolska, A.; Morylowska-Topolska, J.; Gałęcka, M.; Juchnowicz, D.; Krukow, P.; Lasik, Z. The role of IgG hypersensitivity in the pathogenesis and therapy of depressive disorders. *Nutr. Neurosci.* **2017**, *20*, 110–118. [CrossRef] [PubMed]
20. Lovell, R.M.; Ford, A.C. Global prevalence of and risk factors for irritable bowel syndrome: A meta-analysis. *Clin. Gastroenterol. Hepatol.* **2012**, *10*, 712–721.e714. [CrossRef] [PubMed]
21. Sinagra, E.; Pompei, G.; Tomasello, G.; Cappello, F.; Morreale, G.C.; Amvrosiadis, G.; Rossi, F.; Monte, A.I.L.; Rizzo, A.G.; Raimondo, D. Inflammation in irritable bowel syndrome: Myth or new treatment target? *World J. Gastroenterol.* **2016**, *22*, 2242. [CrossRef] [PubMed]
22. Spiller, R.C. Infection, immune function, and functional gut disorders. *Clin. Gastroenterol. Hepatol.* **2004**, *2*, 445–455. [CrossRef]
23. Li, F.X.; Patten, S.B.; Hilsden, R.J.; Sutherland, L.R. Irritable bowel syndrome and health-related quality of life: A population-based study in Calgary, Alberta. *Can. J. Gastroenterol. Hepatol.* **2003**, *17*, 259–263. [CrossRef]
24. Longstreth, G.F.; Thompson, W.G.; Chey, W.D.; Houghton, L.A.; Mearin, F.; Spiller, R.C. Functional bowel disorders. *Gastroenterology* **2006**, *130*, 1480–1491. [CrossRef] [PubMed]
25. Jeffery, I.B.; O'toole, P.W.; Öhman, L.; Claesson, M.J.; Deane, J.; Quigley, E.M.; Simrén, M. An irritable bowel syndrome subtype defined by species-specific alterations in faecal microbiota. *Gut* **2012**, *61*, 997–1006. [CrossRef] [PubMed]
26. Foxx-Orenstein, A.E. New and emerging therapies for the treatment of irritable bowel syndrome: An update for gastroenterologists. *Ther. Adv. Gastroenterol.* **2016**, *9*, 354–375. [CrossRef] [PubMed]
27. Atkinson, W.; Sheldon, T.; Shaath, N.; Whorwell, P. Food elimination based on IgG antibodies in irritable bowel syndrome: A randomised controlled trial. *Gut* **2004**, *53*, 1459–1464. [CrossRef] [PubMed]
28. Shih, D.Q.; Kwan, L.Y. All roads lead to Rome: Update on Rome III criteria and new treatment options. *Gastroenterol. Rep.* **2007**, *1*, 56. [PubMed]
29. Marsh, A.; Eslick, E.M.; Eslick, G.D. Does a diet low in FODMAPs reduce symptoms associated with functional gastrointestinal disorders? A comprehensive systematic review and meta-analysis. *Eur. J. Nutr.* **2016**, *55*, 897–906. [CrossRef] [PubMed]
30. McKenzie, Y.; Bowyer, R.; Leach, H.; Gulia, P.; Horobin, J.; O'sullivan, N.; Pettitt, C.; Reeves, L.; Seamark, L.; Williams, M. British Dietetic Association systematic review and evidence-based practice guidelines for the dietary management of irritable bowel syndrome in adults (2016 update). *J. Hum. Nutr. Diet.* **2016**, *29*, 549–575. [CrossRef] [PubMed]
31. Barmeyer, C.; Schumann, M.; Meyer, T.; Zielinski, C.; Zuberbier, T.; Siegmund, B.; Schulzke, J.-D.; Daum, S.; Ullrich, R. Long-term response to gluten-free diet as evidence for non-celiac wheat sensitivity in one third of patients with diarrhea-dominant and mixed-type irritable bowel syndrome. *Int. J. Colorectal Dis.* **2017**, *32*, 29–39. [CrossRef] [PubMed]
32. Catassi, C.; Alaedini, A.; Bojarski, C.; Bonaz, B.; Bouma, G.; Carroccio, A.; Castillejo, G.; De Magistris, L.; Dieterich, W.; Di Liberto, D. The Overlapping Area of Non-Celiac Gluten Sensitivity (NCGS) and Wheat-Sensitive Irritable Bowel Syndrome (IBS): An Update. *Nutrients* **2017**, *9*, 1268. [CrossRef] [PubMed]
33. Böhmer, C.J.; Tuynman, H.A. The effect of a lactose-restricted diet in patients with a positive lactose tolerance test, earlier diagnosed as irritable bowel syndrome: A 5-year follow-up study. *Eur. J. Gastroenterol. Hepatol.* **2001**, *13*, 941–944. [CrossRef] [PubMed]
34. Defrees, D.N.; Bailey, J. Irritable Bowel Syndrome: Epidemiology, Pathophysiology, Diagnosis, and Treatment. *Prim. Care Clin. Off. Pract.* **2017**, *44*, 655–671. [CrossRef] [PubMed]
35. Halmos, E.P. When the low FODMAP diet does not work. *J. Gastroenterol. Hepatol.* **2017**, *32*, 69–72. [CrossRef] [PubMed]
36. Hill, P.; Muir, J.G.; Gibson, P.R. Controversies and Recent Developments of the Low-FODMAP Diet. *Gastroenterol. Hepatol.* **2017**, *13*, 36.
37. Zar, S.; Mincher, L.; Benson, M.J.; Kumar, D. Food-specific IgG4 antibody-guided exclusion diet improves symptoms and rectal compliance in irritable bowel syndrome. *Scand. J. Gastroenterol.* **2005**, *40*, 800–807. [CrossRef] [PubMed]

38. Drisko, J.; Bischoff, B.; Hall, M.; McCallum, R. Treating irritable bowel syndrome with a food elimination diet followed by food challenge and probiotics. *J. Am. Coll. Nutr.* **2006**, *25*, 514–522. [CrossRef] [PubMed]
39. Monsbakken, K.; Vandvik, P.; Farup, P. Perceived food intolerance in subjects with irritable bowel syndrome–etiology, prevalence and consequences. *Eur. J. Clin. Nutr.* **2006**, *60*, 667–672. [CrossRef] [PubMed]
40. Böhn, L.; Störsrud, S.; Törnblom, H.; Bengtsson, U.; Simrén, M. Self-reported food-related gastrointestinal symptoms in IBS are common and associated with more severe symptoms and reduced quality of life. *Am. J. Gastroenterol.* **2013**, *108*, 634–641.
41. Fritscher-Ravens, A.; Schuppan, D.; Ellrichmann, M.; Schoch, S.; Röcken, C.; Brasch, J.; Bethge, J.; Böttner, M.; Klose, J.; Milla, P.J. Confocal endomicroscopy shows food-associated changes in the intestinal mucosa of patients with irritable bowel syndrome. *Gastroenterology* **2014**, *147*, 1012–1020.e1014. [CrossRef] [PubMed]
42. American Psychiatric Association (APA). *Diagnostic and Statistical Manual of Mental Disorders*, 5th ed.; American Psychiatric Publishing: Arlington, VA, USA, 2013.
43. Hossain, M.I.; Nahar, B.; Hamadani, J.D.; Ahmed, T.; Roy, A.K.; Brown, K.H. Intestinal mucosal permeability of severely underweight and nonmalnourished Bangladeshi children and effects of nutritional rehabilitation. *J. Pediatr. Gastroenterol. Nutr.* **2010**, *51*, 638–644. [CrossRef] [PubMed]
44. Gummesson, A.; Carlsson, L.M.; Storlien, L.H.; Backhed, F.; Lundin, P.; Lofgren, L.; Stenlof, K.; Lam, Y.Y.; Fagerberg, B.; Carlsson, B. Intestinal permeability is associated with visceral adiposity in healthy women. *Obesity* **2011**, *19*, 2280–2282. [CrossRef] [PubMed]
45. Genton, L.; Cani, P.D.; Schrenzel, J. Alterations of gut barrier and gut microbiota in food restriction, food deprivation and protein-energy wasting. *Clin. Nutr.* **2015**, *34*, 341–349. [CrossRef] [PubMed]
46. Karakula-Juchnowicz, H.; Pankowicz, H.; Juchnowicz, D.; Valverde Piedra, J.L.; Malecka-Massalska, T. Intestinal microbiota—A key to understanding the pathophysiology of anorexia nervosa? *Psychiatr. Pol.* **2017**, *51*, 859–870. [CrossRef] [PubMed]
47. Seganfredo, F.B.; Blume, C.A.; Moehlecke, M.; Giongo, A.; Casagrande, D.S.; Spolidoro, J.V.N.; Padoin, A.V.; Schaan, B.D.; Mottin, C.C. Weight-loss interventions and gut microbiota changes in overweight and obese patients: A systematic review. *Obes. Rev.* **2017**, *18*, 832–851. [CrossRef] [PubMed]
48. Alpay, K.; Ertaş, M.; Orhan, E.K.; Üstay, D.K.; Lieners, C.; Baykan, B. Diet restriction in migraine, based on IgG against foods: A clinical double-blind, randomised, cross-over trial. *Cephalalgia* **2010**, *30*, 829–837. [CrossRef] [PubMed]
49. Zeng, Q.; Dong, S.Y.; Wu, L.X.; Li, H.; Sun, Z.J.; Li, J.B.; Jiang, H.X.; Chen, Z.H.; Wang, Q.B.; Chen, W.W. Variable food-specific IgG antibody levels in healthy and symptomatic Chinese adults. *PLoS ONE* **2013**, *8*, e53612. [CrossRef] [PubMed]
50. Lacouture, Y.; Cousineau, D. How to use MATLAB to fit the ex-Gaussian and other probability functions to a distribution of response times. *Tutor. Quant. Methods Psychol.* **2008**, *4*, 35–45. [CrossRef]
51. Field, A.; Hole, G. *How to Design and Report Experiments*; Sage: Newcastle, UK, 2002.
52. Zuo, X.; Li, Y.; Li, W.; Guo, Y.; Lu, X.; Li, J.; Desmond, P. Alterations of food antigen-specific serum immunoglobulins G and E antibodies in patients with irritable bowel syndrome and functional dyspepsia. *Clin. Exp. Allergy* **2007**, *37*, 823–830. [CrossRef] [PubMed]
53. Isolauri, E.; Rautava, S.; Kalliomäki, M. Food allergy in irritable bowel syndrome: New facts and old fallacies. *Gut* **2004**, *53*, 1391–1393. [CrossRef] [PubMed]
54. Whorwell, P.; Lea, R. Dietary treatment of the irritable bowel syndrome. *Curr. Treat. Opt. Gastroenterol.* **2004**, *7*, 307–316. [CrossRef]
55. Anthoni, S.; Savilahti, E.; Rautelin, H.; Kolho, K.-L. Milk protein IgG and IgA: The association with milk-induced gastrointestinal symptoms in adults. *World J. Gastroenterol. WJG* **2009**, *15*, 4915. [CrossRef] [PubMed]
56. Aydinlar, E.I.; Dikmen, P.Y.; Tiftikci, A.; Saruc, M.; Aksu, M.; Gunsoy, H.G.; Tozun, N. IgG-based elimination diet in migraine plus irritable bowel syndrome. *Headache J. Head Face Pain* **2013**, *53*, 514–525. [CrossRef] [PubMed]
57. Guo, H.; Jiang, T.; Wang, J.; Chang, Y.; Guo, H.; Zhang, W. The value of eliminating foods according to food-specific immunoglobulin G antibodies in irritable bowel syndrome with diarrhoea. *J. Int. Med. Res.* **2012**, *40*, 204–210. [CrossRef] [PubMed]
58. Vazquez-Roque, M.I.; Camilleri, M.; Smyrk, T.; Murray, J.A.; Marietta, E.; O'Neill, J.; Carlson, P.; Lamsam, J.; Janzow, D.; Eckert, D. A controlled trial of gluten-free diet in patients with irritable bowel syndrome-diarrhea: Effects on bowel frequency and intestinal function. *Gastroenterology* **2013**, *144*, 903–911.e903. [CrossRef] [PubMed]

59. Mansueto, P.; D'Alcamo, A.; Seidita, A.; Carroccio, A. Food allergy in irritable bowel syndrome: The case of non-celiac wheat sensitivity. *World J. Gastroenterol. WJG* **2015**, *21*, 7089. [CrossRef] [PubMed]
60. Li, H.; Sun, J.; Du, J.; Wang, F.; Fang, R.; Yu, C.; Xiong, J.; Chen, W.; Lu, Z.; Liu, J. Clostridium butyricum exerts a neuroprotective effect in a mouse model of traumatic brain injury via the gut-brain axis. *Neurogastroenterol. Motil.* **2017**. [CrossRef] [PubMed]
61. Stevens, B.R.; Goel, R.; Seungbum, K.; Richards, E.M.; Holbert, R.C.; Pepine, C.J.; Raizada, M.K. Increased human intestinal barrier permeability plasma biomarkers zonulin and FABP2 correlated with plasma LPS and altered gut microbiome in anxiety or depression. *Gut* **2017**. gutjnl-2017-314759. [CrossRef] [PubMed]
62. Katzenberger, R.J.; Ganetzky, B.; Wassarman, D.A. The gut reaction to traumatic brain injury. *Fly* **2015**, *9*, 68–74. [CrossRef] [PubMed]
63. Ma, E.L.; Smith, A.D.; Desai, N.; Cheung, L.; Hanscom, M.; Stoica, B.A.; Loane, D.J.; Shea-Donohue, T.; Faden, A.I. Bidirectional brain-gut interactions and chronic pathological changes after traumatic brain injury in mice. *Brain Behav. Immun.* **2017**, *66*, 56–69. [CrossRef] [PubMed]
64. Torres-Platas, S.G.; Cruceanu, C.; Chen, G.G.; Turecki, G.; Mechawar, N. Evidence for increased microglial priming and macrophage recruitment in the dorsal anterior cingulate white matter of depressed suicides. *Brain Behav. Immun.* **2014**, *42*, 50–59. [CrossRef] [PubMed]
65. Setiawan, E.; Wilson, A.A.; Mizrahi, R.; Rusjan, P.M.; Miler, L.; Rajkowska, G.; Suridjan, I.; Kennedy, J.L.; Rekkas, P.V.; Houle, S. Role of translocator protein density, a marker of neuroinflammation, in the brain during major depressive episodes. *JAMA Psychiatry* **2015**, *72*, 268–275. [CrossRef] [PubMed]
66. Hart, G.R. Food-specific IgG guided elimination diet; a role in mental health? *BAOJ Nutr.* **2017**, *3*, 045.
67. Okusaga, O.; Fuchs, D.; Reeves, G.; Giegling, I.; Hartmann, A.M.; Konte, B.; Friedl, M.; Groer, M.; Cook, T.B.; Stearns-Yoder, K.A. Kynurenine and Tryptophan Levels in Patients With Schizophrenia and Elevated Antigliadin Immunoglobulin G Antibodies. *Psychosom. Med.* **2016**, *78*, 931–939. [CrossRef] [PubMed]
68. Severance, E.G.; Gressitt, K.L.; Yang, S.; Stallings, C.R.; Origoni, A.E.; Vaughan, C.; Khushalani, S.; Alaedini, A.; Dickerson, F.B.; Yolken, R.H. Seroreactive marker for inflammatory bowel disease and associations with antibodies to dietary proteins in bipolar disorder. *Bipolar Disord.* **2014**, *16*, 230–240. [CrossRef] [PubMed]
69. Rudzki, L.; Pawlak, D.; Pawlak, K.; Waszkiewicz, N.; Małus, A.; Konarzewska, B.; Gałęcka, M.; Bartnicka, A.; Ostrowska, L.; Szulc, A. Immune suppression of IgG response against dairy proteins in major depression. *BMC Psychiatry* **2017**, *17*, 268. [CrossRef] [PubMed]
70. Köhler, C.; Freitas, T.; Maes, M.; Andrade, N.; Liu, C.; Fernandes, B.; Stubbs, B.; Solmi, M.; Veronese, N.; Herrmann, N. Peripheral cytokine and chemokine alterations in depression: A meta-analysis of 82 studies. *Acta Psychiatr. Scand.* **2017**, *135*, 373–387. [CrossRef] [PubMed]
71. Coutinho, A.E.; Chapman, K.E. The anti-inflammatory and immunosuppressive effects of glucocorticoids, recent developments and mechanistic insights. *Mol. Cell. Endocrinol.* **2011**, *335*, 2–13. [CrossRef] [PubMed]
72. Zunszain, P.A.; Anacker, C.; Cattaneo, A.; Carvalho, L.A.; Pariante, C.M. Glucocorticoids, cytokines and brain abnormalities in depression. *Prog. Neuro-Psychopharmacol. Biol. Psychiatry* **2011**, *35*, 722–729. [CrossRef] [PubMed]
73. Pariante, C.M. Why are depressed patients inflamed? A reflection on 20 years of research on depression, glucocorticoid resistance and inflammation. *Eur. Neuropsychopharmacol.* **2017**, *27*, 554–559. [CrossRef] [PubMed]
74. Lamers, F.; Vogelzangs, N.; Merikangas, K.; De Jonge, P.; Beekman, A.; Penninx, B. Evidence for a differential role of HPA-axis function, inflammation and metabolic syndrome in melancholic versus atypical depression. *Mol. Psychiatry* **2013**, *18*, 692–699. [CrossRef] [PubMed]
75. Cai, C.; Shen, J.; Zhao, D.; Qiao, Y.; Xu, A.; Jin, S.; Ran, Z.; Zheng, Q. Serological investigation of food specific immunoglobulin G antibodies in patients with inflammatory bowel diseases. *PLoS ONE* **2014**, *9*, e112154. [CrossRef] [PubMed]
76. Lee, H.S.; Lee, K.J. Alterations of Food-specific Serum IgG4 Titers to Common Food Antigens in Patients With Irritable Bowel Syndrome. *J. Neurogastroenterol. Motil.* **2017**, *23*, 578. [CrossRef] [PubMed]
77. Ikechi, R.; Fischer, B.D.; DeSipio, J.; Phadtare, S. *Irritable Bowel Syndrome: Clinical Manifestations, Dietary Influences, and Management*; Healthcare, Multidisciplinary Digital Publishing Institute: Basel, Switzerland, 2017; p. 21.

78. Hayes, P.; Corish, C.; Vny, E.; Quigley, E.M.M. A dietary survey of patients with irritable bowel syndrome. *J. Hum. Nutr. Dietet.* **2014**, *27*, 36–47. [CrossRef] [PubMed]
79. Ligaarden, S.C.; Lydersen, S.; Farup, P.G. IgG and IgG4 antibodies in subjects with irritable bowel syndrome: A case control study in the general population. *BMC Gastroenterol.* **2012**, *12*, 166. [CrossRef] [PubMed]
80. Rees, T.; Watson, D.; Lipscombe, S.; Speight, H.; Cousins, P.; Hardman, G.; Dowson, A.J. A prospective audit of food intolerance among migraine patients in primary care clinical practice. *Headache Care* **2005**, *2*, 105–110.
81. Wilders-Truschnig, M.; Mangge, H.; Lieners, C.; Gruber, H.-J.; Mayer, C.; März, W. IgG antibodies against food antigens are correlated with inflammation and intima media thickness in obese juveniles. *Exp. Clin. Endocrinol. Diabet.* **2008**, *116*, 241–245. [CrossRef] [PubMed]
82. Bentz, S.; Hausmann, M.; Piberger, H.; Kellermeier, S.; Paul, S.; Held, L.; Falk, W.; Obermeier, F.; Fried, M.; Schölmerich, J. Clinical relevance of IgG antibodies against food antigens in Crohn's disease: A double-blind cross-over diet intervention study. *Digestion* **2010**, *81*, 252–264. [CrossRef] [PubMed]
83. Piche, T. Tight junctions and IBS-the link between epithelial permeability, low-grade inflammation, and symptom generation? *Neurogastroenterol. Motil.* **2014**, *26*, 296–302. [CrossRef] [PubMed]
84. Sentsova, T.; Vorozhko, I.; Isakov, V.; Morozov, S.; Shakhovskaia, A. Immune status estimation algorithm in irritable bowel syndrome patients with food intolerance. *Exp. Clin. Gastroenterol.* **2014**, *7*, 13–17.
85. Stapel, S.O.; Asero, R.; Ballmer-Weber, B.; Knol, E.; Strobel, S.; Vieths, S.; Kleine-Tebbe, J. Testing for IgG4 against foods is not recommended as a diagnostic tool: EAACI Task Force Report. *Allergy* **2008**, *63*, 793–796. [CrossRef] [PubMed]
86. Carr, S.; Chan, E.; Lavine, E.; Moote, W. CSACI Position statement on the testing of food-specific IgG. *Allergy Asthma Clin. Immunol.* **2012**, *8*, 12. [CrossRef] [PubMed]
87. Sicherer, S.H.; Allen, K.; Lack, G.; Taylor, S.L.; Donovan, S.M.; Oria, M. Critical Issues in Food Allergy: A National Academies Consensus Report. *Pediatrics* **2017**, *140*, e20170194. [CrossRef] [PubMed]
88. Chabane, H.; Doyen, V.; Bienvenu, F.; Adel-Patient, K.; Vitte, J.; Mariotte, D.; Bienvenu, J. Les dosages d'IgG anti-aliments: Méthodes et pertinence clinique des résultats. Position du groupe de travail de biologie de la Société française d'allergologie. *Revue Française d'Allergologie* **2018**. Available online: https://www.sciencedirect.com/science/article/pii/S1877032018300289 (accessed on 11 April 2018). [CrossRef]
89. Engelhart, S.; Glynn, R.J.; Schur, P.H. Disease associations with isolated elevations of each of the four IgG subclasses. *Semin. Arthritis and Rheum.* **2017**, *47*, 276–280. [CrossRef] [PubMed]
90. Aljada, A.; Mohanty, P.; Ghanim, H.; Abdo, T.; Tripathy, D.; Chaudhuri, A.; Dandona, P. Increase in intranuclear nuclear factor κB and decrease in inhibitor κB in mononuclear cells after a mixed meal: Evidence for a proinflammatory effect. *Am. J. Clin. Nutr.* **2004**, *79*, 682–690. [CrossRef] [PubMed]
91. Abautret-Daly, Á.; Dempsey, E.; Parra-Blanco, A.; Medina, C.; Harkin, A. Gut-brain actions underlying comorbid anxiety and depression associated with inflammatory bowel disease. *Acta Neuropsychiatr.* **2017**, 1–22. [CrossRef] [PubMed]
92. Powell, N.; Walker, M.M.; Talley, N.J. The mucosal immune system: Master regulator of bidirectional gut-brain communications. *Nat. Rev. Gastroenterol. Hepatol.* **2017**, *14*, 143–159. [CrossRef] [PubMed]
93. Delaney, S.; Hornig, M. Environmental Exposures and Neuropsychiatric Disorders: What Role Does the Gut–Immune–Brain Axis Play? *Curr. Environ. Health Rep.* **2018**, *5*, 158–169. [CrossRef] [PubMed]
94. Rios-Covian, D.; Ruas-Madiedo, P.; Margolles, A.; Gueimonde, M.; de Los Reyes-Gavilan, C.G.; Salazar, N. Intestinal Short Chain Fatty Acids and their Link with Diet and Human Health. *Front. Microbiol.* **2016**, *7*, 185. [CrossRef] [PubMed]
95. Quigley, E.M.M. The Gut-Brain Axis and the Microbiome: Clues to Pathophysiology and Opportunities for Novel Management Strategies in Irritable Bowel Syndrome (IBS). *J. Clin. Med.* **2018**, *7*, 6. [CrossRef] [PubMed]

14

Effects of a Lutein and Zeaxanthin Intervention on Cognitive Function: A Randomized, Double-Masked, Placebo-Controlled Trial of Younger Healthy Adults

Lisa M. Renzi-Hammond [1,2], Emily R. Bovier [1,3], Laura M. Fletcher [1], L. Stephen Miller [1], Catherine M. Mewborn [1], Cutter A. Lindbergh [1], Jeffrey H. Baxter [4] and Billy R. Hammond Jr. [1,*]

1 Department of Psychology, The University of Georgia, Athens, GA 30602-3013, USA; lrenzi@uga.edu (L.M.R.-H.); emily.bovier@oswego.edu (E.R.B.); fletcher.lauram@gmail.com (L.M.F.); lsmiller@uga.edu (L.S.M.); mewborn@uga.edu (C.M.M.); cal@uga.edu (C.A.L.)
2 Institute of Gerontology, Department of Health Promotion and Behavior, College of Public Health, The University of Georgia, Athens, GA 30602, USA
3 Department of Psychology, State University of New York, Oswego Campus, Oswego, NY 13126, USA
4 Abbott Nutrition, Global Research and Development, Columbus, OH 43219, USA; jeffrey.baxter@abbott.com
* Correspondence: bhammond@uga.edu

Abstract: Background: Past studies have suggested that higher lutein (L) and zeaxanthin (Z) levels in serum and in the central nervous system (as quantified by measuring macular pigment optical density, MPOD) are related to improved cognitive function in older adults. Very few studies have addressed the issue of xanthophylls and cognitive function in younger adults, and no controlled trials have been conducted to date to determine whether or not supplementation with L + Z can change cognitive function in this population. **Objective:** The purpose of this study was to determine whether or not supplementation with L + Z could improve cognitive function in young (age 18–30), healthy adults. **Design:** A randomized, double-masked, placebo-controlled trial design was used. Fifty-one young, healthy subjects were recruited as part of a larger study on xanthophylls and cognitive function. Subjects were randomized into active supplement ($n = 37$) and placebo groups ($n = 14$). MPOD was measured psychophysically using customized heterochromatic flicker photometry. Cognitive function was measured using the CNS Vital Signs testing platform. MPOD and cognitive function were measured every four months for a full year of supplementation. **Results:** Supplementation increased MPOD significantly over the course of the year, vs. placebo ($p < 0.001$). Daily supplementation with L + Z and increases in MPOD resulted in significant improvements in spatial memory ($p < 0.04$), reasoning ability ($p < 0.05$) and complex attention ($p < 0.04$), above and beyond improvements due to practice effects. **Conclusions:** Supplementation with L + Z improves CNS xanthophyll levels and cognitive function in young, healthy adults. Magnitudes of effects are similar to previous work reporting correlations between MPOD and cognition in other populations.

Keywords: xanthophylls; cognition; reasoning; visual memory; attention

---

1. Introduction

A wide body of research, across disciplines, has shown a direct effect of diet on nearly every aspect of brain function [1]. One big category of effect appears to be simply prophylactic. The brain is a strongly lipid-based, highly oxygenated structure prone to inflammatory stress. Dietary intake, good or bad, can influence the oxidative and inflammatory state of the brain and, hence, its function [2]. Another category is acute effects on cellular metabolism [3]. Dietary intake is involved in every aspect of a neuron's function, ranging from influencing the basic structure of the cell itself (e.g., phospholipid composition [4]); to resting and action potentials; to neurotransmitter synthesis from amino acid and vitamin precursors (e.g., pyridoxal 5′-phosphate, a form of Vitamin B_6, is a coenzyme required for the biosynthesis of gamma-aminobutyric acid (GABA), norepinephrine and serotonin from glutamic acid, tyrosine and tryptophan, respectively). B_6, B_{12} and folate are required to support methylation reactions, some of which are noted above, and are also important in gene regulation. It is interesting to note that methylation is the sole method for regulation of genes in mitochondrial DNA, and that these vitamins are critical for mitochondrial function.

Like many areas of nutrition, most research on the diet–brain connection has focused on micronutrient deficiencies, such as the role of B vitamins in cognitive decline or diseases such as Korsakoff's and dementia [5,6]. Much less is known about the many other phytochemicals that are commonly found in food (i.e., not yet defined as essential or even as nutrients). Even less is known about how those components of diet influence the brains of young healthy adults. One exception to this general trend is a growing interest in a possible role for the xanthophylls, specifically lutein (L), zeaxanthin (Z) and meso-zeaxanthin (MZ) [7]. These dietary carotenoids concentrate in neural tissue (particularly, the macula or central retina, there termed macular pigment (MP)). Unlike many dietary components, the amount of retinal L, Z and MZ can be measured directly and non-invasively [8]. MPOD has been shown to be highly correlated to L + Z accumulation in brain [9]. This allows the concentration of these xanthophylls in neural tissue to be correlated with dependent measures of interest. Using this technique, a number of cross-sectional studies have correlated the macular xanthophylls with many aspects of both visual and cognitive function in both young and older subjects [10–15].

The ability to directly measure the macular pigments also provides the additional advantage of being able to monitor the results of an intervention; to wit, one can supplement L, Z or MZ, measure changes in MP, and then assess any possible functional changes that result (and how those changes relate to the actual change in tissue levels). Using this strategy, a number of studies have now shown that supplementing L and Z is related to both increases in the amount of L + Z measured in the retina and alteration in behaviors that are thought to be primarily mediated by the brain. For example, supplementation with carotenoid-rich avocados causes increases in both the macular pigments and spatial working memory [16]. This improvement was not found for control subjects whose carotenoid levels did not increase. L + Z supplementation in healthy older adults produces improvements in cognitive function on a variety of domains [17–19]. Such effects have even been found in young healthy subjects (i.e., those seemingly less likely to change). For example, Bovier et al. [14,15] supplemented young subjects and found changes in visual temporal processing speed in subjects whose MP increased by 0.1 log units of optical density or more, versus those that did not, using a placebo-controlled design. Visual processing speed was chosen because, although it is a lower level visual function (basically, the fusion of square-and sine wave modulated light), it is thought to be mediated by central brain mechanisms (e.g., [20]). Indeed, some have argued that processing speed in general underlies many more complex cognitive traits [21] and should be considered a cognitive fundamental [22]. The results by Bovier et al. implied the possibility that supplementing xanthophylls could change other aspects of cognition (such as memory) even in young healthy subjects at the (apparent) peak of their cognitive life (e.g., college students). The present study was a first test of this hypothesis.

2. Materials and Methods

2.1. Subjects

This sub-study was part of a larger clinical trial on xanthophyll supplementation and cognitive function. For the young adult sub-study, a total of 79 potential participants (college students from the Athens-Clarke County, GA area) were screened for enrollment between August 2012 and December 2013, with follow-up lasting through December 2014. Of those 79 potential participants, three participants were initially excluded for failure to meet the inclusion criteria.

Randomization to either the active supplement group or the placebo group was accomplished as follows: a set of numerical codes was created that corresponded to either the active supplement or the intervention. The codes were placed into an opaque envelope. After informed consent was signed and inclusion/exclusion criteria were verified (see below), a code was drawn from the envelope by the clinical coordinator, who had no data collection responsibilities. From the 76 participants who were deemed eligible for participation, 30 participants were randomized into the placebo group, and 46 total participants were randomized into the intervention group. Of those participants, two members of the placebo group and three members of the intervention group withdrew from the trial due to scheduling conflicts prior to completion of baseline measurements and allocation of supplements. Given the fact that students enrolled in the trial occasionally graduated and moved away during the study, 14 total placebo participants and 9 total intervention participants were lost to follow-up during the course of the year-long intervention.

The final analyzable data set included 51 healthy subjects ranging in age from 18 to 30 ($M = 21.21 \pm 2.52$) years. Approximately equal numbers of males and females ($n = 29$ males, 22 females) were analyzed, with a total of $n = 14$ participants in the placebo group, and $n = 37$ participants who received the intervention. The active supplement contained 10 mg L + 2 mg Z (DSM Nutritional Products; Kaiseraugst, Switzerland), and the placebo was visually identical to the active supplement. Supplement and placebo containers were visually identical, with the exception of the numerical code on the bottle contents label. Participants were instructed to take one tablet per day with their highest fat meal. Compliance with the supplement regime was monitored by bi-monthly phone calls as well as pill counts.

The baseline characteristics of the entire analyzable young adult sample, as well as the two sub-groups, are shown in Table 1. The majority of the subjects were students from the University of Georgia, and placebo and active supplement groups were not significantly different from each other in demographic characteristics. Inclusion criteria included good overall and ocular/refractive (20:40 best corrected acuity) health and no supplement use in the previous six months (excluding a multivitamin containing less than 1 mg LZ/day).

Table 1. Baseline characteristics of placebo participants vs. those on the active supplement.

Group	Age (Years)	Body Mass Index	Gender	Ethnicity	Race	Years of Education	MP Optical Density
Active, Mean ± SD	21.50 ± 2.69	24.15 ± 3.86	21 M, 16 F	$n = 35$ non-Hispanic $n = 2$ Hispanic	$n = 30$ White $n = 4$ Black $n = 1$ pan-Asian $n = 2$ Latino	12+	0.47 ± 0.18
Placebo, Mean ± SD	20.50 ± 1.91	23.03 ± 3.98	8 M, 6 F	$n = 14$ non-Hispanic	$n = 10$ White $n = 2$ Black $n = 2$ pan-Asian	12+	0.39 ± 0.12

None of the differences between the groups were statistically significant at baseline ($p > 0.05$). SD = standard deviation. M = male; F = female.

2.2. Ethics

The tenets of the Declaration of Helsinki were adhered to at all times during the course of this study. All participants both verbally consented to participation and provided written informed consent prior to participation. The protocol was approved by the University of Georgia Institutional Review Board (2012105172).

2.3. Methods

2.3.1. Retinal L + Z Levels

Retinal L + Z levels (as macular pigment optical density, MPOD) was measured at 30-min of retinal eccentricity along the horizontal meridian of the temporal retina, using customized heterochromatic flicker photometry (cHFP) [23,24]. Briefly, a macular densitometer (Macular Metrics; Rehoboth, MA, USA) was used to present participants with a one-degree test stimulus composed of light generated by two narrow-band LEDs, peaking at 460 nm (strongly absorbed by MP) and 570 nm (not absorbed by MP), respectively. Each waveband was presented in counter-phase orientation at two different starting intensities, which, when combined, appeared to participants as a single, uniform, flickering disk. The stimulus was presented on a 470 nm background.

Participants were required to centrally view the stimulus, and to adjust the intensity of the 460 nm test light relative to the 570 nm reference light until the appearance of flicker was minimized. The participants then viewed a larger (two-degree) stimulus while fixating on a point at 7-degrees of retinal eccentricity. This placed the stimulus on the parafovea, where MPOD is negligible. Participants completed five trials at each locus. The two loci were compared to yield MPOD at 30-min of eccentricity. MPOD was measured at baseline, and after 4-, 8- and 12-month supplementation.

2.3.2. Serum L + Z Levels

In addition to measuring CNS L + Z levels (as MPOD), L + Z were measured in the serum via high performance liquid chromatography (HPLC) to confirm participant compliance. The methods used to collect serum samples and measure L and Z concentration have been presented previously [25].

2.3.3. Cognitive Function

Cognitive function was tested using a computerized test battery (CNS Vital Signs; Morrisville, NC, USA) at baseline, 4-, 8- and 12-month time points [26]. The procedure used to collect cognitive function data was presented previously [18]. Briefly, in order to complete computerized tests, participants were seated in front of a Dell E 2211H 18-inch monitor with a full QWERTY keyboard. A research assistant familiar with the test procedure remained in the room with the participant during the entire test protocol. Visual acuity of 20:40 or better was confirmed prior to enrollment. Prior to each test set, participants were given a practice session to confirm that test instructions were clear.

Individual functional tests and cognitive domains computed by raw scores on these tests are listed in Table 2, and have been presented previously [18]. During the test session, participants were given the same sequence of individual tests, each designed to measure some aspect of cognitive function. Raw scores on these individual tests were used to calculate cognitive domain scores, which were used in statistical analysis. For example, average numbers of taps executed by the right and left hands on the Finger Tapping Test were combined with the number of correct responses on the Symbol-Digit Coding task to compute the Psychomotor Speed domain score. Errors on the Stroop Task, Continuous Performance Task and Shifting Attention Task were combined to compute the Complex Attention domain score. For a complete list of tests administered, domains computed and computation parameters, see Table 2 and [18].

Table 2. Individual tests administered and cognitive domains evaluated in the test battery.

Domain	Corresponding Tests	Computation Procedure
Verbal Memory (VeM)	Verbal Memory Test	Correct hits for presented words + correct passes on distractors for tests immediately after presentation and after a 30-min delay.
Visual Memory (ViM)	Visual Memory Test	Correct hits for presented shapes and symbols + correct passes on distractors for tests immediately after presentation and after a 30-min delay.
Reasoning (R)	Non-Verbal Reasoning Test (NVRT)	Correct responses on the NVRT − commission errors on the NVRT.
Executive Function (EF)	Shifting Attention Test (SAT)	Correct responses on the SAT − errors on the SAT.

Table 2. *Cont.*

Domain	Corresponding Tests	Computation Procedure
Psychomotor Speed (PmS)	Finger Tapping Test (FTT) Symbol-Digit Coding Test (SDC)	Average number of taps on the FTT with the right hand + average number of taps with the left hand + number of correct responses on the SDC
Complex Attention (CA)	Stroop Test (ST) SAT Continuous Performance Task (CPT)	Commission errors on the ST + Errors on the SAT + Commission and omission errors on the CPT
Cognitive Flexibility (CF)	SAT ST	Correct responses on the SAT − errors on the SAT − Commission errors on the ST

Note: Raw scores computed as described above were used in all statistical analyses.

2.3.4. Statistical Analyses and other Considerations

All statistical analyses were performed using SPSS version 23 (IBM) with $p < 0.05$ as the criterion for significance. The following domain scores were compared in statistical analyses: verbal memory, visual memory, reasoning, executive function, psychomotor speed, complex attention and cognitive flexibility. All tests were one-tailed, given the directional nature of the a priori hypotheses, specified below. The relationship between nutritional status and cognitive function was analyzed in two ways, as follows:

First, domain scores from participants on the placebo were directly compared against domain scores from participants taking the active supplement. To make these comparisons, difference scores were computed between baseline and 12-month time points for each cognitive domain tested, and those difference scores were compared between groups receiving placebo and those receiving the active supplement, for each domain. This comparison tests whether or not supplementation with L + Z was able to improve MPOD (the study biomarker of CNS xanthophyll levels) and whether such increases could affect cognitive function.

The second set of comparisons was aimed at addressing two major issues commonly seen in nutritional trials: poor compliance and dietary change. Non-compliance with the study regimen is seen in a number of clinical trials, from drug trials to nutrition trials, and we expected that some participants would not consistently take their nutritional supplement. Those in the active group who did not consistently take their supplements would, we predicted, have performance similar to placebo participants, rather than to other active supplement users.

The issue of dietary change is more complex. Although many nutrition trials (this trial included) are double-masked, to adhere to the tenets of the Declaration of Helsinki, participants should to the extent possible be informed about the nature of the trial. This model is most commonly used in drug trials, where participants either cannot acquire or would have some difficulty acquiring the active agent being tested. In nutrition trials that follow this "gold standard" randomized, double-masked, placebo-controlled trial model, once participants know the identity of the test supplement and the motivation for testing it, they can do individual research on the ingredients within that supplement and actually acquire the test molecules via the diet (or, if available, as is true in this case, in supplement form). In the current study, for example, participants were told at baseline that they would be taking either an active supplement containing L + Z or a visually identical placebo to examine putative benefits of these molecules on cognitive function. Given that fact, we expected that participants who researched the foods that naturally contain L and Z to learn more about the molecules might (even unintentionally) start increasing intakes of L- and Z-containing foods. For placebo group participants, we predicted that these dietary changes (or the frank obtaining of actives in the dietary supplement market) would cause performance to look more like the performance of active supplement users. Finally, it is well known that participants in clinical trials with diet questionnaires will unconsciously improve their diet (and in some cases other aspects of their lifestyle (exercise, alcohol intake and so forth) over the course of the study—perhaps simply because they know someone is "watching".

In an attempt to determine whether or not participants changed dietary intakes, a food frequency questionnaire (FFQ) was collected at baseline and 12-month time points to measure fruit and vegetable intake. Participants in both groups tended to slightly increase the number of servings of fruits and vegetables consumed per day between baseline (3+ servings of fruits + vegetables per day) and 12 months (4+ servings/day). With respect to the compliance issue, compliance calls, pill counts and serum analysis suggested that 6 out of 37 participants in the active group were not fully compliant over the course of the year with the supplement regiment (these participants reported forgetting to take pills in at least three compliance phone calls), and thus would be less likely to show changes in MP optical density, the study biomarker of increased L + Z levels in the CNS. Finally, past research [27] has suggested that a small subset of the population is likely unable to absorb and/or appropriately traffic L and Z, and thus would not show serum and retinal responses even if they were fully compliant with the supplementation regimen.

To address these issues statistically, difference scores between MPOD at baseline and 12 months were computed. All participants who showed an increase of 0.10+ log units of MPOD, regardless of randomized group membership at study entry, were then grouped ($n = 27$) and were compared against participants whose MPOD did not increase ($n = 24$). Cognitive performance was then compared between those whose MPOD increased vs. those who did not increase. This comparison indicates whether or not increases in CNS L + Z (as predicted by MPOD measures) can improve cognitive function, irrespective of what caused the increased L + Z status.

3. Results

3.1. Retinal L + Z Levels

At baseline, MPOD in the study sample was higher ($M = 0.48 \pm 0.18$) than previously published averages for healthy adults (M = approximately 0.3; [28,29]), indicating that the sample was relatively well-nourished. Following one year of supplementation, those on the active supplement increased significantly ($p < 0.001$) between the baseline ($M = 0.47 \pm 0.18$) and 12-month ($M = 0.56 \pm 0.16$) time-points. The participants on placebo did not increase significantly (baseline: 0.40 ± 0.12, 12-month: 0.44 ± 0.18; $p > 0.05$).

3.2. Serum L + Z Levels

At baseline, serum L, Z and L + Z levels were not significantly different between the participants randomized into the active supplement group vs. the placebo group (see Table 3). Following one year of supplementation, serum L ($p = 0.029$), Z ($p = 0.011$) and L + Z ($p = 0.023$) levels were all significantly higher in the active supplement group than the placebo group (see Table 4, Figure 1).

Table 3. Baseline serum levels by supplement group.

Group	Serum Lutein (ng/μL)	Serum Zeaxanthin (ng/μL)	Lutein + Zeaxanthin (ng/μL)
Active, Mean ± SD	0.11 ± 0.07	0.03 ± 0.02	0.14 ± 0.08
Placebo, Mean ± SD	0.10 ± 0.03	0.03 ± 0.02	0.13 ± 0.04

None of the differences between the groups were statistically significant at baseline.

Table 4. Serum levels following one year of supplementation.

Group	Serum Lutein (ng/μL)	Serum Zeaxanthin (ng/μL)	Lutein + Zeaxanthin (ng/μL)
Active, Mean ± SD	0.38 ± 0.28	0.08 ± 0.05	0.46 ± 0.32
Placebo, Mean ± SD	0.19 ± 0.19	0.04 ± 0.04	0.23 ± 0.23

Note: Statistically significant differences were seen between the placebo group and the control group for serum L (p = 0.029), Z (p = 0.011), and L + Z (p = 0.023) following one year of supplementation.

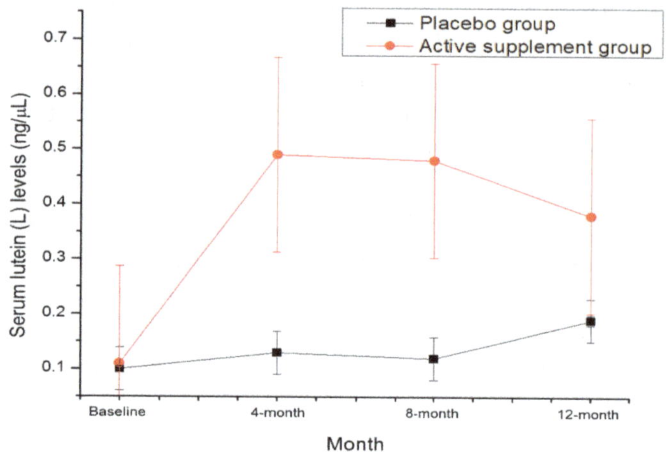

(**a**) Serum L changes across time.

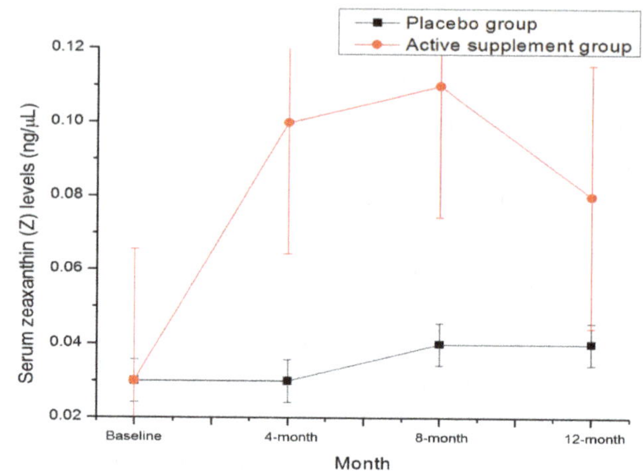

(**b**) Serum Z changes across time.

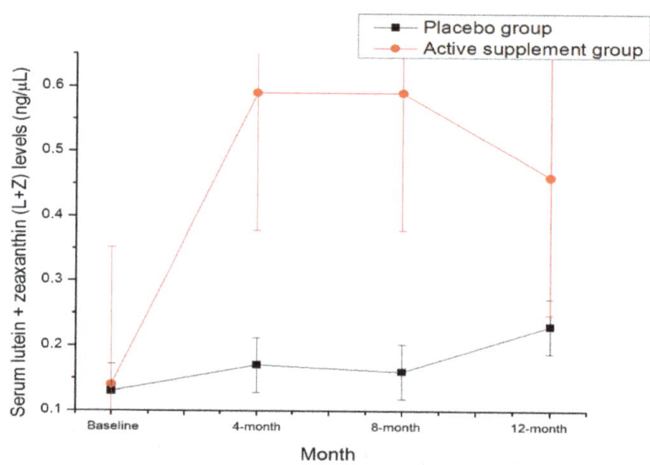

(**c**) Combined serum L + Z changes over time.

Figure 1. Serum changes from baseline to 12-month time points in: (**a**) lutein (L); (**b**) zeaxanthin (Z); and (**c**) and lutein + zeaxanthin (L + Z). Error bars represent the standard deviation of the mean at each time point.

3.3. Cognitive Function

At baseline, participants were not significantly different from each other on any of the cognitive domains tested. Given the fact that participants were tested four times throughout the course of the study, practice effects were anticipated, and seen, regardless of group identity (see Table 5).

As mentioned previously, not all members of the supplement group were compliant with the intervention, and some of the members of the placebo group also had increases in MPOD (likely due to dietary changes since the intervention was an entire year). Consequently, analyses were conducted in two ways: by supplement group, and by percent increase in MPOD, regardless of group membership. With respect to supplement status, after 12 months of supplementation, participants taking the active supplement had significantly higher performance on visual memory tasks ($p < 0.04$) than those participants taking the placebo (see Figure 2). Analysis of the Reliable Change Index (RCI) using a standard criterion of 1.96 for both groups suggested that the effects seen in the active supplement group were not simply due to practice effects (RCI active = 6.77; RCI placebo = 1.88).

Table 5. Practice effects demonstrated by improvement in cognitive function across domains, regardless of supplementation status.

Group	Verbal Memory	Visual Memory	Reasoning Ability	Executive Function	Complex Attention *	Cognitive Flexibility
Baseline Mean, all subjects	54.22	41.04	9.06	53.73	7.38	52.02
12-Month Mean, all subjects	56.26	49.24	10.20	62.59	5.98	60.65
Average change between baseline and 12 months, placebo group participants	3.57	4.93	1.64	8.86	0.46	8.43

* Lower score = fewer errors; for all other scores, an increase indicates improved performance.

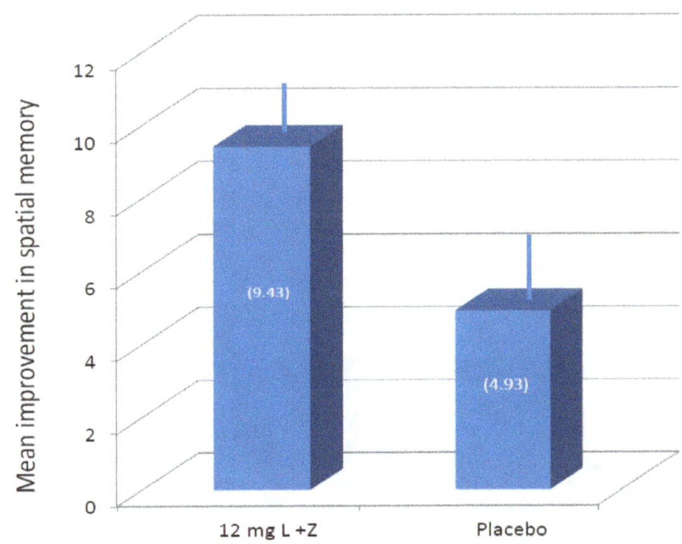

Figure 2. Average (with standard error of the mean, SEM) improvement in spatial memory following one-year supplementation. L, lutein; Z, zeaxanthin.

With respect to percent increase in MPOD, baseline MPOD was subtracted from 12-month MPOD scores. Participants who had numerical increases of 0.10 or greater were classified as "increasers", and participants who did not increase by a minimum of 0.10 were classified as "flat liners", regardless of supplement group assignment. Compared to "flat liners", participants with improvements of at least 0.10 for MPOD not only maintained significant differences in visual memory ($p < 0.05$) also scored significantly higher in the complex attention ($p < 0.04$) and reasoning ability ($p < 0.05$) tasks (see Figures 3 and 4). Analysis of the RCIs for each task suggested, again, that the differences seen in complex attention (RCI for "increasers" = 2.02; RCI for "flat liners" = 0.00) and likely reasoning ability (RCI for "increasers" = 1.94; RCI for "flat liners" = 0.18) were not due simply to practice effects.

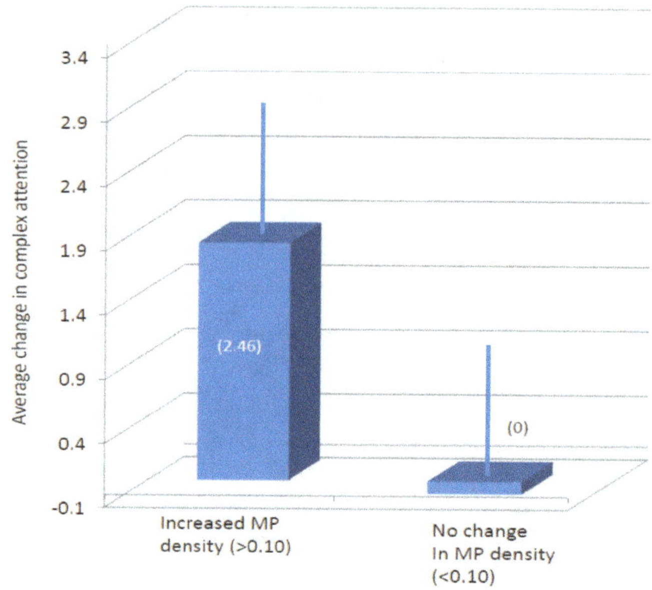

Figure 3. Average (and standard error of the mean (SEM)) change in complex attention segregated according to changes in macular pigment (MP) density.

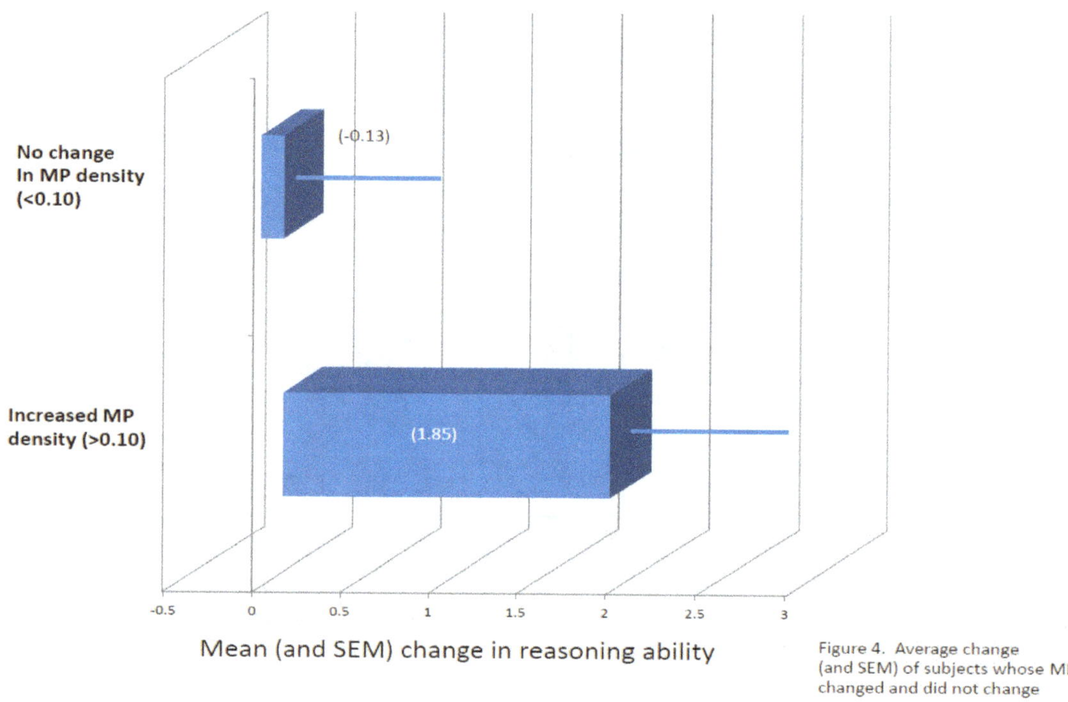

Figure 4. Average change (and SEM) of subjects whose MP changed and did not change.

4. Discussion

This randomized, double-masked, placebo-controlled study tested the effects of one year of nutritional supplementation (10 mg of L and 2 mg of Z) on the cognitive function of healthy, well-nourished college students. L and Z were picked because they are commonly available in supplement form (often marketed for eye health) and the xanthophylls are commonly found in food (e.g., supplementing spinach will directly increase retinal levels [27]). They can also be easily measured in central nervous tissue (neural retina) [8] and are found in some key locations in the brain, such as hippocampus, and frontal and occipital cortex [9]. We originally speculated that changing cognitive function via a simple dietary intervention in young well-nourished college students was unlikely. Past studies, such as the companion older adult sample tested in the larger study from which these data were drawn [18], and others (e.g., [19]) have shown improvements in cognitive function in older adults. Older adult samples tend to have baseline cognitive function that is more variable (e.g., [10,11,13]), with a higher proportion of individuals who are at risk for dementia. Consequently, the older adult population is likely to an easier population in which to demonstrate change. This young adult, highly educated sample was selected deliberately to isolate treatment effects that were not likely to be confounded by education status, underlying nutritional deficiency, or progression toward cognitive impairment. Nonetheless, we were able to measure several distinct cognitive benefits that were directly tied to increasing central nervous system levels of L and Z, as shown by increased MPOD, even though the starting MPOD levels were substantially higher than those previously reported for the general population.

The most significant effect according to treatment was visual memory: the treated group changed but the placebos did not. In a recent study that tested retinal and brain L and Z levels in human decedents, L tended to be relatively highly concentrated in occipital cortex, and L + Z levels in neural retina tended to be highly ($r = 0.78$) correlated to brain levels of the macular carotenoids in occipital lobe [9]. This current study represents the first of its kind that suggests that increasing CNS L + Z can also improve performance in a function that is mediated in large part by occipital cortex, which preferentially accumulates L + Z relative to the other carotenoids more commonly consumed in the diet [30] in young, otherwise healthy, high performing subjects.

Visual memory is a relatively low-level cognitive function. Sometimes referred to as stimulus memory [31], it reflects dynamic cortical changes resulting from the storage or processing of visual stimuli. It is the stage that precedes processing by other structures such as the hippocampus which encodes more complex visual memories such as maps or scenes. Visual memory is hard to distinguish from attention since some aspects of the stimulus must be attended to in order to enter visual memory in the first place [32]. Characteristics such as visual memory, attention and processing speed have all, in turn, been related to improved reasoning ability [22,33].

In our study, the xanthophyll intervention was related to all three of these variables: visual memory, complex attention and reasoning ability. Specifically, improved visual memory was related to the treatment; complex attention and reasoning ability were improved only if significant increases in MP were also achieved. The fact that L + Z supplementation was related specifically to these variables in the younger adults may not be coincidence. As noted, these three cognitive functions are, in some ways, related to each other. Our results further suggest, however, that they are physiologically connected in a way that xanthophylls could improve, even in the young, who are, theoretically, also near ceiling in these functions. Earlier data from our lab has indicated that speed of processing in young subjects can also be changed by changing MPOD [14,15]. It is important to note that the intervention was not related to change in any of the other cognitive functions tested, and some of the functions that improved in the companion older adult sample [18] did not also improve in the young adult sample. Additional neuroimaging analyses of the entire study sample, including the older adult sample, suggests that L + Z supplementation improves white matter integrity in regions of brain known to show white matter declines in older age, and in those at risk for dementia [34]. Supplementation with L + Z also buffers against age-related declines in verbal learning and memory and improves cerebral perfusion in older adults [17]. Consequently, L + Z might be serving multiple functions in the CNS, some of which are more important in older age.

One common factor that could affect all of these functions is a general improvement in neural efficiency, a hypothesis proposed for L + Z in 2010 [35]. Hence, increasing central levels of L + Z could improve neural efficiency, which would both speed neural conduction while simultaneously reducing the likelihood of cross-talk between axons. Such basic effects can influence higher functions. The latter, for instance, could lower interference allowing multiple representations within the brain to be maintained and operated upon. We are currently using neuroimaging methods to assess these possibilities.

In the current study, several limitations should be considered with respect to generalizability. As mentioned previously, this sample was selected with the intention of avoiding both underlying nutritional deficiency that can contribute to poor cognitive performance, and cognitive differences between subjects that are due to differences in education level. Consequently, we ended up with a sample that should have been difficult to improve. The fact that these participants were well-nourished and cognitively high performing at baseline may limit generalizability to those with, for example, cognitive and neurological disease states.

Acknowledgments: The authors would like to acknowledge Matthew Tankersley and Medina Bello for their assistance with study coordination and data management, and Joanne Curran-Celentano and Karen Semo for assistance with serum analysis. This work was supported by Abbott Nutrition; Columbus, OH. Active supplements and placebos were supplied by DSM Nutritional Products; Basel, Switzerland.

Author Contributions: L.M.R.-H., B.R.H. and L.S.M. contributed to research study design; L.M.R.-H., B.R.H., E.R.B., L.M.F., L.S.M., C.M.M. and C.A.L. collected study data; J.H.B. provided study materials; L.M.R.-H., B.R.H. and L.S.M. contributed to data analysis; L.M.R.-H. and B.R.H. drafted the initial manuscript; L.M.R.-H., B.R.H., J.H.B. and L.S.M. primarily edited the manuscript; and L.M.R.-H., E.R.B., L.M.F., L.S.M., J.H.B., C.A.L., C.M.M. and B.R.H. assume responsibility for the final content of the manuscript.

Abbreviations

L	lutein
Z	zeaxanthin
MPOD	macular pigment optical density
MZ	meso-zeaxanthin
CNS	central nervous system
MP	macular pigment
HPLC	high-performance liquid chromatography
FFQ	food frequency questionnaire
RCI	reliable change index
VeM	verbal memory
ViM	visual memory
R	reasoning
EF	executive function
PmS	psychomotor speed
CA	complex attention
CF	cognitive flexibility
NVRT	non-verbal reasoning test
SAT	shifting attention test
FTT	finger tapping test
SDC	symbol-digit coding
ST	Stroop test
CPT	continuous performance task

References

1. Gomez-Pinilla, F. Brain foods: The effects of nutrients on brain function. *Nat. Rev. Neurosci.* **2008**, *9*, 568–578. [CrossRef] [PubMed]
2. Joseph, J.A.; Shukitt-Hale, B.; Casadesus, G.; Fisher, D. Oxidative stress and inflammation in brain aging: Nutritional considerations. *Neurochem. Res.* **2005**, *30*, 927–935. [CrossRef] [PubMed]

3. Bourre, J.M. Effects of nutrients (in food) on the structure and function of the nervous system: Update on dietary requirements for brain. Part 1: Micronutrients. *J. Nutr. Health Aging* **2006**, *10*, 377–385. [PubMed]
4. Carlson, S.E.; Carver, J.D.; House, S.G. High fat diets varying in ratios of polyunsaturated to saturated fatty acid and linoleic to linolenic acid: A comparison of rat neural and red cell membrane phospholipids. *J. Nutr.* **1986**, *116*, 718–725. [PubMed]
5. Cook, C.C.; Thomson, A.D. B-complex vitamins in the prophylaxis and treatment of Wernicke-Korsakoff syndrome. *Br. J. Hosp. Med.* **1997**, *57*, 461–465. [PubMed]
6. McCaddon, A.; Regland, B.; Hudson, P.; Davies, G. Functional vitamin B12 deficiency and Alzheimer disease. *Neurology* **2002**, *58*, 1395–1399. [CrossRef] [PubMed]
7. Erdman, J.W.; Smith, J.W.; Kuchan, M.J.; Mohn, E.S.; Johnson, E.J.; Rubakhin, S.S.; Wang, L.; Sweedler, J.V.; Neuringer, M. Lutein and Brain Function. *Foods* **2015**, *4*, 547–564. [CrossRef] [PubMed]
8. Hammond, B.R.J.; Wooten, B.R.; Smollon, B. Assessment of the validity of in vivo methods of measuring human macular pigment optical density. *Optom. Vis. Sci.* **2005**, *82*, 387–404. [CrossRef] [PubMed]
9. Vishwanathan, R.; Schalch, W.; Johnson, E.J. Macular pigment carotenoids in the retina and occipital cortex are related in humans. *Nutr. Neurosci.* **2015**, *19*, 95–101. [CrossRef] [PubMed]
10. Renzi, L.M.; Dengler, M.J.; Puente, A.; Miller, L.S.; Hammond, B.R.J. Relationships between macular pigment optical density and cognitive function in unimpaired and mildly cognitively impaired older adults. *Neurobiol. Aging* **2014**, *35*, 1695–1699. [CrossRef] [PubMed]
11. Feeney, J.; Finucane, C.; Savva, G.M.; Cronin, H.; Beatty, S.; Nolan, J.M.; Kenny, R.A. Low macular pigment optical density is associated with lower cognitive performance in a large, population-based sample of older adults. *Neurobiol. Aging* **2013**, *34*, 2449–2456. [CrossRef] [PubMed]
12. Kelly, D.; Coen, R.F.; Akuffo, K.O.; Beatty, S.; Dennison, J.; Moran, R.; Stack, J.; Howard, A.N.; Mulcahy, R.; Nolan, J.M. Cognitive Function and Its Relationship with Macular Pigment Optical Density and Serum Concentrations of its Constituent Carotenoids. *J. Alzheimers Dis.* **2015**, *48*, 261–277. [CrossRef] [PubMed]
13. Vishwanathan, R.; Iannaccone, A.; Scott, T.M.; Kritchevsky, S.B.; Jennings, B.J.; Carboni, G.; Forma, G.; Satterfield, S.; Harris, T.; Johnson, K.C.; et al. Macular pigment optical density is related to cognitive function in older people. *Age Ageing* **2014**, *43*, 271–275. [CrossRef] [PubMed]
14. Bovier, E.R.; Renzi, L.M.; Hammond, B.R. A double-blind, placebo-controlled study on the effects of lutein and zeaxanthin on neural processing speed and efficiency. *PLoS ONE* **2014**, *9*, e108178. [CrossRef] [PubMed]
15. Bovier, E.R.; Hammond, B.R. A randomized placebo-controlled study on the effects of lutein and zeaxanthin on visual processing speed in young healthy subjects. *Arch. Biochem. Biophys.* **2015**, *572*, 54–57. [CrossRef] [PubMed]
16. Johnson, E.; Vishwanathan, R.; Mohn, E.; Haddock, J.; Rasmussen, H.; Scott, T. Avocado Consumption Increases Neural Lutein and Improves Cognitive Function. *FASEB J.* **2015**, *29*, 32.8.
17. Lindbergh, C.A.; Renzi-Hammond, L.M.; Hammond, B.R.; Terry, D.P.; Mewborn, C.M.; Puente, A.N.; Miller, L.S. Lutein and Zeaxanthin Influence Brain Function in Older Adults: A Randomized Controlled Trial. *J. Int. Neuropsychol. Soc.* **2017**, 1–14. [CrossRef] [PubMed]
18. Hammond, B.R.; Miller, L.S.; Bello, M.O.; Lindbergh, C.A.; Mewborn, C.; Renzi-Hammond, L.M. Effects of Lutein/Zeaxanthin Supplementation on the Cognitive Function of Community Dwelling Older Adults: A Randomized, Double-Masked, Placebo-Controlled Trial. *Front. Aging Neurosci.* **2017**, *9*, 254. [CrossRef] [PubMed]
19. Johnson, E.J.; McDonald, K.; Caldarella, S.M.; Chung, H.-Y.; Troen, A.M.; Snodderly, D.M. Cognitive findings of an exploratory trial of docosahexaenoic acid and lutein supplementation in older women. *Nutr. Neurosci.* **2008**, *11*, 75–83. [CrossRef] [PubMed]
20. Zlody, R.L. The Relationship between Critical Flicker Frequency (CFF) and Several Intellectual Measures. *Am. J. Psychol.* **1965**, *78*, 596. [CrossRef] [PubMed]
21. Owsley, C. Visual processing speed. *Vis. Res.* **2013**, *90*, 52–56. [CrossRef] [PubMed]
22. Satlhouse, D.J.; Timothy, A.; Madden, D.J. Information Processing Speed and Aging. In *Information Processing Speed in Clinical Populations*; DeLuca, J., Kalmar, J.H., Eds.; Taylor and Frances: New York, NY, USA, 2008; pp. 221–242.
23. Stringham, J.M.; Hammond, B.R.; Nolan, J.M.; Wooten, B.R.; Mammen, A.; Smollon, W.; Snodderly, D.M. The utility of using customized heterochromatic flicker photometry (cHFP) to measure macular pigment in patients with age-related macular degeneration. *Exp. Eye Res.* **2008**, *87*, 445–453. [CrossRef] [PubMed]

24. Wooten, B.R.; Hammond, B.R.; Land, R.I.; Snodderly, D.M. A practical method for measuring macular pigment optical density. *Investig. Ophthalmol. Vis. Sci.* **1999**, *40*, 2481–2489.
25. Lindbergh, C.A.; Mewborn, C.M.; Hammond, B.R.; Renzi-Hammond, L.M.; Curran-Celentano, J.M.; Miller, L.S. Relationship of Lutein and Zeaxanthin Levels to Neurocognitive Functioning: An fMRI Study of Older Adults. *J. Int. Neuropsychol. Soc.* **2017**, *23*, 11–22. [CrossRef] [PubMed]
26. Gualtieri, C.T.; Johnson, L.G. Reliability and validity of a computerized neurocognitive test battery, CNS Vital Signs. *Arch. Clin. Neuropsychol.* **2006**, *21*, 623–643. [CrossRef] [PubMed]
27. Hammond, B.R., Jr.; Johnson, E.J.; Russell, R.M.; Krinsky, N.I.; Yeum, K.J.; Edwards, R.B.; Snodderly, D.M. Dietary modification of human macular pigment density. *Investig. Ophthalmol. Vis. Sci.* **1997**, *38*, 1795–1801.
28. Hammond, B.R.; Caruso-Avery, M. Macular pigment optical density in a Southwestern sample. *Investig. Ophthalmol. Vis. Sci.* **2000**, *41*, 1492–1497.
29. Curran-Celentano, J.; Hammond, B.R.; Ciulla, T.A.; Cooper, D.A.; Pratt, L.M.; Danis, R.B. Relation between dietary intake, serum concentrations, and retinal concentrations of lutein and zeaxanthin in adults in a Midwest population. *Am. J. Clin. Nutr.* **2001**, *74*, 796–802. [PubMed]
30. Craft, N.; Dorey, C.K. Carotenoid, tocopherol, and retinal concentrations in elderly human brain. *J. Nutr. Health Aging* **2004**, *8*, 156–162. [PubMed]
31. Murray, E.A. What have ablation studies told us about the neural substrates of stimulus memory? *Semin. Neurosci.* **1996**, *8*, 13–22. [CrossRef]
32. Downing, P.E. Interactions between visual working memory and selective attention. *Psychol. Sci.* **2000**, *11*, 467–473. [CrossRef] [PubMed]
33. Lean, G.; (Ken) Clements, M.A. Spatial ability, visual imagery, and mathematical performance. *Educ. Stud. Math.* **1981**, *12*, 267–299. [CrossRef]
34. Mewborn, C.; Terry, D.; Lindbergh, C.; Renzi-Hammond, L.; Hammond, B.; Miller, L. Aging and Dementia-2Retinal and Serum Lutein and Zeaxanthin: Relation to white Matter Integrity in Younger and Older Adults. *Arch. Clin. Neuropsychol.* **2016**, *31*, 573. [CrossRef]
35. Renzi, L.M.; Hammond, B.R. The relation between the macular carotenoids, lutein and zeaxanthin, and temporal vision. *Ophthalmic Physiol. Opt.* **2010**, *30*, 351–357. [CrossRef] [PubMed]

15

The Macular Carotenoids are Associated with Cognitive Function in Preadolescent Children

Sarah E. Saint [1,2,*], Lisa M. Renzi-Hammond [1,2], Naiman A. Khan [3], Charles H. Hillman [4], Janet E. Frick [1] and Billy R. Hammond Jr. [1]

1 Department of Psychology, The University of Georgia, Athens, GA 30602, USA; lrenzi@uga.edu (L.M.R.-H.); jfrick@uga.edu (J.E.F.); bhammond@uga.edu (B.R.H.J.)
2 Institute of Gerontology, Department of Health Promotion and Behavior, College of Public Health, The University of Georgia, Athens, GA 30602, USA
3 The University of Illinois at Urbana-Champaign, Department of Kinesiology and Community Health, Champaign, IL 61820, USA; nakhan2@illinois.edu
4 Departments of Psychology and Physical Therapy, Movement & Rehabilitation Sciences, Northeastern University, Boston, MA 02115, USA; c.hillman@northeastern.edu
* Correspondence: saints@uga.edu

Abstract: The macular carotenoids lutein (L) and zeaxanthin (Z) are obtained via diet and accumulate in the central retina where they are referred to as macular pigment. The density of this biomarker (macular pigment optical density; MPOD) has been positively correlated with cognitive functioning via measures of global cognition, processing speed, and visual-spatial abilities, among others. Although improvements in cognitive function have been found in adults, much less is known about how L and Z intake may support or improve cognitive functioning during periods of rapid developmental change, such as childhood and pre-adolescence. This study examined the relationship between MPOD and cognitive functioning in 51 7–13-year-old children (51% female). MPOD was measured using heterochromatic flicker photometry (HFP) optimized for this age group. Cognitive function was assessed using the Woodcock-Johnson III (composite standard scores were obtained for Brief Intellectual Ability, Verbal Ability, Cognitive Efficiency, Processing Speed, and Executive Processes). In this sample, MPOD was significantly related to Executive Processes, $r(47) = 0.288$, $p < 0.05$, and Brief Intellectual Ability, $r(47) = 0.268$, $p < 0.05$. The relationship to Cognitive Efficiency was positive and trending but not significant, $r(49) = 0.206$, $p = 0.074$. In general, these data are consistent with those of adults showing a link between higher carotenoid status and improved cognitive functioning.

Keywords: macular pigment; lutein; cognition; children

---

1. Introduction

The carotenoids lutein (L) and zeaxanthin (Z) are found in highest concentrations in dark green leafy vegetables (e.g., kale and spinach) and, when present in the diet, accumulate in the central retina where they are referred to collectively as macular pigment. In the retina, these pigments (along with their isomer, meso-zeaxanthin) serve as intraocular light filters, absorbing short-wavelength "blue" light (peak absorption at 460 nm) before it can reach the macula and damage the photoreceptors responsible for central vision. L and Z are also potent antioxidants and anti-inflammatory agents that help to protect the central nervous system from oxidative and inflammatory stress [1,2]. The brain and eye are particularly susceptible to free radical damage because they both have very high concentrations of polyunsaturated fatty acids and a high metabolic load.

Like many naturally derived compounds, the effects of L and Z on human biology are pleiotropic [3]; emerging research, for instance, has demonstrated a relationship between the macular carotenoids and cognitive performance in adults (see [4] for a review). There is reason to believe that these molecules may also be important for cognitive development in early life, but the relationship between L and Z status, measured directly in the central nervous system, and cognitive performance has only recently been examined in children [5–7].

An effect of L and Z on the developing retina/brain is biologically feasible [8]. L is the predominant carotenoid in the developing fetal and infant brain, despite relatively low dietary intake, and makes up 59% of the carotenoids in the infant brain [9] compared to 34% in geriatric adults [10]. It has been suggested that such high concentrations of L in the developing brain are an indication that it may be necessary during periods of rapid neural development [8,11,12]. Development is a time characterized by increased vulnerability to oxidative and inflammatory stress [13] and children tend to have significantly lower intake of L and Z compared to adults [14]. When studied in model cell cultures, carotenoids have been shown to promote the formation of gap junctions between cells [15]. Promoting gap junction communication would allow neurons to communicate laterally via direct ion exchange. This may improve cell-to-cell communication and could lead to faster and more efficient processing within the visual system, as well as throughout the central nervous system (i.e., the neural efficiency hypothesis [16,17]). Evidence showing that L and Z supplementation increases visual processing speed [18,19] is consistent with this possibility.

A number of studies have shown that higher L and Z predict better cognitive outcomes [5,7,20–23]. For example, low macular pigment optical density (MPOD) in a sample of older adults was associated with significantly lower performance on global measures of cognitive functioning (mini-mental status exam (MMSE) and Montreal Cognitive Assessment (MoCA)), as well as prospective memory and processing speed tasks [21]. MPOD has also been associated with attention and cognitive flexibility (as assessed by task switching), as well as visual memory and learning (paired associate learning task) in both healthy adults and those with retinal disease [24]. Older adults with higher MPOD exhibited less brain activation to complete a verbal learning task in a recent fMRI study [25].

Intervention trials with L and Z have yielded similar findings. For example, healthy older women who were supplemented with L, docosahexaeonic acid (DHA, an omega-3 fatty acid), or a combination of L and DHA showed improved verbal fluency in all three groups, as well as improvements in performance on several delayed recall memory tests in the L + DHA group [20]. A recent placebo-controlled trial involving older adults found that supplementation with L and Z improved performance on measures of complex attention and executive functions (i.e., cognitive flexibility) [23].

Similar observations have been made even in the very young. For example, infant recognition memory, tested using an event-related potential (ERP) oddball paradigm, has been positively associated with the amount of L and choline in mother's breastmilk [26]. MPOD, measured in preadolescent children, has been shown to associate positively with educational achievement (math and written comprehension) [5], aspects of relational memory on a spatial reconstruction task [7], as well as cognitive control performance and ERP outcomes on an attentional inhibition task [6].

These past studies have shown that MPOD can predict academic performance (math and written comprehension) and lab-based cognitive outcomes in preadolescent children. Whether MPOD can also predict outcomes on standardized tests of cognition, as it has been shown to do in adults [27], has yet to be determined. The present study tests the hypothesis that MPOD will positively correlate with performance on standardized cognitive assessments of global intelligence, verbal ability, cognitive efficiency, processing speed, and executive processes using the standardized Woodcock Johnson III Tests of Cognitive Abilities [28].

2. Materials and Methods

2.1. Participants

Fifty-four children (45.5% female) were recruited from the Athens, Georgia community. Data from three of these children were excluded from all analyses for the following reasons: (a) $n = 2$ participants had diagnoses that made testing (cognitive and/or MPOD) challenging (i.e., sensory processing disorder, ADHD), and (b) $n = 1$ participant was an outlier on the cognitive outcomes and complained of excessive fatigue (not characteristic of other subjects) during testing. The final sample consisted of 51 children (49% female). Children ranged in age from 7 to 13 and were largely white (non-Hispanic; 76.5%) and from well-educated families (90.2% of children had at least one parent with some level of post-secondary education). See Table 1 for complete demographic information. All participants had normal (or corrected-to-normal) vision while completing the tasks. Informed consent was obtained prior to participation from each participant's accompanying parent/guardian, in addition to the participant's assent, which was given verbally and/or in writing after an age-appropriate discussion of the study and what is meant by "voluntary participation". All study activities were carried out in accordance with the Declaration of Helsinki, and the study protocol was approved by the Ethics Committee of the University of Georgia (Study ID: 2013100730).

Table 1. Descriptive statistics for all participants included in analyses.

	N (%)
Age (years)	
7	16 (31.4)
8	5 (9.8)
9	9 (17.6)
10	6 (11.8)
11	8 (15.7)
12	6 (11.8)
13	1 (2.0)
Sex	
Male	26 (51.0)
Female	25 (49.0)
Race	
White (Non-Hispanic)	39 (76.5)
Hispanic	1 (2.0)
>1 Race Listed	11 (21.6)
Parent Highest Education	
High School or less	3 (5.9)
College Degree (AS, BS, BA)	18 (35.3)
Graduate Degree	28 (54.9)

2.2. Measures

2.2.1. Macular Pigment Optical Density (MPOD)

MPOD was measured using customized heterochromatic flicker photometry (HFP) via a Macular Densitometer™ (Macular Metrics Corporation, Rehoboth, MA, USA) as described in [29]. Measurement of MPOD in children using HFP has been demonstrated to be possible with a moderate degree of reliability (Cronbach's $\alpha = 0.72$) [30]. The standard one-degree and 460 nm test stimulus was used and the procedure largely followed that described in [30]. One difference from [30] in the present study is that testing was confined to only two experimenters who had extensive experience working with children, and the method of adjustment was used.

2.2.2. Cognitive Testing

Selected tests from the Woodcock-Johnson III (WJ-III) Tests of Cognitive Abilities [28] were used to assess children's cognitive functioning. The WJ-III is a norm-referenced set of tests designed to measure intellectual abilities in 2- to 90+-year-olds. The WJ-III was designed using the Cattell-Horn-Carroll Theory of Cognitive Abilities and has been standardized on over 8000 individuals who are representative of the demographics and communities of the general United States population [31]. All subtests of interest for this study have median reliability scores of 0.8 or higher, with the exception of the Planning subtest (median reliability = 0.75) [31]. All Cognitive Performance Composite scores of interest have median reliability scores of 0.9 or higher [31].

Participants completed the following WJ-III standard battery subtests: Verbal Comprehension, Concept Formation, Visual Matching 2, Numbers Reversed, Decision Speed, Planning, and Pair Cancellation. These subtests were chosen so that the following cognitive performance cluster scores could be calculated: Brief Intellectual Ability (BIA), Verbal Ability, Cognitive Efficiency, Processing Speed, and Executive Processes. Time constraints prevented the administration of the entire WJ-III standard battery, therefore these cluster scores were selected as being most likely to be related to levels of L and Z in the CNS based on previous work with adults, children, and infants [20–23,26].

One trained experimenter was responsible for testing all of the participants to reduce potential inter-rater reliability confounds. Participants were allowed to take breaks between subtests, and the order in which subtests were completed was altered as needed to maintain attention. For example, the Concept Formation subtest is particularly challenging, and participants frequently feel cognitively fatigued by the time that test is administered. On occasion, that subtest was moved to a later point in the testing session to allow participants to recover their attention during the more hands-on tasks (e.g., Visual Matching 2, Decision Speed, Planning, and Pair Cancellation) before attempting the more challenging Concept Formation task. Completion of these WJ-III subtests took 90 min to two hours. The decision to alter the order of subtest administration was made during the testing session based on experimenter judgment of the participant's level of fatigue.

2.3. Statistical Analyses

Statistical analyses were performed using SPSS version 24 (IBM, Armonk, NY, USA) and $\alpha = 0.05$ was used as the cutoff value for statistical significance. Bivariate correlations were calculated between MPOD and all cognitive variables, and one-tailed test values are reported (unless otherwise specified) given the directional nature of all a priori hypotheses (i.e., higher MPOD is associated with higher cognitive functioning). Partial correlations were calculated when necessary to control for sex or age differences. The distributional shapes of the MPOD and cognitive composite score variables were examined and found to meet the assumption of normality ($S\text{-}W \geq 0.967$, $df = 49$, $p \geq 0.181$ for all variables).

3. Results

The standard scores for the WJ-III Brief Intellectual Ability, Processing Speed, Cognitive Efficiency, and Executive Processes composite measures were used to assess specific components of cognitive functioning to control for age differences among participants. Four of the children tested were born prematurely (<37 weeks gestation). Given that prematurity has been linked to deficits in processing speed and academic achievement into adolescence [32,33], independent-samples *t*-tests were conducted to determine whether any differences in cognitive or visual performance existed based on prematurity. No significant differences were found for either measure (visual or cognitive), therefore these children were kept in the data set. Sex differences in WJ-III performance were detected for the Processing Speed composite score and Visual-Auditory Learning subtest; female participants demonstrated higher performance on both measures, $t(49) = -2.795$, $p = 0.007$ and $t(49) = -2.119$, $p = 0.039$ (two-tailed), respectively. Sex differences were not detected for MPOD or any other cognitive variables.

Two participants (7- and 10-years-old) were unwilling to complete the Concept Formation subtest of the WJ-III, which is required to calculate the BIA and Executive Processes composite scores, resulting in missing data for those variables. Additionally, one 7-year-old was unwilling to complete the Spatial Relations subtest. Final sample size and descriptive statistics for all measures can be found in Table 2.

MPOD was significantly related to global intelligence (Brief Intellectual Ability; BIA) and Executive Processes composite scores (age-normed; see Table 3 and Figure 1). In addition, the relationship between MPOD and Cognitive Efficiency approached significance, $r(49) = 0.206$, $p = 0.074$ (one-tailed). The Verbal Learning and Processing Speed measures were not significantly related to MPOD (see Table 3; both $ps > 0.10$, one-tailed).

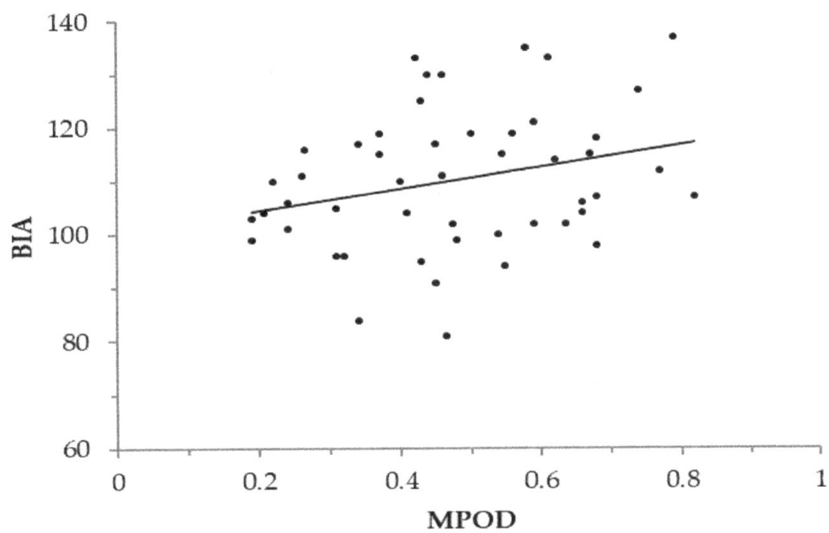

(a)

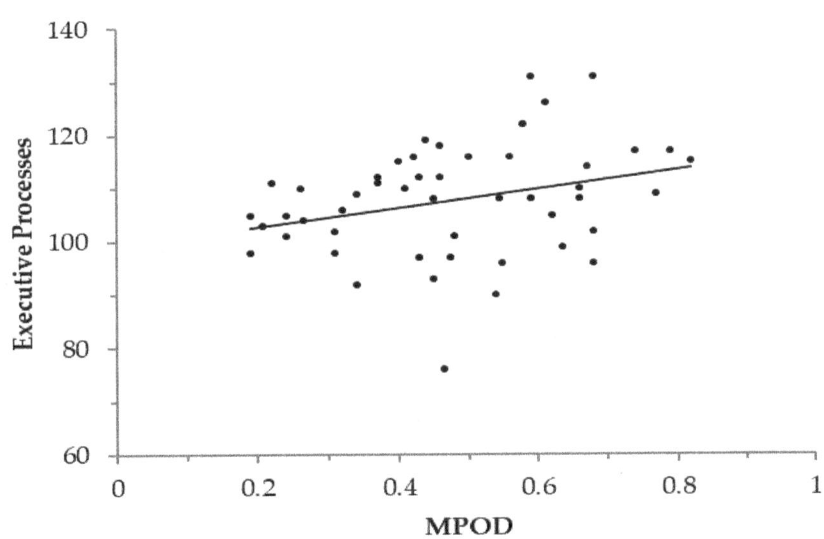

(b)

Figure 1. The relationship between macular pigment optical density (MPOD) and the following WJ-III Cognitive Composite scores: (**a**) Brief Intellectual Ability (BIA), regression line constant = 100.295, $\beta = 20.523$, $R^2(47) = 0.072$, and (**b**) Executive Processes, regression line constant = 99.234, $\beta = 17.705$, $R^2(47) = 0.083$. Standard scores were used for all cognitive variables to control for age. Note: Regression equations were calculated with MPOD predicting cognitive performance, though it should be noted that the correlational design of the present study does not allow for causal interpretations.

Exploratory analyses were performed using MPOD and two WJ-III subtests that were not included in the calculation of the cluster scores reported above. Performance on the Spatial Relations subtest (a measure of visual-spatial thinking abilities) was positively related to MPOD, $r(48) = 0.299$, $p = 0.035$ (two-tailed; see Figure 2), while the partial correlation controlling for sex between MPOD and performance on the Visual-Auditory Learning subtest (a measure of paired-associate learning) did not reach significance, $r(48) = 0.236$, $p = 0.099$ (two-tailed; see Table 4).

Table 2. Descriptive statistics for all measures.

	Mean	SD	Range	*N*
MPOD	**0.476**	**0.167**	**0.190–0.820**	**51**
Cognitive Measures (All Standard Scores)				
WJ-III Composite Scores				
Brief Intellectual Ability (BIA)	110.10	13.012	81–137	49
Verbal Ability	112.41	12.420	89–144	51
Cognitive Efficiency	104.02	15.909	65–132	51
Processing Speed	100.10	17.258	75–151	51
Executive Processes	107.69	10.453	76–131	49
Select WJ-III Subtests				
Visual-Auditory Learning	100.84	13.249	75–132	51
Spatial Relations	108.48	13.526	72–132	50

Note: MPOD = Macular Pigment Optical Density. SD: standard deviation.

Table 3. Correlations among MPOD and WJ-III cognitive cluster scores. All correlations are bivariate with the exception of Processing Speed, which was calculated as a partial correlation controlling for sex, given that sex differences were evident in the Processing Speed variable.

	BIA	Verbal Ability	Cognitive Efficiency	Processing Speed	Executive Processes
MPOD	0.268 * (*N* = 49)	0.159 (*N* = 51)	0.206 † (*N* = 51)	0.099 (*N* = 51)	0.288 * (*N* = 49)

* $p < 0.05$, † $p \leq 0.10$ (one-tailed). Note: MPOD = Macular Pigment Optical Density. BIA = Brief Intellectual Ability. The number of subjects who completed each set of measures is reported in parentheses below each correlation.

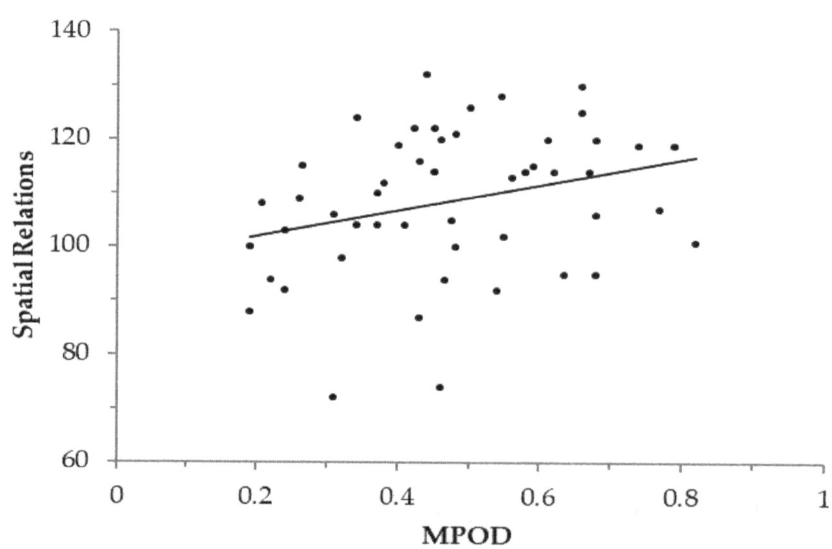

Figure 2. The relationship between macular pigment optical density (MPOD) and the WJ-III Spatial Relations subtest, regression line constant = 97.073, β = 24.081, $R^2(48) = 0.090$. Standard scores were used for Spatial Relations variable to control for age. Note: Regression equation was calculated with MPOD predicting cognitive performance, though it should be noted that the correlational design of the present study does not allow for causal interpretations.

Table 4. Correlations among MPOD and two WJ-III cognitive subtests of interest. The correlation between MPOD and Visual-Auditory Learning was calculated as a partial correlation controlling for sex, given that sex differences were evident in that cognitive subtest.

	Spatial Relations	Visual-Auditory Learning
MPOD	0.299 * ($N = 50$)	0.236 † ($N = 51$)

* $p < 0.05$, † $p \leq 0.10$ (two-tailed). Note: MPOD = Macular Pigment Optical Density. The number of subjects who completed each set of measures is reported in parentheses below each correlation.

4. Discussion

The present study tested whether MPOD, a marker of macular pigments L and Z concentration in the retina, related to standardized measures of cognitive functioning in pre-adolescent children. MPOD correlates highly with levels of lutein in the brain [34] and is therefore considered a reliable biomarker of overall central nervous system carotenoid status. Our findings further demonstrate that the ability to measure these carotenoids directly within neural tissue is a unique and powerful approach to assess the role these phytochemicals play in that very tissue: MPOD was positively related to global intelligence (BIA), executive functioning, and visuo-spatial thinking abilities in this sample of preadolescent children. In addition, the relationship between MPOD and cognitive efficiency approached significance.

These cognitive processes are founded in networks involving the frontal and parietal cortices, with input from the occipital cortex (as well as other regions), and the frontal and occipital cortices are brain regions that contain particularly high concentrations of L and Z, when they are present in diet [34]. Our results are in general agreement with data collected from adult and aging populations, as well as recent studies of other samples of preadolescent children [5–7,20–23]. Higher MPOD has been associated with higher cognitive performance in a number of areas. For example, MPOD relates to measures of global cognitive functioning and executive functioning in older adults [21,23]. These types of cognitive effects have also been manifest when using neuroimaging tools. For example, studies using fMRI have shown that higher MPOD is related to greater efficiency in the form of reduced brain activation during task execution in adults [25], and EEG work has demonstrated better cognitive control in both young children and adults [6,22].

Children's scores on the WJ-III Processing Speed composite measure were not related to MPOD in the present study. The tests that make up the WJ-III Processing Speed Composite score require children to circle items on a page (given various rules, such as "circle the two items in each row that are most alike" or "circle the two numbers in each row that are the same") as fast as they can until they reach the end or three minutes has passed. Despite the "speed" designation, this test is unlike other measures of processing speed, such as critical flicker fusion frequency (CFF), that are significantly related to MPOD in young adults [16–18]. Tasks such as CFF are atomistic in nature. They are limited by the transmission speed of neurons within the visual cortex and do not reflect the additional processing necessary for decision-making and understanding relationships between items in categories, which are largely frontal lobe phenomena [35].

These results highlight the importance of diet in supporting cognitive health in preadolescent children. It is likely that the participants tested in our study (similar to those tested in [30]) may reflect less deficiency than is often seen in the average American diet given the sample was collected in a large public university-based community (our average MPOD was relatively high). The latest National Health and Nutrition Examination Survey (NHANES) fruit and vegetable intake report reveals that dark green vegetables were consumed by only 10.7% of US children between the ages of 6–11 on a given day in 2009–2010 [36]. This dietary behavior is reflected in relatively low average intake of L and Z (about three times lower than adults) [14] and suggest that this dietary behavior may be worsening over time. Children under the age of 12 decreased their yearly vegetable intake between 2009 and 2015 by 12 servings per capita [37]. The present study was not designed to establish a causal relationship between MPOD (or L and Z intake) and cognition, but given the cross-sectional relationships between L and Z with cognitive outcomes in children, future studies should attempt to do so. This could be done by increasing L and Z intake in children via supplementation or dietary interventions to determine whether children also exhibit the same positive benefits that adult supplementation studies have demonstrated [18,20,23].

Acknowledgments: The authors would like to thank Lloyd Stephen Miller for his feedback and suggestions. Funding Source: Research support was provided by Abbott Nutrition through the Center for Nutrition, Learning, and Memory (CNLM) at the University of Illinois, Urbana-Champaign.

Author Contributions: L.M.R.-H., B.R.H.J., N.A.K. and C.H.H. conceived and designed the experiments; S.E.S. and L.M.R.-H. performed the experiments; S.E.S. analyzed the data; S.E.S., B.R.H.J., L.M.R.-H., C.H.H., N.A.K. and J.E.F. wrote the paper.

References

1. Stahl, W.; Sies, H. Antioxidant activity of carotenoids. *Mol. Asp. Med.* **2003**, *24*, 345–351. [CrossRef]
2. Ozawa, Y.; Sasaki, M.; Takahashi, N.; Kamoshita, M.; Miyake, S.; Tsubota, K. Neuroprotective Effects of Lutein in the Retina. *Curr. Pharm. Des.* **2012**, *18*, 51–56. [CrossRef] [PubMed]
3. Hammond, B. Lutein's Influence on Neural Processing Speed. In Proceedings of the 114th Abbott Nutrition Research Conference, Cognition and nutrition, Columbus, OH, USA, 8–9 April 2013; pp. 1–6.
4. Jia, Y.P.; Sun, L.; Yu, H.S.; Liang, L.P.; Li, W.; Ding, H.; Song, X.B.; Zhang, L.J. The pharmacological effects of lutein and zeaxanthin on visual disorders and cognition diseases. *Molecules* **2017**, *22*, 610. [CrossRef] [PubMed]
5. Barnett, S.M.; Khan, N.A.; Walk, A.M.; Raine, L.B.; Moulton, C.; Cohen, N.J.; Kramer, A.F.; Hammond, B.R.; Renzi-Hammond, L.; Hillman, C.H. Macular pigment optical density is positively associated with academic performance among preadolescent children. *Nutr. Neurosci.* **2017**, *8305*, 1–9. [CrossRef] [PubMed]
6. Walk, A.M.; Khan, N.A.; Barnett, S.M.; Raine, L.B.; Kramer, A.F.; Cohen, N.J.; Moulton, C.J.; Renzi-Hammond, L.M.; Hammond, B.R.; Hillman, C.H. From neuro-pigments to neural efficiency: The relationship between retinal carotenoids and behavioral and neuroelectric indices of cognitive control in childhood. *Int. J. Psychophysiol.* **2017**, *118*, 1–8. [CrossRef] [PubMed]
7. Hassevoort, K.M.; Khazoum, S.E.; Walker, J.A.; Barnett, S.M.; Raine, L.B.; Hammond, B.R.; Renzi-Hammond, L.M.; Kramer, A.F.; Khan, N.A.; Hillman, C.H.; et al. Macular Carotenoids, Aerobic Fitness, and Central Adiposity Are Associated Differentially with Hippocampal-Dependent Relational Memory in Preadolescent Children. *J. Pediatr.* **2017**, *183*, 108–114. [CrossRef] [PubMed]
8. Hammond, B.R. The Dietary Carotenoids Lutein and Zeaxanthin in Pre-and-Postnatal Development. *Funct. Food Rev.* **2012**, *4*, 130–137. [CrossRef]
9. Vishwanathan, R.; Kuchan, M.J.; Sen, S.; Johnson, E.J. Lutein and preterm infants with decreased concentrations of brain carotenoids. *J. Pediatr. Gastroenterol. Nutr.* **2014**, *59*, 659–665. [CrossRef] [PubMed]
10. Johnson, E.J.; Vishwanathan, R.; Johnson, M.A.; Hausman, D.B.; Davey, A.; Scott, T.M.; Green, R.C.; Miller, L.S.; Gearing, M.; Woodard, J.; et al. Relationship between serum and brain carotenoids, α-tocopherol, and retinol concentrations and cognitive performance in the oldest old from the Georgia centenarian study. *J. Aging Res.* **2013**, *2013*, 951786. [CrossRef] [PubMed]
11. Hammond, B.R. Possible role for dietary lutein and zeaxanthin in visual development. *Nutr. Rev.* **2008**, *66*, 695–702. [CrossRef] [PubMed]
12. Johnson, E.J. Role of lutein and zeaxanthin in visual and cognitive function throughout the lifespan. *Nutr. Rev.* **2014**, *72*, 605–612. [CrossRef] [PubMed]
13. Holt, E.M.; Steffen, L.M.; Moran, A.; Basu, S.; Steinberger, J.; Ross, J.A.; Hong, C.P.; Sinaiko, A.R. Fruit and Vegetable Consumption and Its Relation to Markers of Inflammation and Oxidative Stress in Adolescents. *J. Am. Diet. Assoc.* **2009**, *109*, 414–421. [CrossRef] [PubMed]
14. Johnson, E.J.; Maras, J.E.; Rasmussen, H.M.; Tucker, K.L. Intake of Lutein and Zeaxanthin Differ with Age, Sex, and Ethnicity. *J. Am. Diet. Assoc.* **2010**, *110*, 1357–1362. [CrossRef] [PubMed]

15. Stahl, W.; Sies, H. Effects of carotenoids and retinoids on gap junctional communication. *BioFactors* **2001**, *15*, 95–98. [CrossRef] [PubMed]
16. Hammond, B.R.; Wooten, B.R. CFF thresholds: Relation to macular pigment optical density. *Ophthalmic Physiol. Opt.* **2005**, *25*, 315–319. [CrossRef] [PubMed]
17. Renzi, L.M.; Hammond, B.R. The relation between the macular carotenoids, lutein and zeaxanthin, and temporal vision. *Ophthalmic Physiol. Opt.* **2010**, *30*, 351–357. [CrossRef] [PubMed]
18. Bovier, E.R.; Renzi, L.M.; Hammond, B.R. A double-blind, placebo-controlled study on the effects of lutein and zeaxanthin on neural processing speed and efficiency. *PLoS ONE* **2014**, *9*, e108178. [CrossRef] [PubMed]
19. Bovier, E.R.; Hammond, B.R. A randomized placebo-controlled study on the effects of lutein and zeaxanthin on visual processing speed in young healthy subjects. *Arch. Biochem. Biophys.* **2015**, *572*, 54–57. [CrossRef] [PubMed]
20. Johnson, E.; McDonald, K.; Caldarella, S.; Chung, H.-Y.; Troen, A.; Snodderly, D. Cognitive findings of an exploratory trial of docosahexaenoic acid and lutein supplementation in older women. *Nutr. Neurosci.* **2008**, *11*, 75–83. [CrossRef] [PubMed]
21. Feeney, J.; Finucane, C.; Savva, G.M.; Cronin, H.; Beatty, S.; Nolan, J.M.; Kenny, R.A. Low macular pigment optical density is associated with lower cognitive performance in a large, population-based sample of older adults. *Neurobiol. Aging* **2013**, *34*, 2449–2456. [CrossRef] [PubMed]
22. Walk, A.M.; Edwards, C.G.; Baumgartner, N.W.; Curran, M.R.; Covello, A.R.; Reeser, G.E.; Hammond, B.R.; Renzi, L.M.; Khan, N.A. The Role of Retinal Carotenoids and Age on Neuroelectric Indices of Attentional Control among early to middle-aged adults. *Front. Aging Neurosci.* **2017**, *9*, 1–13. [CrossRef] [PubMed]
23. Hammond, B.R.; Stephen Miller, L.; Bello, M.O.; Lindbergh, C.A.; Mewborn, C.; Renzi-Hammond, L.M. Effects of lutein/zeaxanthin supplementation on the cognitive function of community dwelling older adults: A randomized, double-masked, placebo-controlled trial. *Front. Aging Neurosci.* **2017**, *9*, 1–9. [CrossRef] [PubMed]
24. Kelly, D.; Coen, R.F.; Akuffo, K.O.; Beatty, S.; Dennison, J.; Moran, R.; Stack, J.; Howard, A.N.; Mulcahy, R.; Nolan, J.M. Cognitive function and its relationship with macular pigment optical density and serum concentrations of its constituent carotenoids. *J. Alzheimer's Dis.* **2015**, *48*, 261–277. [CrossRef] [PubMed]
25. Lindbergh, C.A.; Mewborn, C.M.; Hammond, B.R.; Renzi-Hammond, L.M.; Curran-Celentano, J.M.; Miller, L.S. Relationship of lutein and zeaxanthin levels to neurocognitive functioning: An fMRI study of older adults. *J. Int. Neuropsychol. Soc.* **2016**, *22*, 1–12. [CrossRef] [PubMed]
26. Cheatham, C.L.; Sheppard, K.W. Synergistic effects of human milk nutrients in the support of infant recognition memory: An observational study. *Nutrients* **2015**, *7*, 9079–9095. [CrossRef] [PubMed]
27. Renzi, L.M.; Dengler, M.J.; Puente, A.; Miller, L.S.; Hammond, B.R. Relationships between macular pigment optical density and cognitive function in unimpaired and mildly cognitively impaired older adults. *Neurobiol. Aging* **2014**, *35*, 1695–1699. [CrossRef] [PubMed]
28. Woodcock, R.W.; McGrew, K.S.; Mather, N. *Woodcock-Johnson III Tests of Cognitive Abilities*; Riverside: Rolling Meadows, IL, USA, 2001.
29. Wooten, B.R.; Hammond, B.R.; Land, R.I.; Snodderly, D.M. A practical method for measuring macular pigment optical density. *Investig. Ophthalmol. Vis. Sci.* **1999**, *40*, 2481–2489.
30. McCorkle, S.; Raine, L.; Hammond, B.; Renzi-Hammond, L.; Hillman, C.; Khan, N. Reliability of heterochromatic flicker photometry in measuring macular pigment optical density among preadolescent children. *Foods* **2015**, *4*, 594–604. [CrossRef] [PubMed]
31. Mather, N.; Woodcock, R.W. *Examiner's Manual: Woodcock-Johnson III Tests of Cognitive Abilities*; Riverside: Rolling Meadows, IL, USA, 2001.
32. Rose, S.; Feldman, J.; Jankowski, J.; Van Rossem, R. Basic information processing abilities at 11years account for deficits in IQ associated with preterm birth. *Intelligence* **2011**, *39*, 198–209. [CrossRef] [PubMed]
33. Rose, S.; Feldman, J.; Jankowski, J. Implications of infant cognition for executive functions at age 11. *Psychol. Sci.* **2012**, *23*, 1345–1355. [CrossRef] [PubMed]
34. Vishwanathan, R.; Neuringer, M.; Snodderly, D.M.; Schalch, W.; Johnson, E.J. Macular lutein and zeaxanthin are related to brain lutein and zeaxanthin in primates. *Nutr. Neurosci.* **2013**, *16*, 21–29. [CrossRef] [PubMed]
35. Mishkin, M.; Weiskrantz, L. Effects of cortical lesions in monkeys on critical flicker frequency. *J. Comp. Physiol. Psychol.* **1959**, *52*, 660. [CrossRef] [PubMed]

36. Nielsen, S.J.; Rossen, L.M.; Harris, D.M.; Ogden, C.L. *Fruit and Vegetable Consumption of U.S. Youth, 2009–2010*; U.S. Department of Health and Human Services, Centers for Disease Control and Prevention, National Center for Health Statistics: Hyattsville, MD, USA, 2014.
37. Produce for Better Health Foundation. State of the Plate, 2015 Study on America's Consumption of Fruit and Vegetables. 2015. Available online: http://www.pbhfoundation.org (accessed on 5 December 2017).

Permissions

All chapters in this book were first published by MDPI; hereby published with permission under the Creative Commons Attribution License or equivalent. Every chapter published in this book has been scrutinized by our experts. Their significance has been extensively debated. The topics covered herein carry significant findings which will fuel the growth of the discipline. They may even be implemented as practical applications or may be referred to as a beginning point for another development.

The contributors of this book come from diverse backgrounds, making this book a truly international effort. This book will bring forth new frontiers with its revolutionizing research information and detailed analysis of the nascent developments around the world.

We would like to thank all the contributing authors for lending their expertise to make the book truly unique. They have played a crucial role in the development of this book. Without their invaluable contributions this book wouldn't have been possible. They have made vital efforts to compile up to date information on the varied aspects of this subject to make this book a valuable addition to the collection of many professionals and students.

This book was conceptualized with the vision of imparting up-to-date information and advanced data in this field. To ensure the same, a matchless editorial board was set up. Every individual on the board went through rigorous rounds of assessment to prove their worth. After which they invested a large part of their time researching and compiling the most relevant data for our readers.

The editorial board has been involved in producing this book since its inception. They have spent rigorous hours researching and exploring the diverse topics which have resulted in the successful publishing of this book. They have passed on their knowledge of decades through this book. To expedite this challenging task, the publisher supported the team at every step. A small team of assistant editors was also appointed to further simplify the editing procedure and attain best results for the readers.

Apart from the editorial board, the designing team has also invested a significant amount of their time in understanding the subject and creating the most relevant covers. They scrutinized every image to scout for the most suitable representation of the subject and create an appropriate cover for the book.

The publishing team has been an ardent support to the editorial, designing and production team. Their endless efforts to recruit the best for this project, has resulted in the accomplishment of this book. They are a veteran in the field of academics and their pool of knowledge is as vast as their experience in printing. Their expertise and guidance has proved useful at every step. Their uncompromising quality standards have made this book an exceptional effort. Their encouragement from time to time has been an inspiration for everyone.

The publisher and the editorial board hope that this book will prove to be a valuable piece of knowledge for researchers, students, practitioners and scholars across the globe.

List of Contributors

Meng-Chao Tsai
Department of Psychiatry, Taoyuan General Hospital, Taoyuan 33004, Taiwan

Shyh-Hsiang Lin
School of Nutrition and Health Sciences, Taipei Medical University, Taipei 11042, Taiwan
Master Program in Food Safety, Taipei Medical University, Taipei 11042, Taiwan
Research Center of Geriatric Nutrition, Taipei Medical University, Taipei 11042, Taiwan

Kiswatul Hidayah
School of Nutrition and Health Sciences, Taipei Medical University, Taipei 11042, Taiwan

Ching-I Lin
Department of Nutrition and Health Sciences, Kainan University, Taoyuan 33857, Taiwan

Stephen A. Fleming
Piglet Nutrition and Cognition Laboratory, Department of Animal Sciences, University of Illinois, Urbana, IL 61801, USA
Department of Animal Sciences, University of Illinois, Urbana, IL 61801, USA
Neuroscience Program, University of Illinois Urbana-Champaign, Urbana, IL 61801, USA

Maciej Chichlowski
Mead Johnson Pediatric Nutrition Institute, Evansville, IL 61142, USA

Brian M. Berg
Mead Johnson Pediatric Nutrition Institute, Evansville, IL 61142, USA
Division of Nutritional Sciences, University of Illinois, Urbana, IL 61801, USA

Sharon M. Donovan
Division of Nutritional Sciences, University of Illinois, Urbana, IL 61801, USA
Department of Food Science and Human Nutrition, University of Illinois Urbana-Champaign, Urbana, IL 61801, USA

Wei Wang, Daisuke Tanokashira, Yusuke Fukui, Megumi Maruyama, Chiemi Kuroiwa and Akiko Taguchi
Department of Integrative Aging Neuroscience, National Center for Geriatrics and Gerontology, Obu, Aichi 474-8511, Japan

Takashi Saito
Laboratory for Proteolytic Neuroscience, RIKEN Center for Brain Science, Wako, Saitama 351-0106, Japan
Department of Neurocognitive Science, Nagoya City University Graduate School of Medical Science, Nagoya, Aichi 467-8601, Japan

Takaomi C. Saido
Laboratory for Proteolytic Neuroscience, RIKEN Center for Brain Science, Wako, Saitama 351-0106, Japan

Yasuhisa Ano, Tatsuhiro Ayabe, Rena Ohya and Keiji Kondo
Research Laboratories for Health Science & Food Technologies, Kirin Company Ltd, Kanazawa-ku, Yokohama-shi, Kanagawa 236-0004, Japan

Shiho Kitaoka and Tomoyuki Furuyashiki
Division of Pharmacology, Kobe University Graduate School of Medicine, Kobe 650-0017, Japan
AMED-CREST, Chiyoda-ku 100-0004, Tokyo, Japan

Stephanie Bull-Larsen and M. Hasan Mohajeri
Institute of Anatomy, Department of medicine, University of Zurich, Winterthurerstrasse 190, 8057 Zürich, Switzerland

Anca Zanfirescu, Aurelia Nicoleta Cristea, George Mihai Nitulescu, Bruno Stefan Velescu and Daniela Gradinaru
Faculty of Pharmacy, "Carol Davila" University of Medicine and Pharmacy, TraianVuia 6, 020956 Bucharest, Romania

Muhammad Ikram, Kamran Saeed, Amjad Khan, Tahir Muhammad, Muhammad Sohail Khan, Min Gi Jo, Shafiq Ur Rehman and Myeong Ok Kim
Division of Applied Life Science (BK 21), College of Natural Sciences, Gyeongsang National University, Jinju 52828, Korea

Anica Klockars, Erin L. Wood, Sarah N. Gartner and Laura K. McColl
Faculty of Science and Engineering, University of Waikato, Hamilton 3240, New Zealand

Laura M. Fletcher, L. Stephen Miller, Catherine M. Mewborn, Cutter A. Lindbergh and Billy R. Hammond Jr.
Department of Psychology, The University of Georgia, Athens, GA 30602-3013, USA

Elizabeth A. Carpenter and Colin G. Prosser
Dairy Goat Cooperative (NZ) Ltd., Hamilton 3206, New Zealand

Pawel K. Olszewski
Faculty of Science and Engineering, University of Waikato, Hamilton 3240, New Zealand
Department of Food Science and Nutrition, University of Minnesota, St. Paul, MN 55113, USA

Luis G. Bermúdez-Humarán
INRA, Micalis Institute, INRA, AgroParisTech, Université Paris-Saclay, 78352 Jouy-en-Josas, France

Eva Salinas
Department of Microbiology, Center of Basic Science, Universidad Autónoma de Aguascalientes, Aguascalientes 20131, Mexico

Genaro G. Ortiz, Luis J. Ramirez-Jirano and Oscar K. Bitzer-Quintero
Neurosciences Division, Centro de Investigación Biomédica de Occidente, Instituto Mexicano del Seguro Social, Guadalajara 44340, Jalisco, Mexico

J. Alejandro Morales
Department of Computer Sciences, Universidad de Guadalajara, Guadalajara 44430, Jalisco, Mexico

Austin T. Mudd and Joanne E. Fil
Piglet Nutrition & Cognition Laboratory, University of Illinois Urbana-Champaign, Urbana, IL 61801, USA
Neuroscience Program, University of Illinois Urbana-Champaign, Urbana, IL 61801, USA

Laura C. Knight
Piglet Nutrition & Cognition Laboratory, University of Illinois Urbana-Champaign, Urbana, IL 61801, USA
Division of Nutrition Sciences, University of Illinois Urbana-Champaign, Urbana, IL 61801, USA

Fan Lam
Beckman Institute for Advanced Science & Technology, University of Illinois Urbana-Champaign, Urbana, IL 61801, USA

Zhi-Pei Liang
Beckman Institute for Advanced Science & Technology, University of Illinois Urbana-Champaign, Urbana, IL 61801, USA
Department of Electrical & Computer Engineering, University of Illinois Urbana-Champaign, Urbana, IL 61801, USA

Kristi A. Clark
Department of Neurology, Keck School of Medicine of the University of Southern California, Los Angeles, CA 90033, USA

Jasmin M. Alves, Sabrina Jones, Alexandra G. Yunker, Brendan Angelo and Kathleen A. Page
Department of Internal Medicine; Division of Endocrinology, Keck School of Medicine of the University of Southern California, Los Angeles, CA 90033, USA
Diabetes and Obesity Research Institute of the University of Southern California, Los Angeles, CA 90033, USA

Shan Luo
Department of Internal Medicine; Division of Endocrinology, Keck School of Medicine of the University of Southern California, Los Angeles, CA 90033, USA
Diabetes and Obesity Research Institute of the University of Southern California, Los Angeles, CA 90033, USA

Ryan P. Cabeen
Laboratory of Neuro Imaging (LONI), USC Stevens Neuroimaging and Informatics Institute, Keck School of Medicine of USC, Los Angeles, CA 90033, USA

Anny H. Xiang
Department of Research and Evaluation, Kaiser Permanente Southern California, Pasadena, CA 91101, USA

Minsang Kim
Graduate School of Interdisciplinary Program of Biomodulation Collage of Natural Science, Myongji University, Yongin 17058, Korea

Minah Song, Hee-Jin Oh, Woori Bae, Jihwan Shin and Sungho Maeng
Graduate School of East-West Medical Science, Kyung Hee University, Yongin 17104, Korea

Jin Hui and Joo Won Suh
Center for Nutraceutical and Pharmaceutical Materials, Myongji University, Yongin 17058, Korea

Sang-Dock Ji
Department of Agricultural Biology, National Academy of Agricultural Science, Rural Development Administration, Wanju-gun, Jeollabuk-do 55365, Korea

Young Ho Koh
ILSONG Institute of Life Science, Hallym University, Anyang 14066, Korea
Department of Bio-Medical Gerontology, Hallym University Graduate School, Chuncheon 24252, Korea

Hyunwoo Park
Health Park Co., Ltd., #2502, Gangnam-dae-Ro 305, Sucho-gu, Seoul 06628, Korea

Hanna Karakula-Juchnowicz
1st Department of Psychiatry, Psychotherapy and Early Intervention Medical University of Lublin, Gluska Street 1, 20-439 Lublin, Poland
Department of Clinical Neuropsychiatry Medical University of Lublin, Gluska Street 1, 20-439 Lublin, Poland

Mirosława Gałęcka, Anna Bartnicka and Zuzanna Łukaszewicz
Institute of Microecology, Sielska Street 10, 60-129 Poznan, Poland

Janet E. Frick
Department of Psychology, The University of Georgia, Athens, GA 30602, USA

Pawel Krukow and Justyna Morylowska-Topolska
Department of Clinical Neuropsychiatry Medical University of Lublin, Gluska Street 1, 20-439 Lublin, Poland

Karolina Skonieczna-Zydecka
Department of Biochemistry and Human Nutrition, Pomeranian Medical University in Szczecin, Broniewskiego Street 24, 71-460 Szczecin, Poland

Tomasz Krajka
Faculty of Mechanical Engineering, Department of Mathematics, Lublin University of Technology, Nadbystrzycka Street 36, 20-618 Lublin, Poland

Kamil Jonak
1st Department of Psychiatry, Psychotherapy and Early Intervention Medical University of Lublin, Gluska Street 1, 20-439 Lublin, Poland
Department of Biomedical Engineering, Lublin University of Technology, Nadbystrzycka Street 38D, 20-618 Lublin, Poland

Dariusz Juchnowicz
Department of Psychiatric Nursing Medical University of Lublin, Szkolna Street 18, 20-124 Lublin, Poland

Emily R. Bovier
Department of Psychology, The University of Georgia, Athens, GA 30602-3013, USA
Department of Psychology, State University of New York, Oswego Campus, Oswego, NY 13126, USA

Allen S. Levine
Department of Food Science and Nutrition, University of Minnesota, St. Paul, MN 55113, USA

Jeffrey H. Baxter
Abbott Nutrition, Global Research and Development, Columbus, OH 43219, USA

Sarah E. Saint and Lisa M. Renzi-Hammond
Department of Psychology, The University of Georgia, Athens, GA 30602, USA
Institute of Gerontology, Department of Health Promotion and Behavior, College of Public Health, The University of Georgia, Athens, GA 30602, USA

Naiman A. Khan
The University of Illinois at Urbana-Champaign, Department of Kinesiology and Community Health, Champaign, IL 61820, USA

Charles H. Hillman
Departments of Psychology and Physical Therapy, Movement & Rehabilitation Sciences, Northeastern University, Boston, MA 02115, USA

Joanna Rog
1st Department of Psychiatry, Psychotherapy and Early Intervention Medical University of Lublin, Gluska Street 1, 20-439 Lublin, Poland

Paolo Caffarra
Dipartimento di Medicina e Chirurgia, Unità di Neuroscienze, Università degli Studi di Parma, via Gramsci 14, 43126 Parma, Italy

Andrea Zini
Dipartimento di Neuroscienze, Nuovo Ospedale Civile "S.Agostino-Estense", Azienda Ospedaliera Universitaria, via Giardini 1355, 41100 Modena, Italy

Index

www.ingramcontent.com/pod-product-compliance
Lightning Source LLC
LaVergne TN
LVHW060527210926
848485LV00005B/1159
* 9 7 8 1 6 3 9 2 7 6 2 6 4 *